Ultrasound

Editor

MARK E. LOCKHART

RADIOLOGIC CLINICS OF NORTH AMERICA

www.radiologic.theclinics.com

Consulting Editor
FRANK H. MILLER

January 2025 • Volume 63 • Number 1

ELSEVIER

1600 John F. Kennedy Boulevard • Suite 1800 • Philadelphia, Pennsylvania, 19103-2899

http://www.theclinics.com

RADIOLOGIC CLINICS OF NORTH AMERICA Volume 63, Number 1
January 2025 ISSN 0033-8389, ISBN 13: 978-0-443-29376-4

Editor: John Vassallo (j.vassallo@elsevier.com)
Developmental Editor: Malvika Shah

© **2025 Elsevier Inc. All rights are reserved, including those for text and data mining, AI training, and similar technologies.**

This periodical and the individual contributions contained in it are protected under copyright by Elsevier, and the following terms and conditions apply to their use:

Photocopying
Single photocopies of single articles may be made for personal use as allowed by national copyright laws. Permission of the Publisher and payment of a fee is required for all other photocopying, including multiple or systematic copying, copying for advertising or promotional purposes, resale, and all forms of document delivery. Special rates are available for educational institutions that wish to make photocopies for non-profit educational classroom use. For information on how to seek permission visit www.elsevier.com/permissions or call: (+44) 1865 843830 (UK)/(+1) 215 239 3804 (USA).

Derivative Works
Subscribers may reproduce tables of contents or prepare lists of articles including abstracts for internal circulation within their institutions. Permission of the Publisher is required for resale or distribution outside the institution. Permission of the Publisher is required for all other derivative works, including compilations and translations (please consult www.elsevier.com/permissions).

Electronic Storage or Usage
Permission of the Publisher is required to store or use electronically any material contained in this periodical, including any article or part of an article (please consult www.elsevier.com/permissions). Except as outlined above, no part of this publication may be reproduced, stored in a retrieval system or transmitted in any form or by any means, electronic, mechanical, photocopying, recording or otherwise, without prior written permission of the Publisher.

Notice
No responsibility is assumed by the Publisher for any injury and/or damage to persons or property as a matter of products liability, negligence or otherwise, or from any use or operation of any methods, products, instructions or ideas contained in the material herein. Because of rapid advances in the medical sciences, in particular, independent verification of diagnoses and drug dosages should be made.

Although all advertising material is expected to conform to ethical (medical) standards, inclusion in this publication does not constitute a guarantee or endorsement of the quality or value of such product or of the claims made of it by its manufacturer.

Radiologic Clinics of North America (ISSN 0033-8389) is published bimonthly by Elsevier Inc., 360 Park Avenue South, New York, NY 10010-1710. Months of issue are January, March, May, July, September, and November. Periodicals postage paid at New York, NY and additional mailing offices. Subscription prices are USD 566 per year for US individuals, USD 100 per year for US students and residents, USD 649 per year for Canadian individuals, USD 761 per year for international individuals, USD 100 per year for Canadian students/residents, and USD 315 per year for international students/residents. For institutional access pricing please contact Customer Service via the contact information below. To receive student and resident rate, orders must be accompanied by name of affiliated institution, date of term and the signature of program/residency coordinatior on institution letterhead. Orders will be billed at individual rate until proof of status is received. Foreign air speed delivery is included in all *Clinics* subscription prices. All prices are subject to change without notice. Orders, claims, and journal inquiries: Please visit our Support Hub page https://service.elsevier.com for assistance.

Reprints. For copies of 100 or more of articles in this publication, please contact the Commercial Reprints Department, Elsevier Inc., 360 Park Avenue South, New York, New York 10010-1710. Tel.: +1-212-633-3874; Fax: +1-212-633-3820; E-mail: reprints@elsevier.com.

Radiologic Clinics of North America also published in Greek Paschalidis Medical Publications, Athens, Greece.

Radiologic Clinics of North America is covered in MEDLINE/PubMed (Index Medicus), EMBASE/Excerpta Medica, Current Contents/Life Sciences, Current Contents/Clinical Medicine, RSNA Index to Imaging Literature, BIOSIS, Science Citation Index, and ISI/BIOMED.

Printed in the United States of America.

Contributors

CONSULTING EDITOR

FRANK H. MILLER, MD, FACR
Lee F. Rogers, MD, Professor of Medical Education, Chief, Body Imaging Section, Medical Director, MRI, Professor, Department of Radiology, Northwestern Memorial Hospital, Northwestern University, Feinberg School of Medicine, Chicago, Illinois, USA

EDITOR

MARK E. LOCKHART, MD, MPH
Professor, Department of Radiology, University of Alabama at Birmingham, Birmingham, Alabama, USA

AUTHORS

SANDRA J. ALLISON, MD
Associate Professor of Radiology, Georgetown University School of Medicine, Director of Ultrasound, Washington Radiology, Washington, DC, USA

RICHARD G. BARR, MD, PhD
Professor of Radiology, Northeastern Ohio Medical University, Southwoods Imaging, Youngstown, Ohio, USA

WUI K. CHONG, MBBS
Professor, Department of Abdominal Radiology, University of Texas MD Anderson Medical Center, Houston, Texas, USA

CORINNE DEURDULIAN, MD, FSRU
Professor of Radiology, Department of Radiological Sciences, David Geffen School of Medicine at UCLA, Adjunct Associate Professor, USC Keck School of Medicine, Chief, Abdominal MRI, Department of Radiology, Greater Los Angeles VA Medical Center, Los Angeles, California, USA

RICK FELD, MD
Professor, Department of Radiology, Sidney Kimmel Medical College, Thomas Jefferson University Hospital, Thomas Jefferson University, Philadelphia, Pennsylvania, USA

DAVID T. FETZER, MD
Associate Professor, Director of Ultrasound, Department of Radiology, Director of Ultrasound, UT Southwestern Medical Center, Dallas, Texas, USA

PAMELA GARZA-BÁEZ, MD
Fellow, Department of Radiology, Hospital of the University of Pennsylvania, Philadelphia, Pennsylvania, USA

GOWTHAMAN GUNABUSHANAM, MD
Associate Professor, Department of Radiology and Biomedical Imaging, Yale University School of Medicine, New Haven, Connecticut, USA

JENNIFER HUANG, MD
Resident, Division of Internal Medicine, Department of Dermatology, Brigham and Women's Hospital; Associate Professor of Dermatology, Boston Children's Hospital, Boston, Massachusetts, USA; Assistant Professor Radiology & Radiological Sciences, Vanderbilt University Medical Center, Nashville, Tennessee, USA

KATERINA S. KONSTANTINOFF, MD
Assistant Professor of Radiology, Mallinckrodt Institute of Radiology, Washington University School of Medicine, Saint Louis, Missouri, USA

Contributors

CATALINA LE CACHEUX, MD
Assistant Professor, Department of Radiology, UPMC Children's Hospital of Pittsburgh, University of Pittsburgh School of Medicine, Pittsburgh, Pennsylvania, USA

MARK E. LOCKHART, MD, MPH
Professor, Department of Radiology, University of Alabama at Birmingham, Birmingham, Alabama, USA

DANIEL R. LUDWIG, MD
Assistant Professor of Radiology, Mallinckrodt Institute of Radiology, Washington University School of Medicine, Saint Louis, Missouri, USA

KATHERINE E. MATUREN, MD, MS
Clinical Professor, Departments of Radiology, and Obstetrics and Gynecology, Michigan Medicine, Ann Arbor, Michigan, USA

ALEXANDRA MEDELLIN, MD
Clinical Assistant Professor, Department of Radiology, Cumming School of Medicine, University of Calgary, Calgary, Alberta, Canada

LEVON N. NAZARIAN, MD
Professor, Department of Radiology, Hospital of the University of Pennsylvania, Philadelphia, Pennsylvania, USA

LAURENCE NEEDLEMAN, MD
Professor, Department of Radiology, Sidney Kimmel Medical College, Thomas Jefferson University Hospital, Thomas Jefferson University, Philadelphia, Pennsylvania, USA

MAITRAYA K. PATEL, MD
Professor of Radiology, Department of Radiological Sciences, David Geffen School of Medicine at UCLA, UCLA Ronald Reagan Medical Center, Los Angeles, California, USA

KRUPA PATEL-LIPPMANN, MD
Associate Professor, Department of Radiology and Radiological Sciences, Vanderbilt University Medical Center, Nashville, Tennessee, USA

JOHN S. PELLERITO, MD, FSRU, FAIUM
Vice Chairman, Clinical Affairs Director, Peripheral Vascular Laboratory Former Chief, Division of US, CT and MRI Department of Radiology North Shore - Long Island Jewish Health System, New Hyde Park, New York, USA Professor of Radiology, Zucker School of Medicine at Hofstra/ Northwell, Hofstra University Hempstead, New York

CATHERINE H. PHILLIPS, MD
Associate Professor, Department of Radiology and Radiological Sciences, Vanderbilt University Medical Center, Nashville, Tennessee, USA

MARGARITA V. REVZIN, MD, MS, FAIUM, FSRU, FSAR, FACR
Associate Professor of Radiology, Department of Radiology and Biomedical Imaging, Yale School of Medicine, New Haven, Connecticut, USA

MICHELLE LAVONNE ROBBIN, MD
Professor, Department of Radiology, University of Alabama at Birmingham, Birmingham, Alabama, USA

LESLIE MILLAR SCOUTT, MD
Professor, Department of Radiology and Biomedical Imaging, Yale University School of Medicine, New Haven, Connecticut, USA

TYLER J. SEVCO, MD
Assistant Clinical Professor of Radiology, Department of Radiological Sciences, David Geffen School of Medicine at UCLA, UCLA Ronald Reagan Medical Center, Los Angeles, California, USA

JUDY H. SQUIRES, MD, FSRU
Chief of Ultrasound, Associate Professor, Department of Radiology, UPMC Children's Hospital of Pittsburgh, University of Pittsburgh School of Medicine, Pittsburgh, Pennsylvania, USA

BENJAMIN SRIVASTAVA
Wilton Public High School, Wilton, Connecticut, USA

LORI M. STRACHOWSKI, MD
Clinical Professor, Department of Radiology and Biomedical Imaging and Obstetrics, Clinical Professor, Department of Gynecology and Reproductive Sciences, University of California San Francisco, San Francisco, California, USA

Contributors

BENJAMIN S. STRNAD, MD
Assistant Professor of Radiology, Mallinckrodt Institute of Radiology, Washington University School of Medicine, Saint Louis, Missouri, USA

FRANKLIN N. TESSLER, MD, CM
Senior Medical Officer, Health System Information Services, Emeritus Professor, Department of Radiology, University of Alabama at Birmingham, Senior Medical Officer, Health System Information Services, Birmingham, Alabama, USA

JEFFREY J. TUTMAN, MD
Assistant Professor, Department of Radiology, University of Colorado School of Medicine, Director of Ultrasound, Department of Radiology, Children's Hospital of Colorado, Aurora, Colorado, USA

STEPHANIE R. WILSON, MD
Clinical Professor, Department of Radiology, Division of Gastroenterology, Cumming School of Medicine, University of Calgary, Calgary, Alberta, Canada

Contents

Preface: For Many Questions, Ultrasound Is the Answer! xv

Mark E. Lockhart

Achieving and Maintaining Excellence: A Roadmap for Ultrasound Practices 1

Michelle L. Robbin, David T. Fetzer, Franklin N. Tessler, Wui K. Chong, and Mark E. Lockhart

> This article outlines a roadmap to achieving and maintaining excellence in an ultrasound (US) practice. We present constructive advice on how US practices can achieve and maintain quality, patient and referring physician satisfaction, and efficiency in the setting of rising examination volumes. Accreditation, sonographer and resident/fellow physician training, advanced practice sonographers, and Picture Archiving and Communication System/Artificial Intelligence in US are discussed. Advice for how to begin offering new US examinations, begin a practice at new US locations, improve quality assurance, and enhance marketing are covered.

Multiparametric Ultrasound for Chronic Liver Disease 13

Richard G. Barr

> Diffuse liver disease is a substantial world-wide problem. With the combination of conventional ultrasound of the abdomen, fat quantification and elastography, appropriate staging of the patient can be assessed. This information allows for the diagnosis of steatosis and detection of fibrosis as well as prognosis, surveillance, and prioritization for treatment. With the potential for reversibility with appropriate treatment accurate assessment for the stage of chronic liver disease is critical.

Ovarian-Adnexal Reporting and Data System Ultrasound v2022: From Origin to Everyday Use 29

Catherine H. Phillips, Krupa Patel-Lippmann, Jennifer Huang, Lori M. Strachowski, and Katherine E. Maturen

> This review of the American College of Radiology Ovarian-Adnexal Reporting and Data System (O-RADS) ultrasound (US) v2022 will familiarize the reader with the updated O-RADS US system, highlight new updates, and outline key technical and reporting components. Additionally, this review will outline how to approach and incorporate the system into clinical practice, with reporting and real-world examples. Future directions will focus on addressing knowledge gaps and expanding on research opportunities.

Challenges in Ultrasound of the Gallbladder and Bile Ducts: A Focused Review and Update 45

Benjamin S. Strnad, Katerina S. Konstantinoff, and Daniel R. Ludwig

> Although ultrasound is the initial imaging modality of choice in patients with right upper quadrant pain or suspected biliary obstruction, a number of challenges in clinical practice limit its utility as a stand-alone imaging modality. This article presents a focused review of gallbladder and biliary ultrasound, highlighting current knowledge gaps, emerging applications, and directions for further study. The authors cover

selected topics including acute cholecystitis, cystic artery velocity, gallbladder polyps, contrast-enhanced ultrasound, and incidental biliary duct dilatation.

Ultrasound of the Upper Urinary Tract 57

Margarita V. Revzin, Benjamin Srivastava, and John S. Pellerito

Ultrasound (US) plays a primary role in the assessment and diagnosis of renal and ureteral pathologies and their management. It is considered the first-line imaging modality for evaluation of urinary obstruction, nephrolithiasis, and urinary retention among other indications. US is also essential for evaluation of renal vasculature and assessment of renal transplantation. Contrast-enhanced US is an advanced application of US gaining its acceptance in evaluation of the renal masses.

Bowel Ultrasound 83

Alexandra Medellin and Stephanie R. Wilson

 Video content accompanies this article at http://www.radiologic.theclinics.com.

Sonographic evaluation of the intestine is increasing in popularity due to its safety, noninvasive nature, accessibility, and high acceptability by patients. It is now recognized as one of the most valuable imaging modalities in the assessment of patients with inflammatory bowel disease. In addition, recent technical advances in ultrasound (US), especially contrast-enhanced US and shear wave elastography, have given US a competitive edge allowing for subjective and objective measurements of mural and mesenteric inflammation. The dynamic performance and high resolution of US allow for functional and morphologic assessment of the bowel, making it a desirable technique.

Emerging Techniques in Pediatric Ultrasound, with Emphasis on Infants 97

Jeffrey J. Tutman, Catalina Le Cacheux, and Judy H. Squires

 Video content accompanies this article at http://www.radiologic.theclinics.com.

Ultrasound is an important modality to assess pediatric patients and uses continue to increase. In this review, several emerging applications of ultrasound in pediatric patients are detailed, focusing on diseases impacting infants, including necrotizing enterocolitis, malrotation with midgut volvulus, and liver lesion characterization.

Approach to Evaluating Superficial Soft Tissue Masses by Ultrasound 109

Pamela Garza-Báez, Sandra J. Allison, and Levon N. Nazarian

 Video content accompanies this article at http://www.radiologic.theclinics.com.

The purpose of this article is to give a systematic approach to the ultrasound evaluation of superficial soft-tissue masses. The knowledge of proper technique in image acquisition, the characteristic sonographic appearances of the most common masses, their potential pitfalls, and the location of the lesions can help establish a confident diagnosis. Where the sonographic features of the masses are inconclusive, a percutaneous biopsy is effective in establishing the definitive diagnosis.

Ultrasound Evaluation of the Abdominal Aorta and Mesenteric Arteries 123

Gowthaman Gunabushanam, Michelle LaVonne Robbin, and Leslie Millar Scoutt

> The authors review ultrasound (US) imaging findings of the abdominal aorta and mesenteric arteries, with a focus on screening for abdominal aortic aneurysm (AAA) and posttreatment follow-up. US is the primary imaging modality used to screen for AAA and for surveillance of aneurysms for growth after initial diagnosis. US and contrast-enhanced US may play a greater role in patient follow-up status post-endovascular aneurysm repairs. US is also the initial recommended imaging modality for suspected chronic mesenteric ischemia.

Carotid Ultrasound 137

Tyler J. Sevco, Maitraya K. Patel, and Corinne Deurdulian

> Carotid ultrasound is the primary noninvasive method for detecting, grading, and monitoring internal carotid artery (ICA) stenosis. Major components of carotid Doppler ultrasound include assessment of ICA stenosis using Doppler velocity criteria, spectral waveform analysis, and assessment of ICA stenosis. Recently, the Intersocietal Accreditation Commission Vascular Testing put forth new modified Society of Radiologists in Ultrasound criteria with a higher peak systolic velocity threshold of 180 cm/s for 50% to 69% ICA stenosis. Additional emerging techniques, including 3D imaging, contrast-enhanced ultrasound, and superb microvascular imaging, may help identify vulnerable plaque and thus help further risk-stratify patients in the future.

Peripheral Arterial Ultrasound 153

Laurence Needleman and Rick Feld

> Peripheral arterial ultrasound is an important technique to evaluate vascular disease. Protocols include grayscale, color Doppler and spectral Doppler. Arterial duplex is used to evaluate patients with claudication to characterize atherosclerotic disease. Stenoses have characteristic findings which can help profile lesions accurately. Other nonatherosclerotic obstructive processes are also evaluable by duplex Doppler. Traumatic injuries can also be studied in the stable patient. Attention to protocols helps ensure optimal results.

Peripheral Venous Ultrasound 165

Laurence Needleman and Rick Feld

> After clinical evaluation, especially clinical prediction rules, appropriately ordered venous duplex has become the standard test for evaluating and excluding deep vein thrombosis (DVT). Ultrasound is useful for lower- and upper-extremity veins. Protocols include grayscale, color Doppler, and spectral Doppler. Recommended lower-extremity protocols include central leg and calf veins. Duplex Doppler is widely used to evaluate patients with chronic venous disease, especially with suspected venous reflux. Mapping to identify adequate veins before surgery is another widely used indication for venous ultrasound. Ultrasound for thrombosis can be characterized as normal, acute DVT, superficial thrombosis, or chronic postthrombotic changes in most patients.

JOURNAL TITLE: Radiologic Clinics
ISSUE: 63.1

PROGRAM OBJECTIVE
The objective of the *Radiologic Clinics of North America* is to keep practicing radiologists and radiology residents up to date with current clinical practice in radiology by providing timely articles reviewing the state of the art in patient care.

TARGET AUDIENCE
Practicing radiologists, radiology residents, and other healthcare professionals who provide patient care utilizing radiologic findings.

LEARNING OBJECTIVES
Upon completion of this activity, participants will be able to:
1. Describe the next steps when inconclusive or suspicious findings by ultrasound are identified.
2. Discuss clinical practice challenges limiting ultrasound utility as a stand-alone imaging modality.
3. Recognize ultrasound is an important and common modality for evaluating various disease processes.

ACCREDITATION
The Elsevier Office of Continuing Medical Education (EOCME) is accredited by the Accreditation Council for Continuing Medical Education (ACCME) to provide continuing medical education for physicians.

The EOCME designates this journal-based CME activity for a maximum of 12 *AMA PRA Category 1 Credit*(s)™. Physicians should claim only the credit commensurate with the extent of their participation in the activity.

All other healthcare professionals requesting continuing education credit for this enduring material will be issued a certificate of participation.

DISCLOSURE OF RELEVANT FINANCIAL RELATIONSHIPS
The EOCME assesses conflict of interest with its instructors, faculty, planners, and other individuals who are in a position to control the content of CME activities. All relevant conflicts of interest that are identified are thoroughly vetted by EOCME for fair balance, scientific objectivity, and patient care recommendations. EOCME is committed to providing its learners with CME activities that promote improvements or quality in healthcare and not a specific proprietary business or a commercial interest.

The authors and editors listed below have identified no financial relationships or relationships to products or devices they have with ineligible companies related to the content of this CME activity:
Sandra J. Allison, MD; Wui K. Chong, MBBS; Corinne Deurdulian, MD, FSRU; Rick Feld, MD; Pamela Garza-Báez, MD; Gowthaman Gunabushanam, MD; Jennifer Huang, MD; Katerina S. Konstantinoff, MD; Catalina Le Cacheux, MD; Mark E. Lockhart, MD, MPH; Daniel R. Ludwig, MD; Katherine E. Maturen, MD, MS; Alexandra Medellin, MD; Levon N. Nazarian, MD; Laurence Needleman, MD; Krupa Patel-Lippmann, MD; John S. Pellerito, MD, FSRU, FAIUM; Catherine H. Phillips, MD; Margarita V. Revzin, MD, MS, FAIUM, FSRU, FSAR; Leslie Millar Scoutt, MD; Tyler Sevco, MD; Judy H. Squires, MD, FSRU; Benjamin Srivastava; Lori Strachowski, MD; Benjamin S. Strnad, MD; Franklin N. Tessler, MD, CM; Jeffrey J. Tutman, MD; Stephanie R. Wilson, MD

The authors and editors listed below have identified financial relationships or relationships to products or devices they have with ineligible companies related to the content of this CME activity:
Richard G. Barr, MD, PhD: *Speaker*: Canon Medical Systems, Philips Ultrasound, Siemen Healthineers, Mindray, Samsung Ultrasound, Hologic Ultrasound; *Researcher*: Philips Ultrasound, Canon Ultrasound, Canon MRI, Samsung, Siemens Healthineers, Hologic, Mindray; *Advisor*: Bracco Diagnostics, Lantheus

David T. Fetzer, MD: *Researcher*: GE HealthCare, Philips Healthcare, Siemens Healthineers; *Advisor*: GE HealthCare, Philips Healthcare, Bracco Diagnostics; *Speaker*: GE HealthCare, Siemens Healthineers

Maitraya K. Patel, MD: *Researcher*: Philips Healthcare

Michelle L. Robbin, MD, MS: *Independent contractor*: Philips Medical; *Advisor*: Philips Medical, Jazz Pharmaceuticals

The Clinics staff listed below have identified no financial relationships or relationships to products or devices they have with ineligible companies related to the content of this CME activity:
Kothainayaki Kulanthaivelu; Michelle Littlejohn; Patrick J. Manley; Malvika Shah; John Vassallo

UNAPPROVED/OFF-LABEL USE DISCLOSURE
The EOCME requires CME faculty to disclose to the participants:
1. When products or procedures being discussed are off-label, unlabelled, experimental, and/or investigational (not US Food and Drug Administration [FDA] approved); and
2. Any limitations on the information presented, such as data that are preliminary or that represent ongoing research, interim analyses, and/or unsupported opinions. Faculty may discuss information about pharmaceutical agents that is outside of

FDA-approved labelling. This information is intended solely for CME and is not intended to promote off-label use of these medications. If you have any questions, contact the medical affairs department of the manufacturer for the most recent prescribing information.

TO ENROLL
To enroll in the *Radiologic Clinics of North America* Continuing Medical Education program, call customer service at 1-800-654-2452 or sign up online at http://www.theclinics.com/home/cme. The CME program is available to subscribers for an additional annual fee of USD 340.00.

METHOD OF PARTICIPATION
In order to claim credit, participants must complete the following:
1. Complete enrolment as indicated above.
2. Read the activity.
3. Complete the CME Test and Evaluation. Participants must achieve a score of 70% on the test. All CME Tests and Evaluations must be completed online.

CME INQUIRIES/SPECIAL NEEDS
For all CME inquiries or special needs, please contact elsevierCME@elsevier.com.

RADIOLOGIC CLINICS OF NORTH AMERICA

FORTHCOMING ISSUES

March 2025
Pulmonary Vascular Disease
Jeffrey P. Kanne, *Editor*

May 2025
Imaging of the Small Bowel and Colon
Shannon P. Sheedy and Kevin J. Chang, *Editors*

July 2025
Pearls and Pitfalls in Thoracic Disease Imaging
Mylene T. Truong and Girish S. Shroff, *Editors*

RECENT ISSUES

November 2024
Current Controversies in Diagnostic and Interventional Radiology
Douglas S. Katz and John J. Hines, *Editors*

September 2024
Imaging in Rheumatology
Alberto Bazzocchi and Giuseppe Guglielmi, *Editors*

July 2024
Breast Imaging Essentials
Yiming Gao and Samantha L. Heller, *Editors*

SERIES OF RELATED INTEREST

Advances in Clinical Radiology
Available at: https://www.advancesinclinicalradiology.com/
Magnetic Resonance Imaging Clinics
Available at: https://www.mri.theclinics.com/
Neuroimaging Clinics
Available at: www.neuroimaging.theclinics.com
PET Clinics
Available at: www.pet.theclinics.com

THE CLINICS ARE AVAILABLE ONLINE!
Access your subscription at:
www.theclinics.com

Preface
For Many Questions, Ultrasound Is the Answer!

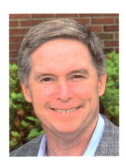

Mark E. Lockhart, MD, MPH
Editor

This collection should be an extremely interesting read for anyone involved in ultrasound for patient care. These twelve articles cover some of the newest concepts in sonography from true experts in the field. It covers a wide range of organ systems and provides information that is immediately useful for daily practice.

We start with a bigger picture discussion in which experts provide suggestions for improving the efficiency of an ultrasound practice and use of physician extenders. Specific diagnostic areas are then covered in subsequent articles. For example, the next article addresses liver imaging opportunities using conventional techniques, elastography, and ultrasound contrast. An update on ACR O-RADS gives more guidance on this useful paradigm, which continues to gain momentum in its use. Next, the new guidelines and recommendations related to biliary dilatation and also gallbladder polyps are covered in detail. For the retroperitoneum, our authors have provided a beautiful tour of upper tract urinary ultrasound. An article devoted to cutting-edge contrast-enhanced imaging of bowel is illustrated with exquisite images. Next, an article on pediatric ultrasound emphasizes an underappreciated area of ultrasound of imaging in infant patients. In the musculoskeletal article, the stepwise approach to soft tissue masses is very logical and easy to follow. A review of aortomesenteric ultrasound covers a wide variety of sonographic diagnoses. Within the neck, recent carotid Doppler recommendations for diagnosis of stenosis have been addressed. In two articles of extremity ultrasound (arteries and veins), the authors provide an excellent description of the basics behind the waveforms and detail the diagnostic findings.

On a personal note, I am thankful for the dedication of this array of experts in sonography and to you as the reader for taking the time to improve your skills in this modality, which is seeing a resurgence due to new applications, such as CEUS and elastography. I hope you enjoy and learn from the experience of our authors and the time they have dedicated to this issue.

DISCLOSURES

The authors declares the following: salary, Deputy Editor, *Journal of Ultrasound in Medicine*; Book royalties, Elsevier Publishing; Book royalties, Jay-Pee Brothers Medical Publishers; Special Governmental Employee, US FDA Medical Devices Panel member; Executive Committee member, Society of Radiologists in Ultrasound; Research Committee Chair, American Institute of Ultrasound in Medicine Future Fund.

Mark E. Lockhart, MD, MPH
Department of Radiology
University of Alabama at Birmingham
619 19th Street South
JTN 344
Birmingham, AL 35249, USA

E-mail address:
mlockhart@uabmc.edu

Achieving and Maintaining Excellence
A Roadmap for Ultrasound Practices

Michelle L. Robbin, MD, MS[a,*], David T. Fetzer, MD[b],
Franklin N. Tessler, MD, CM[c], Wui K. Chong, MBBS[d],
Mark E. Lockhart, MD, MPH[a]

KEYWORDS

- Ultrasound • Physician extender • Contrast-enhanced ultrasound
- Picture archiving and communication system • Artificial intelligence • Accreditation
- Advanced practice

KEY POINTS

- Excellence in ultrasound (US) practice can be achieved with attention to sonographer and physician training, and standardized facility-wide scanner-based protocols.
- Accreditation conveys a practice's commitment to a national standard of excellence, establishing a framework for sonographer certification and US examination rigor.
- Advanced practice sonographers are helpful to provide high-quality, efficient care in busy US facilities.
- Strong information technology support is essential for operating a modern US practice, and AI promises to enhance workflow from image acquisition through interpretation.
- Offering novel sonographic examinations in existing facilities and providing US services at new practice locations are vital to enhancing the value of sonography across the care continuum.

INTRODUCTION

Ultrasound (US) continues to be a rapidly evolving modality with well-known benefits including portability, widespread availability, relatively low-cost, and lack of ionizing radiation associated with computed tomography (CT) and angiography. In the United States, an additional advantage is that US studies generally do not require insurance pre-authorization. Newer capabilities such as contrast-enhanced ultrasound (CEUS), and quantitative techniques such as elastography and fat quantification decrease the need for biopsy or more expensive noninvasive studies such as MRI with their associated longer wait times. In this article, we present practical advice on how US practices can achieve and maintain quality, patient and referring physician satisfaction, and efficiency in the setting of rising examination volumes.[1,2]

ACCREDITATION

Accreditation conveys commitment to a national standard of excellence and can increase provider and patient confidence in the quality of the US examinations performed. Additionally, specific sonographer certification and physician qualifications, as well as submission of high-quality images, inevitably

[a] Department of Radiology, University of Alabama at Birmingham, 619 19th Street South, Birmingham, AL 35294, USA; [b] Department of Radiology, UT Southwestern Medical Center, 5323 Harry Hines Boulevard, EB 1.346, Dallas, TX 75390-9065, USA; [c] Health System Information Services, and Department of Radiology, University of Alabama at Birmingham, 625 19th Street South, Birmingham, AL 35233, USA; [d] Department of Abdominal Radiology, University of Texas MD Anderson Medical Center, Unit 1473, 1515 Hocombe Boulevard, Houston, TX 77030-4009, USA
* Corresponding author. Department of Radiology, 619 19th Street South, Birmingham, AL 35294.
E-mail address: mrobbin@uabmc.edu

set a high bar for the US practice to meet. Accreditation is offered by organizations including the American College of Radiology (ACR), American Institute of Ultrasound in Medicine (AIUM), and Intersocietal Accreditation Commission, each with their own benefits and specific requirements. A common theme is submission of complete US studies with requisite image acquisition parameters.

A single or small group of radiologist and sonographer leaders can serve as points of contact for the team, and can help identify, review, and save submission-worthy examinations. These examinations are generally reviewed for quality at multiple levels, with final authorization by a physician leader or the radiologist originally assigned to that case. The stepwise fashion allows for multiple checkpoints to detect problems prior to submission and review by the accrediting body. This also distributes the workload so that no one individual bears the considerable burden. The submission process is also valuable in informing the radiologists and sonographers as to the necessity of consistency, accuracy, and completeness in images and reports, as well as identifying any areas with incomplete imaging as judged by the accrediting organization, in order to achieve a national standard of excellence.

TRAINING

Given the often-discussed "operator dependence" of US, physicians must feel comfortable in a sonographer's ability to obtain requisite diagnostic images. As sonographers are the physician's eyes, ears, and hands, they are essential for an efficient and accurate US practice. Our sonographers must meet departmental educational requirements (in part based on accreditation), including Registered Diagnostic Medical Sonographer, Registered Vascular Technologist, Registered Vascular Specialist, and American Registry of Radiologic Technologists in sonography or vascular sonography, or equivalent certifications, within a set number of years of hiring. Regardless of credentials, each sonographer is evaluated directly within our departments to identify any gaps in knowledge or areas of educational deficiency at hire, and a training plan is created, agreed upon, and implemented.

A detailed checkoff worksheet for each examination performed at a specific clinical site is used to review the sonographer's capability to perform an examination appropriately at one of our institutions (MLR, MEL and FNT). Until they are confirmed, their examinations are "backscanned" by a more experienced sonographer and then reviewed by a sonologist or physician extender for quality and completeness. Aspects reviewed include quality of grayscale images, Doppler technique, and adherence to imaging protocols. Generally, 5 completed examinations that meet minimum standards (3 normal and 2 abnormal) are sufficient to allow independent scanning, acknowledging that more examinations may be required to show proficiency. If an experienced sonographer who commonly performs these examinations is hired, the required number of examinations may be reduced to 1 normal and 1 abnormal to show proficiency in local standards.

Radiology trainees are trained in an apprenticeship fashion, sitting alongside the attending and in proximity to the physician extenders so that they may benefit from all educational opportunities. They are trained in protocols and then expected to provide feedback to sonographers. In their early educational setting, the resident reviews of sonographer studies are closely monitored by faculty. Often the resident will ask for extender guidance; however, the nearby faculty may also "jump in" to the conversation if they sense that the resident is uncertain about an image or examination parameter. For the new faculty who are unfamiliar with local protocols, there is a brief observation period, and subsequently the extenders are readily available to explain the nuances of specific image requirements or parameters specific to a particular institution. This enables faculty from institutions less familiar with complex sonographic scenarios to rapidly ramp up to speed.

ADVANCED PRACTICE SONOGRAPHERS

Many medical specialties have benefitted from adding advanced practice providers to their ranks, including physician assistants and nurse practitioners, extending the breadth of what a single physician may be able to accomplish on their own. Similarly, in US, the concept of a "sonographic physician's extender" has emerged, albeit without a formal training program or certificate despite discussions within societies like the Society of Diagnostic Medical Sonography and AIUM.[3,4] Nevertheless, individual organizations have taken steps to elevate staff sonographers to roles that capitalize on their experience and dedication, enhancing their contribution to a busy US department beyond the limits of US examination performance. These roles, known by various titles such as US or Sonographer Practitioner, Sonographer Radiologist Assistant, Advanced Practice Sonographer (APS), or simply "super tech" or "quality assurance tech," will be referred to as APS throughout this article.

An APS can fulfill several roles within an US department, including: reviewing examinations for completeness, accuracy, and obtaining additional imaging as required before patients leave; serving as a scribe to create detailed sonographer notes or draft dictations for radiologists; assisting with advanced US applications including creating 3-dimensional (3D) reconstructions, performing musculoskeletal examinations, or functioning as the second pair of hands for a CEUS examination; reviewing examinations for site accreditation; and performing sonographer quality assurance. They can also participate in sonographer onboarding and training, assist with training on new technologies, and contribute to resident and fellow education. An APS may also facilitate US-related research and the development of new techniques or protocols. By performing these tasks, subspecialty US radiologists may not be physically needed at every site where high-level US or complex examinations are performed, allowing for greater flexibility in scheduling and site coverage.

US facilities interested in establishing APS positions must develop their own job description and requirements. Details that should be covered include years of experience since training (eg, minimum of 5, 8, or 10 years), number and type of registries held (covering all areas of the practice), and competencies in a variety of techniques (eg, elastography; musculoskeletal or obstetric US). Strong communication skills, teaching aptitude, and the ability to serve as liaison between sonographers and radiologists are essential qualities for prospective candidates. Although there may be theoretic concerns regarding interpersonal relationships between staff sonographers and an APS, this has not been reported in the literature, and in our experience, the sonographers value the APSs as a resource for education and more consistent workflow. Importantly, an APS is a great career opportunity for those with the passion and desire to advance beyond their position as a staff sonographer, allowing an experienced sonographer to continue working in clinically oriented activities, as opposed to seeking a purely administrative career path.

Budget allocation for APS salaries typically depends on their primary roles and responsibilities within the professional practice or imaging department administration. Some professional practices may cover the entire salary, allowing the APS to primarily work with radiologists in quality and report drafting tasks. Alternatively, imaging service lines may fund APS positions when administrative duties such as quality assurance, education, and accreditation are also included. Some institutions may adopt a cost-sharing model between professional and technical practices, tailoring responsibilities to meet both the radiologist and the imaging service line needs. While some institutions may establish specific full-time APS positions distinct from staff sonographers, others may integrate APS responsibilities into existing sonographer roles.

Ideally, an APS would have the depth and breadth of knowledge and experience to function at the level of a radiology senior resident or fellow, able to correlate US findings with other modalities such as CT or MRI, and review the electronic medical record for relevant medical or surgical history, medications, or specific risk factors. An APS can triage phone calls, and can be assigned the task of calling an ordering provider to collect pertinent information or even report critical results, under specific delegation from their supervising radiologist. An APS may also assist with complex or time-consuming examinations, such as those performed in the operating room or neonatal intensive care unit.

Previous studies have shown a very low significant discrepancy rate between an APS's draft dictation and a radiologist's final report.[5] However, an APS cannot function independently as there is no national or even state-level registry or certification at this time. An APS is unlikely to obtain provider credentials within a hospital or organization, and therefore is unable to perform independent billable services. Therefore, all activities must be directly supervised by a radiologist, and no APS draft report may be viewable outside of the radiology department.

Regardless, the value of an APS to the modern US department is substantial. As techniques and technologies become more numerous and advanced, and the number of US-focused radiologists decreases relative to the number of US examinations being performed, an APS can be a critical and necessary solution to maintaining consistent and high-quality care. One author (DF) calculated that when looking at the time saved, 1 APS is equivalent to nearly one-third of a full-time radiologist, with his team of 4 APSs having drafted over 10,000 reports in 6 months, highlighting their significant contribution to departmental efficiency and productivity.

PICTURE ARCHIVING AND COMMUNICATION SYSTEM/ARTIFICIAL INTELLIGENCE
Information Technology in the Ultrasound Facility

Information Technology (IT) plays a pivotal role in all phases of contemporary US. (Scanner-specific technologies such as advanced beamforming and image processing found in modern US platforms are beyond the scope of this discussion.) To understand how to best leverage IT in a US facility, it is instructive to consider the steps from when the patient's examination is ordered and scheduled to when their sonogram is interpreted and a report is entered into the Electronic Health Record. **Table 1** summarizes considerations for pre-scan preparation, image capture, and post scan activities. Additional considerations are as follows.

Image Storage and Export

All general-purpose Picture Archiving and Communication Systems (PACS) enable presentation of both static US images and cinematic (cine) clips for review, in addition to displaying prior sonograms and other imaging studies for comparison. Retrieval should be accomplished with minimal delay. Some departments may further benefit from a dedicated US PACS that offers functions such as simultaneous display of multiple clips (usually displayed in the chronologic order in which they were acquired), US-specific measurements, and tagging images for teaching or research. These systems are typically implemented in conjunction with a facility's main PACS, and may leverage a single archive to avoid duplication of storage. Regardless, the software should allow static images or clips to be exported in common file formats without the patient's name or other Protected Health Information.

Image Interpretation and Reporting

IT needs at this stage largely depend on how sonograms are read. Regardless, ready access to on-line informational databases and rapid access to ambulatory and inpatient notes, operative reports, and pathology results are essential to improve examination interpretation. If possible, these resources should be viewable on a monitor separate from the one used to display US images.

In many US facilities, particularly those associated with radiology departments and imaging centers, reports are generated using voice dictation software. These systems have progressed considerably over the past several decades, and now enable creation of structured reports that can later be mined for teaching, research, or quality control. Also, software that collects and organizes DICOM-SR (Structured Report) elements from the scanner enables automatic transfer of obstetric, vascular, and other US measurements into the structured report, decreasing reporting time and eliminating errors introduced by entering numbers manually. Some systems also apply quality checks during the reporting process. For example, they can automatically flag right/left or gender-related inconsistencies. These capabilities increase productivity by reducing the need to make corrections after the fact.

Artificial Intelligence

Available applications based on machine learning, deep learning, radiomics, and generative artificial intelligence (AI) in medical imaging have grown exponentially in recent years. Most current AI packages are deployed on PACS or other workstations, though some may be integrated into the US scanner itself.

While US has lagged somewhat because of the way sonograms are performed and reported, this is changing rapidly, and platforms that apply AI are beginning to move from proof-of-concept to clinical use in thyroid, liver, ovarian, breast, and vascular sonography. For example, AI software can provide decision support in categorizing nodules based on the ACR TI-RADS (Thyroid Imaging Reporting and Data System), or assist with ovarian follicle tracking in infertility patients, potentially boosting efficiency and accuracy. As well, generative AI is being used to create US reports, and large language models are being applied to mine the discrete data from free text dictations. Increasingly, AI is being used to optimize US scans in real time, including automatically adjusting grayscale or Doppler settings, or identifying and measuring common anatomic structures—these features may both improve a sonographer's efficiency, and decrease inter-operator variability. Eventually, AI may be able to call the operator's attention to abnormalities while a scan is being performed, reducing the likelihood of missing or not adequately imaging pathology. Several issues remain unresolved in AI applications. For example, how will AI be accepted and trusted if its inner workings are not well-understood by patients or physicians? Will inexperienced readers come to rely on the technology too much, and who will be liable if a physician does not accept AI's conclusion, or accepts a spurious result, potentially leading to a poor patient outcome? Despite these challenges, the future of AI in augmenting US workflow and interpretation is bright.

OFFERING NEW ULTRASOUND EXAMINATIONS

Developing new US services are an integral component of keeping up with the latest technology and techniques, and can allow a site to even lead a rapidly developing field. US examinations these authors have brought to their respective US departments include CEUS, hemodialysis access and other innovative vascular studies, advanced 3D techniques, elastography, and fat

Table 1
Information technology-related capabilities and advantages in the ultrasound facility

Phase	Capability	What It Does	Advantages
Pre-scan	Scheduling software	Schedules US examinations based on available resources, patient/referrer preferences, and needs, and enables protocoling in advance	Boosts efficiency and satisfaction
	DICOM modality worklist	Enters order/examination type and other information into scanner	Improves efficiency and reduces patient identification errors
	Display images from PACS on scanner	Enables viewing of prior imaging examinations before scanning	Facilitates localizing small lesions on US
Scan	Annotation	Automatic labeling for protocol images and ad hoc labeling for non-protocol captures	Boosts efficiency
	Transmission	Automatic sending images to PACS via a secure network, wirelessly for bedside examinations	Enables contemporaneous review by a physician, including for remote studies, lessening the need for re-scanning
Post scan	Offline review workstation	Allows the sonographer to re-arrange images, change annotations, generate images from 3-D volumes, and selectively re-measure	Speeds image interpretation

quantification, among others. Importantly, potential referring services should be consulted regarding their interest in any new examination. After a thorough literature review and consulting other expert US departments, the team can establish an imaging protocol and determine the criteria used to evaluate the findings. Generally, at least 2 radiologists should be enthusiastic and knowledgeable about the new examination and interpretation. Thereafter, 2 to 3 sonographers should be identified as "experts" and teaching sessions provided. These sonographers can oversee the performance of the first few critical cases. Afterward, these experts can facilitate training of additional sonographers as needed, to further expand the new service.

Additional considerations include any special patient instructions such as any need to fast, who will place an intravenous line (in the case of CEUS), as well as average length of study. Scheduling review may include limiting new examinations to certain sites while experience is accumulating, or only on certain days when specific individuals are present and available. Where the examination will take place (inpatient vs outpatient), and whether it can be performed at multiple sites are also important considerations. We usually begin a new examination at one location, and then train additional personnel with the ultimate goal of performing a study enterprise-wide (liver elastography, for example). Other examinations that require local on-site expertise, such as availability of musculoskeletal radiologist experts, may still limit some US examinations to a particular site.

How the referring clinician will order the examination should be considered—in the case of an electronic ordering systems, the creation of a unique order, possibly with key words, order entry questions, and/or imbedded information may help passively educate ordering providers. In addition, knowing how an examination will be billed needs to be planned (ie, what Current Procedural Terminology [CPT] code(s) should be linked to the order).

Once the initial team is comfortable with the new technique, formal patient examinations can be scheduled, and the protocol can be refined. An active case review and quality assurance process should be implemented, and informative cases set aside. Thereafter, educational sessions should take place between physicians and sonographers to widen the pool of personnel that can perform and interpret the examination. Marketing and discussion with potential referring clinicians should continue to increase the number of patients referred.

EXPANDING TO NEW ULTRASOUND LOCATIONS (CLINIC/HOSPITAL/ FREESTANDING EMERGENCY ROOM)

The growth and expansion of a medical organization is invariably accompanied by increased imaging. During this growth, an imaging department should strive to provide consistent and high-quality imaging no matter where a patient may present. A patient undergoing imaging at a small, remote community center should receive the same quality service as a patient receiving care at an organization's flagship hospital or central imaging site.

Adding a new site typically involves the prospective construction of a new location or acquisition and incorporation of an existing site. Both scenarios involve their own unique benefits and challenges. For instance, when an organization builds a new site, leaders can plan to purchase identical equipment and implement policies and protocols from existing sites—this facilitates uniformity and consistency. Alternatively, the acquisition of a new site may involve incorporating sonographers with variable levels of training or comfort with an organization's preferred imaging protocols and workflow, as well as variability in scanner models and technological capabilities, which may prohibit certain services, such as liver elastography or 3D pelvic US. Administrators should strive to homogenize technology as much as is practical and feasible, allowing an organization to provide the same services at all locations, not only simplifying patient scheduling but making it more convenient for patients.

A robust sonographer onboarding and quality assurance program is of paramount importance to providing consistent and high-quality imaging across an enterprise. This may include training new sonographers at more central sites with more direct oversite before deploying them to new or remote sites. Completing a competency process where certain examinations are reviewed by a technical supervisor, APS, or radiologist may help ensure sonographers are ready for more independent work, as discussed in the training section aforementioned. Regardless, a central, easily-accessible database of imaging protocols and policies is essential—this "source of truth" can be referenced at any time from any site, and can be easily updated without having each site maintain their own protocol directory or binder, which risks becoming out-of-date.

Communication tools including PACS or institution-based messaging systems are useful for quick and efficient communication between sites. In addition, video chat tools that facilitate communication between a remote sonographer and their supervising radiologist or APS, some even available on the US systems themselves, may allow a radiologist's real-time live review of an imaging study, ultimately improving patient care by ensuring protocol completeness.

QUALITY ASSURANCE
Ultrasound Performance and Review

The quality of an US study relies heavily on the sonographer's experience, technical expertise, and attenuation to detail to a greater degree than for technologists in other imaging modalities. A QA program is a key to ensuring that studies are of consistent, reproducible quality. Physician or physician extender review of the US study prior to the patient leaving the US department is an important quality check. Most radiologists read USs from the PACS workstation regardless of the location where the US was performed.

Scanning Protocols

Standardized US scanning protocols list the required images (and often orientation, labeling, etc) and can reduce variability between sonographers. Facilities should create protocols customized to the needs of their practice. Protocols themselves should undergo periodic review and updates, can include example images of anatomy and pathology, and list diagnostic criteria (if applicable). These protocols should be stored in an easily-accessible location (preferably electronic, such as within an institution's intranet site), such that sonographers at different locations have immediate access to latest updates. The AIUM and ACR practice parameters, and Society of Radiologists in Ultrasound (SRU) consensus documents provide an excellent basis for scanning protocols.

Scanner-based Protocols

Most equipment manufacturers now allow for protocols to be programmed directly into the scanner, allowing the device to guide a sonographer through the requisite images, automatically labeling images and launching features such as color or spectral Doppler at the appropriate point in the protocol. This can be particularly useful for

Table 2
Protocol for interventional procedures

Pre-procedure	Pre-scan, review prior imaging Screen for coagulopathy Determination of sedation requirements
Intra-procedural	Collection, labeling and delivery of specimens to pathology. Immediate assessment of specimen adequacy. Monitoring of vital signs
Post-procedure	Post-procedure scan Vital signs as indicated Correlate radiology-pathology results for quality assurance

examinations that may not be as common, in which images may be inadvertently forgotten. These "on-cart" protocols make it easier for new sonographers to perform US examinations at the expected level for the department and national accrediting standards. Image-based protocols may also decrease the length of time it takes to perform the examination, as standard protocol images are already labeled as per facility requirements.[6] Protocols also make physician review easier as specific images are located in the same point in the examination, making dictation and comparison with prior studies easier.

Infection Control

Outbreaks of infection have resulted from contaminated transducers and US gel. Facilities should develop infection control procedures based on Center for Disease Control and Prevention and Joint Commission guidelines. These should include handwashing, use of gloves, and policies for cleaning US equipment (**Table 2**). The date/time of disinfection for every transducer should be documented. To prevent reinfection, there should be policies regarding storage and separation of clean from dirty transducers. Special protocols are required for interventional procedures (**Table 3**).[7]

Safety

The ALARA (as low as reasonably achievable) principle should be followed when adjusting acoustic output and overall scanning time.[8] In particular, the lowest setting that provides diagnostic quality images should be used when scanning the embryo, neonatal brain, and the eye. For example, pulse Doppler should not be routinely used to document embryonic cardiac activity. Facilities that perform CEUS should screen patients for a history of allergy to US contrast agents or polyethylene glycol (PEG), and be prepared to manage adverse effects (**Table 4**). Sterile gels containing chlorhexidine are contraindicated in patients with associated allergy. PEG can also be a component

Table 3
Infection control

Scenario	Policy	Notes
Transducer contacts intact skin	Low-level disinfection (LLD): Disinfectant wipes Alcohols Quaternary ammonium compounds	Effective against most microorganisms. Exceptions include mycobacteria, bacterial spores.
Transducer contacts non-intact skin or mucous membranes (intracavitary transducers)	High-level disinfection (HLD): Automated (Hydrogen peroxide mist) Liquid soak devices (Glutaraldehyde) Sterile gel Transducer cover optional	Effective against all microorganisms except some bacterial spores. Latex-free covers should be available
Transducer contacts sterile tissue	Sterile gel Transducer cover	
Neonates	Sterile gel	
Suspected or positive Covid-19, or other novel or endemic infectious agents.	Dedicated US units and transducers if possible Low-level disinfection (LLD) Transducer cover Keyboard and console cover	Covid-19 is viable on plastic surfaces for 72 h.

Table 4
Ultrasound contrast agents - adverse effects[9-11]

Serious	Mild
Anaphylaxis 0.006%– 0.01%	Nausea and vomiting
Life-threatening anaphylaxis 0.001%	Taste alteration
	Headache
	Flushing
	Vertigo
	Rash
Resuscitation resources and response plan needed.	Generally, resolves spontaneously. No treatment required in most cases.

of some gels and can therefore cause contact dermatitis. Non-latex gloves and sterile transducer covers should also be available.

Work-related Musculoskeletal Disorders (WRMSD)

Work-related Musculoskeletal Disorders (WRMSD) are musculoskeletal injuries caused by repetitive strain that affect US users, particularly sonographers (Table 5).[12,13] 15% of sonographers experience symptoms 6 months from the start of employment, 45% after 3 years, and 72% after 10 years. Ultimately, these injuries are career-ending for 20%. Portable studies exacerbate WRSMD because they are often performed in non-ergonomic settings.[14] Apart from the personal toll on those affected, WRMSD are a major cause of sonographer absenteeism and attrition, which exacerbates the nationwide sonographer shortage that currently exists. Facilities also must bear costs related to worker's compensation. The Occupational Safety and Health Administration, which holds employers responsible for worker safety, recognizes WRMSD as a significant problem in sonography.

Continuing Education and Peer Learning

A continuing education (CE) program and Peer Learning are integral to QA. CE can be didactic lectures or informal teaching at the workstation. Peer Learning (now preferred over Peer Review) embraces recognition of errors as a teaching opportunity, and can be applied to sonographers and radiologists.[15] Individuals are encouraged to reveal their own or others' mistakes in a non-punitive framework, which avoids blame and responsibility and focuses instead on process improvement and error prevention. Features include confidential, constructive feedback to individuals, peer learning conferences, and linking the peer learning program to process improvement. During a peer learning conference, cases are shared and opportunities for improvement are discussed. Areas of weakness are noted, and a dedicated effort is launched to drive improvement.

Turnaround Times

Turnaround times (TAT) for US studies are key measures of productivity, and can include time from order to appointment, examination initiation to completion, and completion to final interpretive report. QA should aim to reduce TAT, particularly for time-sensitive scenarios such as emergency department or critically ill

Table 5
Work-related musculoskeletal disorders in sonographers

Symptoms	Location and Incidence of Symptoms	Findings	Policies that can Reduce WRMSDs
Pain Joint stiffness/ inflammation Muscle tightness	Shoulder 90% Low back 69% Hand and wrist 54%	Carpal tunnel syndrome Cubital tunnel syndrome Elbow epicondylitis Shoulder capsulitis and tendonitis Neck and back strain	Minimize manual lifting and patient positioning by sonographers. Sonographer education about WRMSD prevention Use of ergonomic US equipment Adopt OSHA ultrasound WRMSD guidelines. https://www.osha.gov/etools/hospitals/clinical-services/sonography

Table 6
Turnaround time

Turnaround Time	Responsible Personnel	Policies that can Reduce TAT
Order entry to study initiation	Scheduling Patient transporters	Radiology staff can modify orders without obtaining approval from ordering provider. Effective transportation system, controlled by Radiology.
Study initiation to completion	Sonographers	Registered, experienced sonographers. Standardized scanning protocols. Minimize number of portable studies. Study review by physician before patient discharge to minimize callback.
Study completion to final report	Radiologists	Electronic worksheets. Structured reports (templates).

hospitalized patients. Portable studies are inefficient given the additional time required for the sonographer to travel to and from the bedside. The elements of TAT in sequential order, and mitigation strategies, are described in **Table 6**. However, TAT should not be the only metric by which a department is evaluated. Unreasonably short examination time slots, for instance, may reduce a sonographer's ability to acquire high-quality studies, increase the number of mistakes (eg, protocol exclusions), and could lead to increased WRMSD.

BILLING AND REIMBURSEMENT

A billing operation should aim to submit claims promptly and receive reimbursement as quickly as possible. Radiologists, technologists, and the institutional billing department should be educated regarding the latest ultrasound billing codes, and how to optimize billing. CPT coding rules list specific criteria that must be met for reimbursement (**Table 7**). For example, it is important for physicians and sonographers to know when a Doppler charge can be added to an abdominal, pelvic, or scrotal US or when a transabdominal and transvaginal pelvic US can be performed together. Failure to perform proper documentation may result in denials, which delay reimbursement, disrupt cash flow, and generate additional work for the billing department.

At one of our institutions (MLR, MEL and FNT), we have worked with our compliance department to have standing orders that allow adding an US examination when pre-defined findings on the primary examination are found. For example, when the top of the lower extremity thrombus cannot be seen in the common femoral/external iliac vein, we have compliance permission to add an inferior vena cava (IVC) US examination to assess for more proximal thrombus in the pelvic veins and IVC. This

Table 7
Billing and coding

Requirements	Coding and Billing Resources

Document medical necessity for exam
Permanent image archive
Document required anatomic elements and measurements for each study.
	ACR ultrasound coding user's guide
	MedLearn® ultrasound coder
	ACR membership benefits:
	   Clinical examples in Radiology – a practical guide with in-depth explanations of coding scenarios and new CPT codes
	   Answers to imaging related coding questions (includes AMA members).

obviates the need to contact the ordering provider by adding the additional IVC US order automatically, following Center for Medicare and Medicaid Services rules governing imaging of adjacent/contiguous body parts. The examination order would then list: "US Lower Extremity Venous Doppler + US IVC, as indicated". A similar order is used in pelvic and scrotal US orders, allowing the addition of an abdominal Doppler US examination in patients with pelvic pain that meet pre-specified criteria.

MARKETING

In a radiologist's report, listing the group's departmental accreditation(s), and referencing applicable contemporary consensus documents and literature (for example, SRU consensus on gallbladder polyps and elastography[16,17]) are methods for conveying a high quality, evidence-based practice. A combination of excellent image quality, use of contemporary technology, good communication between team members and between your department and the referring providers and their patients, and a friendly staff are some of the best forms of local marketing. Even in situations where another department (outside of Radiology) owns US scanners and may offer a similar service, for example, elastography, other providers may still utilize your services, yielding a large patient volume.

Early successes and a willingness to provide the extra effort to develop unique protocols or tackle difficult examinations goes a long way and will increase referrals. For example, many practices may not attempt renal artery Doppler, and may then refer such orders to a facility with the known experience and expertise. Specialized examinations for mesenteric vasculature, or evaluation of organ transplants, may also only be offered by select sites, further helping build a robust referral base.

Moreover, focused marketing may occur in the form of presentations at local meetings or tumor boards, collaborations with other non-radiology clinicians, regional education offerings, national reputation through published research, and word-of-mouth from physicians who have been helped when turned away from other institutions. Calling clinicians to discuss abnormal findings and querying patient disposition for urgent findings such as in patients with a new deep vein thrombosis, or a new liver mass, can help form physician relationships that have lasting effects.

SUMMARY

It should be clear that no two US departments are the same; however, there are many common themes that differentiate a successful department from those who simply offer standard US services as a part of their larger imaging practice, or only offer US for the potential financial benefit. Quality should be top priority, represented by thorough onboarding and continuous learning and training, well-organized structure and workflow, credentialing and accreditation. Many of the other aspects described earlier can contribute greatly to a thriving US department.

CLINICS CARE POINTS

- Uniform facility wide US scanner-based protocols decrease the acquisition time for some US examinations, increasing efficiency with increased uniformity and accreditation guideline adherence.
- Advanced practice sonographers can substantially increase exam consistency and high-quality care in an US department.
- Quality assurance, turn-around time, billing, coding and marketing are the key underpinnings for a successful US practice.

DISCLOSURE

M.L. Robbin: Philips Healthcare, research agreement through ended 2024. Philips Medical Vascular Advisory Board (single session), 2/2023. Jazz Pharmaceuticals, VOD Advisory Board (single session), 6/2023. D.T. Fetzer: Research agreements: GE HealthCare; Philips Healthcare; Siemens Healthineers. Advisory board: GE HealthCare; Philips Healthcare; Bracco Diagnostics. Speakers' bureau: GE HealthCare; Siemens Healthineers. F.N. Tessler: No disclosures. W.K. Chong: No Disclosures. M.E. Lockhart: Journal of Ultrasound, Deputy Editor Salary, ongoing. Elsevier, Book royalties, ongoing. JayPee Brothers Medical Publishers, Book royalties, ongoing. United States FDA Medical Devices Panel, Special Governmental Employee, ongoing.

REFERENCES

1. Robbin ML, Lockhart ME, Weber TM, et al. Ultrasound quality and efficiency: how to make your practice flourish. J Ultrasound Med 2011;30(6): 739–43.
2. Finberg HJ. Whither (wither?) the ultrasound specialist? J Ultrasound Med 2004;23(12):1543–7.
3. Lockhart ME, Robbin ML, Berland LL, et al. The sonographer practitioner: one piece to the radiologist

3. shortage puzzle. J Ultrasound Med 2003;22(9): 861–4.
4. Benacerraf BR, Bromley BS, Shipp TD, et al. The making of an advanced practice sonographer. J Ultrasound Med 2003;22(9):865–7.
5. Bude RO, Fatchett JP, Lechtanski TA. The use of additionally trained sonographers as ultrasound practitioners: our first-year experience. J Ultrasound Med 2006;25(3):321–7 [quiz: 328–7].
6. Sanyal R, Kraft B, Alexander LF, et al. Scanner-based protocol-driven ultrasound: an effective method to improve efficiency in an ultrasound department. AJR Am J Roentgenol 2016;206(4): 792–6.
7. AIUM Official Statement: Guidelines for Cleaning and Preparing External- and Internal-Use Ultrasound Transducers and Equipment Between Patients as Well as Safe Handling and Use of Ultrasound Coupling Gel. J Ultrasound Med 2023;42(7):E13–22.
8. As Low As Reasonably Achievable (ALARA) Principle. AIUM official statement. 2020. Available at: https://www.aium.org/resources/official-statements/view/as-low-as-reasonably-achievable-(alara)-principle. [Accessed 5 September 2024].
9. Tang C, Fang K, Guo Y, et al. Safety of Sulfur Hexafluoride Microbubbles in Sonography of Abdominal and Superficial Organs: Retrospective Analysis of 30,222 Cases. J Ultrasound Med 2017;36(3):531–8.
10. Wei K, Mulvagh SL, Carson L, et al. The safety of deFinity and Optison for ultrasound image enhancement: a retrospective analysis of 78,383 administered contrast doses. J Am Soc Echocardiogr 2008;21(11):1202–6.
11. Piscaglia F, Bolondi L. The safety of Sonovue in abdominal applications: retrospective analysis of 23188 investigations. Ultrasound Med Biol 2006; 32(9):1369–75.
12. Evans K, Roll S, Baker J. Work-Related Musculoskeletal Disorders (WRMSD) Among Registered Diagnostic Medical Sonographers and Vascular Technologists: A Representative Sample. J Diagn Med Sonogr 2009;25(6):287–99.
13. Industry Standards for the Prevention of Work Related Musculoskeletal Disorders in Sonography. J Diagn Med Sonogr 2017;33(5):370–91.
14. Kliewer M, Walker T, Bagley AR. Toward Ergonomic Design in Ultrasound Scanning: Strategies to Mitigate Injurious Forces. Ultrasound Q 2022;38(1):65–71.
15. Donnelly LF, Larson DB, Heller RE III, et al. Practical Suggestions on How to Move From Peer Review to Peer Learning. AJR American journal of roentgenology 2018;210(3):578–82.
16. Barr RG, Wilson SR, Rubens D, et al. Update to the Society of Radiologists in Ultrasound Liver Elastography Consensus Statement. Radiology 2020; 296(2):263–74.
17. Kamaya A, Fung C, Szpakowski JL, et al. Management of Incidentally Detected Gallbladder Polyps: Society of Radiologists in Ultrasound Consensus Conference Recommendations. Radiology 2022; 305(2):277–89.

Multiparametric Ultrasound for Chronic Liver Disease

Richard G. Barr, MD, PhD

KEYWORDS

- Liver • Chronic liver disease • Focal liver lesions • MASLD • NAFLD • Liver steatosis
- Fat quantification • Quantitative ultrasound

KEY POINTS

- Chronic liver disease (CID) is a world-wide epidemic. As treatments for viral hepatitis have become available, fatty liver disease is now the major cause of CID world-wide.
- Shear wave imaging using ultrasound (US) is a non-invasive, inexpensive, widely-available technique to estimate liver stiffness (LS). LS is influenced by fibrosis, inflammation, and congestion.
- Quantitative US is now clinically available to estimate the amount of liver fat.
- For accurate estimates of LS and fat quantification, a strict acquisition protocol needs to be followed.

INTRODUCTION

Chronic liver disease (CLD) is a substantial worldwide problem. Any disease that incites liver inflammation can lead to fibrosis which can progress to cirrhosis. Major etiologies are hepatitis B, hepatitis C, metabolic associated steatohepatitis (MASH), alcoholic liver disease, autoimmune response, and primary biliary cirrhosis. **Box 1** lists major causes of liver inflammation. The primary etiology varies depending on the region of the world with the viral etiologies more prevalent in Asia and Africa[1] while metabolic associated liver disease is more prevalent in Europe and North America although becoming a world-wide epidemic.[2] Chronic liver damage from any etiology results in hepatic fibrosis characterized by an increase in extracellular matrix produced by fibroblast-like cells. The major consequence is increasing deposition of fibrous tissue leading to the development of portal hypertension (PHT), hepatic insufficiency, and hepatocellular carcinoma (HCC). Liver fibrosis (LF) can progress to cirrhosis with distortion of the normal liver architecture and resultant PHT. The time needed to progress to cirrhosis varies with the inciting cause.[3]

Cirrhosis is a diffuse process, characterized by fibrosis and the conversion of normal liver architecture into structurally abnormal nodules.[4] The stage of LF is important to determine prognosis, surveillance, and prioritize for treatment now that it is known that treating the underlying cause may cause regression of the fibrosis.[5]

With increasing fibrosis, the liver becomes stiffer, and this eventually results in PHT. Previously the only method of quantifying the degree of fibrosis was a random liver biopsy, but liver histology is an imperfect reference standard.[5] Conventional ultrasound (US) is limited in the detection of fibrosis until the development of cirrhosis. Shear wave elastography (SWE) has become widely available and can assess and monitor liver stiffness (LS).[5] For accurate stiffness measurements a strict protocol is required and is discussed at length in this document.[6]

Metabolic dysfunction-associated steatotic liver disease (MASLD), previously termed non-alcoholic fatty liver disease, is currently the leading cause of CLD world-wide. Hepatic steatosis can be caused by several pathologic processes. The differential diagnosis for diffuse fatty infiltration of the liver is

Northeastern Ohio Medical University, Southwoods Imaging, 7623 Market Street, Youngstown, OH 44512, USA
E-mail address: Rgbarr525@gmail.com

> **Box 1**
> **Common causes of hepatic inflammation that progress to fibrosis**
>
> Hepatitis B (chronic)
> Hepatitis C
> Nonalcoholic fatty liver disease/nonalcoholic steatohepatitis
> Alcohol abuse
> Drugs (eg, methotrexate and some chemotherapy agents)
> Primary biliary cirrhosis
> Hemochromatosis
> Autoimmune hepatitis
> Wilson's disease
> α1-Antitrypsin deficiency
> Sclerosing cholangitis
> Post gastric bypass
> Schistosomiasis

listed in **Box 2**. The prevalence of the disease has increased over the last few years: it has been estimated that it increased from 25.5% before 2005 to 37.8% in 2016 or later.[7] MASLD is often a silent disease even at the late stage of severe fibrosis and the diagnosis is frequently made incidentally.[8] Patients with MASLD have a risk of cardiovascular disease, liver-related events, and all-cause mortality higher than the general population.[9,10] The steatosis grade predicts mortality and the risk of developing type 2 diabetes mellitus in patients with MASLD.[11] The fatty infiltration of the liver causes inflammation leading to MASH leading to fibrosis and progression to cirrhosis (**Fig. 1**). If fatty liver disease is identified at an early-stage treatment can reverse the process and prevent the development of cirrhosis and liver cancer.

Liver biopsy has been considered the reference standard for detecting and grading liver steatosis. However, it is an invasive procedure with some associated risk of severe complications, and the inter-observer variability in evaluating the specimens is not negligible.[12] In 1 published study, the authors found that there was a poor agreement among pathologists for the assessment of steatosis (intraclass correlation coefficient: 0.57) as well as inconsistent assessment of histologic features of steatohepatitis.[13] Considering the epidemic proportions of fatty liver disease throughout the population, biopsy is not practical for screening purposes due to the large number of affected individuals and invasive procedures should be limited since the tests find only MAFLD with simple steatosis in the majority cases. Furthermore, liver steatosis is a dynamic process that may vary in a short period of time (months); therefore, a non-invasive assessment is crucial.

> **Box 2**
> **Causes of diffuse hepatic steatosis**
>
> Obesity
> Hyperlipidemia
> Nonalcoholic fatty liver disease/Nonalcoholic steatohepatitis
> Chronic alcohol ingestion
> Steroid use
> Amiodarone
> Hepatitis B
> Hepatitis C
> Some chemotherapy agents
> Valproic acid
> Glycogen storage diseases
> Hemochromatosis
> Wilson disease
> Total parenteral nutrition
> Cystic fibrosis

NORMAL ANATOMY AND IMAGING TECHNIQUE

A review of the normal anatomy of the liver can be found elsewhere.[14,15]

IMAGING PROTOCOLS

When evaluating patients with CLD, a complete US evaluation of the liver should be performed. The examination should be performed with a curved linear transducer optimized for abdominal imaging. The frequency of the transducer should be adjusted as needed for the patient's body habitus. Generally, the left lobe of the liver is best imaged in a supine position using a subcostal approach while the right lobe is best imaged using a left lateral decubitus position through an intercostal window. Deep inspiration by the patient may be required to visualize the dome of the liver. A small sector probe can also be helpful in anatomically difficult locations. Vascular landmarks should be included so the position of the images can be identified according to the Couinaud classification.[16] Color or power Doppler is used to evaluate vessel patency and flow dynamics. The biliary system should also be

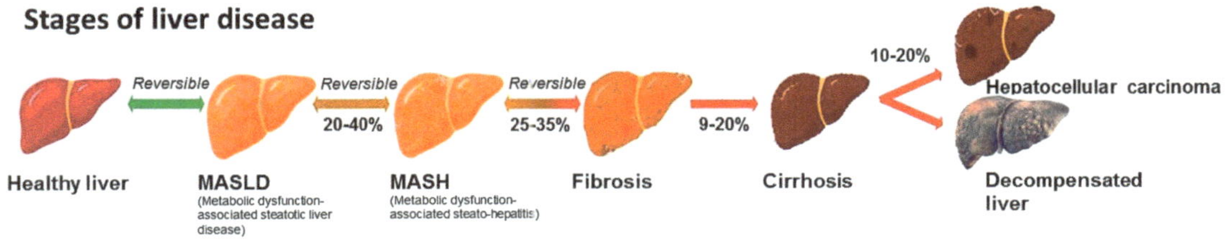

Stages of liver disease

Fig. 1. Stages of Fatty Liver Disease. The progression of fatty liver disease occurs with first deposition of fat within the liver (MASLD). The fat causes inflammation in some patients leading to MASH which progresses to fibrosis. Up to this point, treatment can reverse the progression of the disease. Progression from this point can lead to cirrhosis with its complications of hepatic failure, development of varies and possible development of hepatocellular carcinoma.

evaluated. This examination should include evaluation of the liver echotexture, a high-resolution image of the liver capsule, assessment of the size of the right lobe of the liver and caudate lobe, and portal vein diameter. Doppler evaluation with spectral analysis of the portal vein and hepatic veins should be performed. Detection and characterization of focal liver lesions should be included but is not discussed in this paper. The splenic size and evaluation for varies should also be evaluated, particularly in patients with cirrhosis. **Table 1** lists the conventional US protocol for CID.

LIVER FAT ESTIMATION
B-mode

B-mode US allows a subjective estimation of the degree of LS, which is usually based on a series of US findings including liver echogenicity, hepatorenal echo contrast, visualization of intrahepatic vessels, and visualization of the diaphragm.[17] However, in addition to a substantial inter-observer variability in scoring steatosis, the performance for detecting LS (fat content ≥ 5%) is low, with reported sensitivity of 53.3%–63.6%.[18] Diffuse fatty infiltration results in increased echogenicity of the liver. This leads to poor or non-visualization of the diaphragm, intrahepatic vessels and posterior part of the right hepatic lobe. Grading can be made using a qualitative grading system of mild, moderate, or severe.[19] Mild (Grade 1) has a diffuse slight increase in fine echoes with normal visualization of the diaphragm and intrahepatic vessels borders. Some have mentioned loss of detail of the hepatic vein margins as an early finding. Moderate (Grade 2) has moderate diffuse increase in fine echoes with slightly impaired visualization of the intrahepatic vessels and diaphragm. There may be apparent relative loss of the echogenicity of the fatty portal triads as the echogenicity of the surrounding parenchyma increases alongside them. Marked (Grade 3) is represented by a marked increase in fine echoes with poor or no visualization of the intrahepatic vessel borders, diaphragm and posterior portion of the right lobe of the liver (**Fig. 2**).

Hepatorenal Index

A more qualitative method of staging LS is the hepatorenal index[19–22] (**Fig. 3**). This is based on

Table 1
Typical Scanning protocol for chronic liver disease patients

	Mode	Anatomic Location	Key Findings
B-mode	Curved linear probe	Entire Liver Bile Ducts/Gallbladder	Echo Pattern Capsule Nodularity Liver Size (right lobe and caudate lobe) Focal Liver Lesions
	Linear probe		Liver Capsule–smooth or nodular
Color Doppler with Spectral Analysis		Portal Vein Hepatic Vein Splenic Vein IVC Aorta	Portal Vein Size and Flow Pattern Hepatic Vein Patency Varies (present or not)
Elastography		Liver Stiffness ? Splenic Stiffness	Liver Stiffness ? Spleen Stiffness in cirrhotic patients

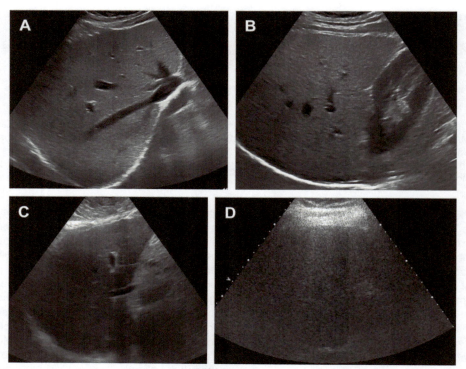

Fig. 2. B-mode images demonstrating increasing fatty deposition in the liver. (A) Normal, (B) mild, (C) moderate, and (D) severe. As the degree of fat increases in the liver, the liver becomes more echogenic. With increasing fat there is a loss of visualization of the blood vessels and diaphragm. The fat causes increased attenuation of the ultrasound beam leading to inability to visualize deep structures.

comparison of the echogenicity of the liver to the normal kidney. This is available on most US systems. Several studies have found this technique has significant correlation to histologic steatosis. A recent study using 3T MRI as the reference standard found that cut-off values of 1.21, 1.28 and 2.15 had 100% sensitivity for diagnosis of greater than 5%, 25% and 50%, respectively with a specificity of greater than 70%.[20]

Quantitative Ultrasound

Currently, 3 different quantitative US parameters can be obtained to estimate liver fat with US: attenuation coefficient (AC), backscatter coefficient (BSC), and speed of sound (SoS). All of them are obtained by analyzing the US signals that return to the transducer before any post-processing is applied, that is, the raw echo (radio-frequency) data. AC estimates the rate of the amplitude loss of the US beam traversing the tissue; it is directly related the amount of fat in the liver. BSC is a measure of US energy scattered by reflectors that are smaller than or equal to the US wavelength and that is returning to the transducer. As with AC, the BSC value increases with

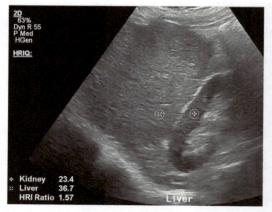

Fig. 3. Hepatorenal Index (HI). A semiquantitative method of estimating liver fat is the HI. The echogenicity of the liver is compared to the echogenicity of the normal renal cortex at the same depth. As the normal renal cortex is not affected by fatty deposition, it can be used as a reference standard. As the degree of fat in the liver increases, the echogenicity of the liver increases leading to an increase in the HI. As each ultrasound vendor calculates this differently it is important to use vendor specific cut-off values.

an increase of liver fat. On the contrary, SoS is inversely related to the amount of liver fat. More details can be found elsewhere.[17]

Controlled attenuation parameter

Controlled attenuation parameter (CAP) is the algorithm available on the FibroScan system (Echosens, France) for the quantification of liver fat content. CAP, which is a non-imaging US-based algorithm performed with a standalone system, is available since more than a decade and has become a point-of-care technique since it does not require imaging expertise. CAP thresholds for detecting and grading liver fat content are highly variable between studies in the literature and also vary depending on the etiology of liver disease.

The system calculates the attenuation slope in decibels per meter (dB/m); results range from 100 to 400 dB/m and is obtained together with the value of LS (**Fig. 4**). The choice of a correct probe is of utmost importance for reliable readings. It has been shown that the use of the M probe in patients with a skin-to-liver capsule distance greater than or equal to 25 mm may overestimate liver steatosis.[23]

The threshold for detecting steatosis (S >0) is quite variable among published studies, ranging from 222 dB/m in a cohort of patients with chronic hepatitis C to 294 dB/m in a meta-analysis that included MASLD patients.[24,25] It has been shown that body mass index, diabetes, and etiology of liver disease may have a significant and relevant impact on the CAP values.[26] A recent meta-analysis has shown that the CAP has a suboptimal performance for grading liver steatosis in patients with MASLD.[25] Given the significant variability of CAP, it is not recommended for longitudinal studies.

Quantification of liver fat with B-mode imaging ultrasound systems

The availability of quantitative US for measuring liver fat on B-mode imaging US systems allows visualizing the area to be sampled while avoiding artifacts; it can be used for the morphologic evaluation of the liver with B-mode, for assessing the portal hemodynamics with the Doppler flowmetry, for the assessment of LS with SWE, and for characterizing a focal liver lesion (if any) with US contrast. 3 methods of quantitative US have been evaluated to estimate the degree of liver steatosis; AC, BSC, and SoS (**Fig. 5**).

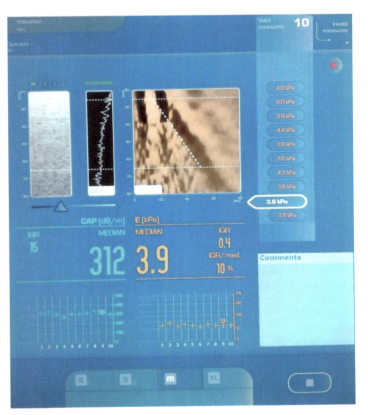

Fig. 4. Example of report from Fibroscan. Ten measurements are obtained, and the median value used. In this case the controlled attenuation parameter is 312 dB/m and the liver stiffness (LS) is 3.9 kPa. The IQR/med is a quality measure for LS and should be less than 30% (for measurements expressed in kPa).

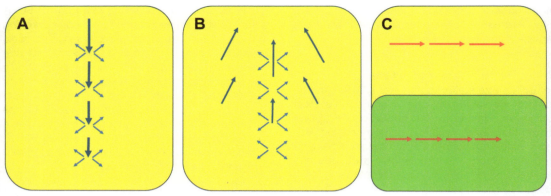

Fig. 5. Illustrations demonstrating the 3 quantitative ultrasound parameters that can be used to estimate the degree of liver fat. (*A*) Attenuation Coefficient (AC). As the ultrasound beam passes through the liver some energy is lost, and the strength of the pulse is decreased resulting in less signal returning to the transducer. In practice the time gain compensation (TGC) setting is used to increase the returning signal at depth to provide an image with uniform signal. The loss of signal (or attenuation) can be measured. With increasing fatty deposition, the AC increases. The AC is measured as dB/cm/MHz. (*B*) Backscatter coefficient (BSC). When the ultrasound beam interacts with tissue, some of the energy is scattered and therefore does not return to transducer. Structures such as fat lobules reflect the ultrasound beam. Some of the scattered signal returns to the transducer and is used to generate the ultrasound image. With increasing fat in the liver, more signals are returned to the transducer leading to increased echogenicity in the image. The amount of returning signal to the transducer is the BSC which is expressed as dB/cm-steradian. (*C*) Speed of Sound (SoS). The speed of the ultrasound beam is dependent on the stiffness of the tissue traversed. The stiffer the tissue the faster the speed of the ultrasound beam. As the degree of fatty deposition in the liver increases, the liver becomes less stiff leading to a decrease in the SoS.

Most of the commercially-available algorithms implemented on US imaging systems are based on the AC estimate. The AC is calculated within a region of interest (ROI) that has a fixed size or is user adjustable. A detailed description of each vendors system can be found elsewhere.[27] The field of view is color-coded in most US systems, allowing the operator to visualize artifacts that should not be included in ROI. These artifacts usually appear in the near field due to reverberation, or sometimes in the far field. In this latter case the artifacts are generally due to low signal-to-noise ratios (**Fig. 6**). Most systems automatically identify artifacts such as blood vessels and do not include them in the fat estimate. The software on the US system calculates the AC in decibel/centimeter/megahertz (dB/cm/MHz).

Combining the AC with the BSC, some manufacturers have obtained a parameter that gives the results in percentage of fat which they correlated with MRI-PDFF. It must be underscored that this percentage does not correspond to the percentage of liver fat at histology. Rather, it is a quantitative estimate that correlates very well, in an almost linear manner, with MRI-PDFF.[28,29] It is expected that other manufacturers will follow this approach. In fact, a percentage is a more practical and intuitive evaluation of liver fat content.

The performance of these new tools has been evaluated using either histology or MR techniques

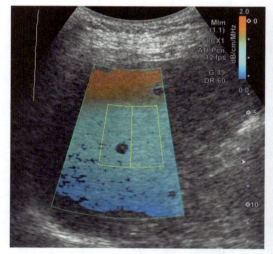

Fig. 6. Example of estimating the AC. The larger rectangular box is the area that AC is measured. The smaller rectangular box is where the AC measurement is made. Note the orange area in the near field which is reverberation artifact and should not be included in the measurement. Therefore, the measurement box needs to be placed below the reverberation artifact (recommended 2 cm). The dark blue area in the far field is artifactual due to loss of signal relative to noise at depth. Also, there is a depth dependance of the AC and standardization of the location of the measurement box below the liver capsule (2 cm depth is recommended) and the size of the measurement box from the near field to the far field needs to be standardized (3 cm is recommended).

as the reference standard. Most of the published studies were conducted using the AC algorithms. Their accuracy in detecting and grading LS showed an AUC above 0.80 for S greater than 0 in most studies.[30–40]

A recent meta-analysis, that included studies performed with the AC algorithm from different manufacturers in 1509 patients, has reported that the pooled sensitivity and specificity of AC were 76% and 84%, respectively, for S greater than or equal to 1, and 87% and 79%, respectively, for S greater than or equal to 2.[41]

However, it must be noted that the AC cutoff values for detecting and grading liver steatosis vary between studies, even when they are carried out using the algorithm of the same manufacturer.[22,42] These differences most likely are due to the lack of a standardized protocol when performing the AC measurement. Indeed, it has been shown that there is a depth dependence of the AC measurement with a progressive decrease of the AC values with the depth.[43] This effect has been observed with different AC algorithms and may account for the differences in the AC cutoff values observed in the published studies. Moreover, the ROI size can also affect the AC value, yielding an AC value that is higher for 1 cm ROI respect to the 3 cm ROI since the larger box includes a greater proportion of deeper samples if both boxes start at a 2 cm depth.[43] On the other hand, the highest repeatability of the AC measurement was observed when the upper edge of the ROI was positioned at 2 cm below the liver capsule, avoiding reverberation artifacts, and using an ROI size of 3 cm.[44] Early guidance has been published for a standardized protocol.[21] However, additional studies are needed to refine this protocol for widespread acceptance by US vendors.

A few studies in small cohorts have assessed the performance of the algorithm that combines the AC with the BSC. In a study that enrolled 56 overweight and obese adolescents and adults, US Derived Fat Fraction (UDFF) was positively associated with MRI-PDFF (Spearman ρ, 0.82) and the mean bias between UDFF and MRI-PDFF was 4.0%.[45] UDFF greater than 5% had 94.1% sensitivity and 63.6% specificity for diagnosing MRI-PDFF greater than 5.5% with an AUC of 0.90. UDFF is available also with the deep abdominal transducer (DAX transducer) that has been specifically designed for the US evaluation of obese individuals. A very recent study in a large series of patients with CLD has shown that the combination of multiple parameters, namely integrated BSC, signal-to-noise ratio, and US-guided attenuation parameter (UGAP), had an accuracy higher than that of the UGAP alone (AUC 0.96 vs 0.92).[39]

Studies evaluating BC or SoS are lacking, and further studies are needed to assess their accuracy alone. Further studies are also needed to assess for confounding factors in the use of quantitative US for fat quantification.

Liver Stiffness Evaluation

B-mode ultrasound

As fibrosis progresses to cirrhosis, the liver becomes nodular. The nodularity can be described as micronodular or macronodular.[46] Nodules less than 3 mm are classified as micronodular while larger ones are classified as macronodular. The end effect of the imaging changes is the same regardless of the inciting etiology. The nodularity of the liver can be best detected by evaluating the liver surface with a high frequency transducer (**Fig. 7**). The surface should be a smooth echogenic line measuring less than 1 mm.[47,48] The presence of ascites may make the surface nodularity more apparent. Interruption of the normal liver capsule line is termed the "dotted-line sign" and has been described as characteristic for micronodular cirrhosis.[47]

The right lobe of the liver tends to be more involved in the changes than the left lobe and caudate lobe. The caudate lobe often becomes hypertrophic to compensate for the cirrhotic right lobe.[49–51] The use of the ratio greater than or equal to 0.65 of the transverse diameter of the caudate to the right lobe has been reported to yield a sensitivity of 84%, specificity of 100% for cirrhosis.[50]

The normal splenic size ranges from 12 to 14 cm in adults and a threshold of 13 cm is often loosely applied although as many as 7% of normal young adults may exceed this limit.[52] Splenomegaly can even be considered if the spleen is greater than 12 cm in longitudinal diameter or greater than 45 cm^2 maximum cross-sectional area, but there is risk of overestimation of disease. In cases of uncertainty, estimation of splenic volume may be helpful if there are no other signs of PHT. Cirrhosis and PHT are associated with splenomegaly.[53]

SHEAR WAVE IMAGING

There are several types of elastography that can assess LF. These include Transient Elastography (TE), Magnetic Resonance Elastography (MRE), and Acoustic Radiation Force Impulse (ARFI) US techniques.[5,54,55] TE is a non-imaging technique that uses a mechanical push to generate shear waves and single line US is used to estimate the shear wave speed. MRE uses a mechanical device to create standing waves in the liver and special

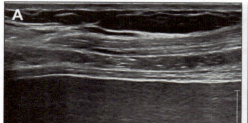
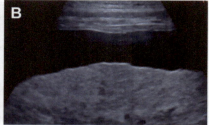

Fig. 7. With the development cirrhosis, the liver capsule becomes nodular. This is best visualized using a higher frequency linear transducer. (*A*) Liver capsule in a normal patient. It is a linear bright line without nodularity. (*B*) Liver capsule in a cirrhotic patient. Note the nodularity of the liver capsule.

sequences are used to calculate the LS. TE and MRE techniques are discussed in detail elsewhere and will not be discussed further.[5,56]

There are 2 ARFI techniques clinically available to estimate LS, point shear wave elastography (p-SWE) and 2D shear wave elastography (2D-SWE). **Fig. 8** shows representative images from p-SWE and 2D-SWE. P-SWE determines the LS in an approximately 1 cc volume where 2D-SWE evaluates a larger area (around 20 cc). A detailed description of the basic science of these 2 techniques can be found elsewhere.[5,55,56] There are differences between systems with reports of approximately 12% variability between systems in the same patient.[57] These difference are greater at higher degrees of fibrosis.[58]

The technique for both p-SWE and 2D-SWE are similar. Adherence to a strict protocol is required for accurate measurements.[5,6] Patients should fast for 4 hours before the examination as food ingestion increases blood flow to the liver via the portal vein, thereby elevating the LS. The examination should be performed in the supine or slight left lateral position with the patient's arm raised above the head to increase the intercostal spaces for better acoustic window. Measurements should be taken through an intercostal approach at the location of the best acoustical window. Measurements taken in the left lobe of the liver or by a substernal approach are usually inaccurate due to motion artifact from cardiac pulsations. Measurements should be taken in a neutral breath hold, since taking deep inspiration and breath holding increases right heart pressure and increases LS as a result. Measurements should be taken 1.5 to 2.0 cm below the liver capsule to avoid reverberation

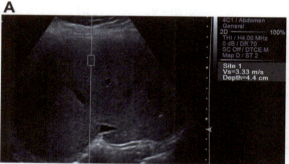
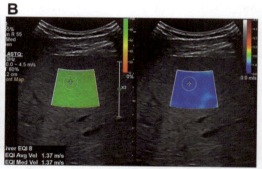

Fig. 8. Examples of the 2 types of acoustic radiation force impulse shear wave elastography methods. (*A*) Point shear wave. In this technique an approximately 1 cm box is placed appropriately in the liver (see text for location and protocol) and a measurement of the stiffness is estimated within that box. The stiffness is measured in meters/second (m/s) or can be converted to a pressure measurement in kiloPascals (kPa). In this case the LS is 3.33 m/s consistent with compensated advanced chronic liver disease. (*B*) 2D-shear wave (2D-SWE). In this technique the measurement is made in a larger area (*large rectangle box*). Then a region of interest (*circle*) is placed at the site of the area free of artifacts to make the measurement. The image on the right is the stiffness (or velocity) map while the image on the left is the confidence or quality map. The stiffness map displays the stiffness values using a color scale where blue is soft and red is stiff. The confidence map evaluates the shear waves and determines the quality of the shear waves with green (go) as high quality, yellow (caution) poor quality, and red (stop) meaning the shear waves are not accurate. In this case the LS was measured in an area of high confidence (*green*) and is 1.37 m/s corresponding to no or mild fibrosis.

artifact (Fig. 9). However, when using 2D-SWE the reverberation artifact can be visualized and avoided allowing for placement of the transducer closer to the optimal position of 4.0 to 4.5 cm from the transducer. The transducer should be placed perpendicular to the liver capsule in both planes. Placement of the ROI should avoid large blood vessels and bile ducts.[6]

Number of Measurements

The results can be reported either as the shear wave speed (which is what is measured on all systems) in meters/second (m/s) or converted to pressure measurements (Young's modulus) in kilo-Pascals (kPa) making some assumptions.[5,55] The number of measurements that should be taken varies with which technique is used. For p-SWE, 10 measurements are recommended with the median value used. For 2D-SWE when a quality measure is used, the number of high-quality measurements recommended is 5 and the median value should be reported for the result.[6,56] For both systems the interquartile range/median (IQR/M) should be used as a quality assessment. An IQR/M of less than 0.3 (30%) for measurements taken in kPa and less than 0.15 (15%) for measurement taken in m/s is suggestive of a good set of measurements. If the IRQ/M is higher than these limits, a statement that the data set are less accurate should be included in the report. A greater IQR/M can occur in patients with cirrhosis due to attenuation of the ARFI pulse. In this scenario, the measurement should be considered accurate if all the measurements are suggestive of cirrhosis.

Confounding factors

There are multiple confounding factors that need to be considered when performing liver elastography. These are listed in Box 3. During breathing the hepatic venous pressure changes leading to changes in LS. This is especially true during a Valsalva maneuver (Fig. 10). Therefore, it is recommended that the patient stop their breath in a neutral position (not inhaling or exhaling) when measurements are being taken. Taking measurements at the same breathing position are necessary for consistent results. After eating there is increased blood flow through the portal vein which also increases the LS. It is recommended that the patient be fasting for 4 hours before measurements are taken, but small amounts of water will not affect the measurements. Note that eating will only increase the LS. So, if the patient ate before the examination and the LS value is normal a repeat examination is not required. Acute inflammation of the liver which can be identified as elevated liver enzymes will also elevate the stiffness of the liver, so the amount of fibrosis will be overestimated in this setting.[59] Usually this is not critical until the transaminase levels are 5 times normal. Other causes of overestimating the degree of LF include increased right heart pressure from

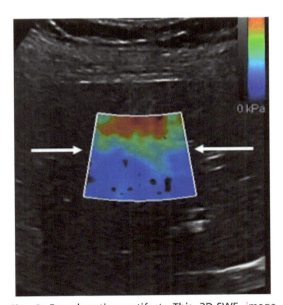

Fig. 9. Reverberation artifact. This 2D-SWE image shows the reverberation artifact from the liver capsule. This can be a few mm or as deep as 2 cm. The reverberation artifact in this image is the red and green colored area (arrows). Measurements should not be taken in this area.

Box 3
Confounding factors for accurate liver stiffness values with elastography

Method of performing examination (MRE, TE, SWE)

Type of equipment (hardware and software)

Patient factors
   Obesity
   Ascites
   Medications
   Fasting

Lab Values (AST. ALT)

Co-morbidities
   Acute on chronic disease
   Vascular congestion (CHF, fluid overload)

Pre-test and post-test probability

Technologist experience

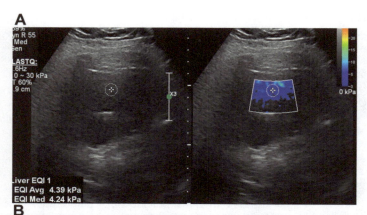
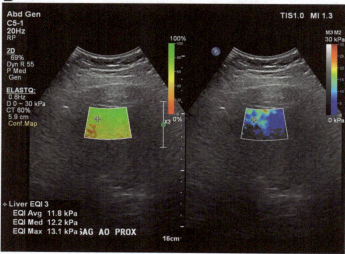

Fig. 10. Effect of increased right heart pressure on LS measurements. (A) LS measurement taken with breath hold in a neutral position. (B) Same patient with measurement taken during a Valsalva. Note the marked changed in the LS from 4.39 kPa (normal) in (A) and 11.8 kPa with a Valsalva maneuver (incorrectly suggesting severe fibrosis).

congestive heart failure or fluid overload and extrahepatic cholestasis.[5,60]

The scanning protocol for liver elastography is summarized in **Box 4**. There are several consensus and guidelines available regarding the use of SWE in the staging of LF.[5,55,61,62]

IMAGING FINDINGS/PATHOLOGY

In addition to the CLDs already discussed, there are several acute diffuse liver diseases. These include viral hepatitis and acute Budd-Chiari syndrome. In acute hepatitis of any cause, there is hepatomegaly and hypoechoic parenchyma which results in apparent increased relative echogenicity of the unaffected periportal triads. Color Doppler and spectral Doppler findings may remain normal. It should be noted that for the viral causes only chronic infections progress to fibrosis. While 5% to 15% of hepatitis B acute infections become chronic, 75% to 85% of acute hepatitis C infections become chronic. In the acute phase, the LS will be increased due to the inflammation (not due to fibrosis). In acute Budd-Chiari syndrome there will be hepatomegaly and heterogeneity of the liver due to congestion. Often, the venous occlusion will be identified on Color Doppler with spectral analysis, and there may be development of small intrahepatic venous collaterals. In chronic Budd-Chiari syndrome, there is usually peripheral liver atrophy with central hypertrophy and regenerating nodules.

Portal Hypertension

As the degree of fibrosis increases, the portal pressures also increase to overcome the increased resistance to flow. Cirrhosis causes intrahepatic PHT. PHT leads to many complications of varies, ascites, hepatic encephalopathy, splenomegaly, thrombocytopenia and anemia.[63] The safest and most reproducible method is measurement of the hepatic venous pressure gradient (HVPG). The wedged hepatic venous pressure correlates well

> **Box 4**
> **Strict protocol for acquiring accurate liver stiffness values**
>
> Patient should fast for at least 4 hours
>
> Examination should be performed in the supine or slight left lateral position with the arm raised above the head to increase the intercostal space
>
> Measurements should be taken through an intercostal approach at the location of the best acoustical window
>
> Measurements should be taken 1.5 to 2.0 cm below the liver capsule to avoid reverberation artifact. However, the reverberation artifact can be identified using the 2D-SWE and avoided so the measurement can be taken closer to the liver capsule. The optimal location for maximum shear wave generation is 4.0 to 4.5 cm from the transducer
>
> The transducer should be perpendicular to the liver capsule in both planes
>
> Placement of the ROI should avoid large blood vessels, bile ducts, and masses
>
> 10 measurements should be obtained from 10 independent images, in the same location, with the median value used for TE and pSWE techniques.
>
> 3 to 5 measurements may be appropriate for 2-D SWE when a quality assessment parameter is used.
>
> The IQR/M should be used as a measure of quality. For kPa measurements the IQR/M should be less than 0.3 and for m/s it should be less than 0.15 for an accurate data set
>
> For TE the appropriate transducer should be selected based on patient's body habitus

with liver biopsy in chronic hepatitis.[64] Clinically significant portal hypertension (CSPH) is defined as an HVPG $\geq$10 mm Hg.[65] This pressure predicts the development of varies and clinical decompensation.[66] In patients with compensated cirrhosis, a reduction in HVPG greater than 10% at 1-year protects against the development of varices.[67]

The normal portal vein diameter is less than 13 mm but a threshold diameter greater than 15 mm correlates better with PHT. The normal portal venous flow is hepatopetal with a velocity of 20 to 33 cm/sec. The normal portal venous flow should always be antegrade and pulsatile. Doppler US is highly accurate for evaluation of the sequelae of PHT and identifying the cause. With PHT the diameter of the portal vein increases while the velocity decreases (Fig. 11). The hepatic artery flow usually increases as a compensatory response to the decreased portal flow. As the PHT increases the portal flow can develop "to-and-fro" flow. Eventually the portal flow becomes hepatofugal (reversed). This is a sign of severe PHT. The slow flow state in PHT can cause portal vein thrombosis. Over time, the portal thrombus fibroses become more echogenic and decreases in caliber. Cavernous thrombosis is the formation of collateral vessels around the small thrombosed portal vein (Fig. 12).

Varices occur at sites of portosystemic communication; common varices are a recanalized umbilical vein, coronary or left gastric, and splenorenal shunt.[68] Varices can enlarge substantially, and variceal bleeding is one of the major causes of death in cirrhotic patients.[69] Upper gastrointestinal endoscopy is the reference standard for diagnosis of esophageal varices. US findings include lower esophageal Doppler signals, left gastric vein hepatofugal flow, paraumbilical vein recanalization, increased spleen diameter, increased splenic vein diameter, increased portal vein diameter, and decreased portal vein velocity. When any of these findings are present, the patient has decompensated cirrhosis.

Preliminary studies have found that splenic stiffness may perform better than LS in diagnosing CSPH.[70–72] However, at the time of this paper there is not a consensus on the cut-off values of splenic stiffness for diagnosis of CSPH.

DIAGNOSTIC CRITERIA

There is significant overlap of stiffness values for the varying degrees of LF.[5,6] The population being evaluated also needs to be taken into consideration. In populations with a high prevalence, it is important to not miss the diagnosis so false negatives are bad and a lower cut-off should be used. In a population with a low prevalence of disease false positives are bad so a higher cut-off is more appropriate. Therefore, it is important to adjust cut-off values obtained from the appropriate population. All techniques have high accuracy for differentiating between the normal patients and most patients with cirrhosis. However, degrees of LS between these 2 extremes overlap substantially.[5,6] 1 approach is to use a cut-off value system as recommended by the Society of Radiologists in Ultrasound (Table 2), with a low cut-off below which there is a high probability of being normal or minimal fibrosis and a separate high cut-off value where there is a high probability of significant fibrosis or cirrhosis.[5,6] Some patients with biopsy proven cirrhosis have had relatively low stiffness values in many studies so correlation with other imaging findings and blood findings

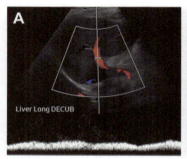 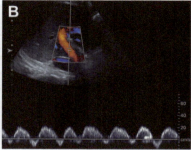 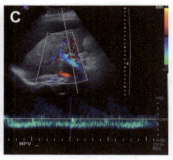

Fig. 11. Doppler evaluation of the portal vein. (*A*) Normal (*B*) antegrade and retrograde biphasic flow (*C*) reversed flow. These images demonstrate the changes in the Doppler signal of the portal vein with increasing LS due to increasing fibrosis. With continued increase in LS, the portal vein can occlude.

should be performed. Therefore, the use of Metavir cut-off values has been discouraged.[5,62] Another clinical approach to interpreting LS values would be in keeping with that recommended for TE by the Baveno VI Conference.[73] The so-called "rule of 5" (Young's modulus 5, 10, 15 and 20 kPa) is recommended when using TE (**Table 3**).

PEARLS, PITFALLS, VARIANTS

It is important to remember that elastography measures LS *but it does not measure LF*. When confounding factors are present, blindly using cut-off values can over or underestimate the degree of LF.

B-mode imaging is used to measure the shear wave speed. Therefore, it is important to have the best B-mode image possible without artifacts to yield an accurate shear wave measurement. A strong B-mode image implies that the optimal acoustical energy is getting to the liver. In this case the ARFI push will also have optimal energy for creating strong shear waves leading to more accurate assessment of their speed.

For accurate LS measurements with elastography, decreasing motion from both the patient and the technologists are important. Resting your arm on the patient while performing the examination is helpful in holding the transducer still. Controlling patient breathing is critical for accurate measurements. Practicing the temporary cessation of breathing with the patient before collecting results is helpful for the patient to understand how to stop their breathing without deep inspiration or

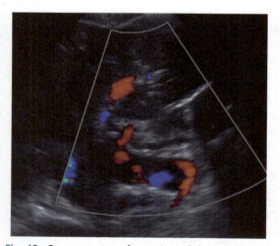

Fig. 12. Cavernous transformation of the portal vein. If the portal vein occludes due to marked increased LS, small vessels may develop to bring blood to the liver. This is called cavernous transformation of the portal vein. Note the small areas of flow surrounding the thrombosed portal vein.

Table 2
Rule of 4 for interpretation of ARFI liver stiffness techniques

ARFI-LSM	Interpretation
≤ 5 kPa (1.3 m/s)	High probability of being normal
< 9 kPa (1.7 m/s)	In the absence of other known clinical signs, rules out cACLD. If there are known clinical signs, may need further test for confirmation
9 kPa–13 kPa (1.7–2.1 m/s)	Suggestive of cACLD but need further test for confirmation
> 13 kPa (2.1 m/s)	Rules in cACLD
> 17 kPa (2.4 m/s)	Suggestive of CSPH

Interpretation of liver stiffness measurement obtained using ARFI-SWE techniques (rule of 4).
Abbreviations: ARFI, acoustic radiation force impulse; cACLD, compensated advanced chronic liver disease; CSPH, clinically significant portal hypertension; kPa, kilopascal; LSM, liver stiffness measurement.

Table 3
Suggested liver stiffness interpretation based on Baveno VI

Liver Stiffness	Interpretation
<5 kPa (1.2 m/s)	High probability of being normal
5 kPa-10 kPa (1.2–1.8 m/s)	In the absence of other known clinical signs, rules out cACLD[a]
10kPa-15 kPa (1.8–2.2 m/s)	Suggestive of cACLD but need further test for confirmation
>15 kPa (2.2 m/s)	Highly suggestive of cACLD
>20–25 kPa (2.6–2.9 m/s)	Can rule in CSPH[b]

[a] Compensated Advanced Chronic Liver Disease.
[b] Clinically Significant Portal Hypertension.

Valsalva for the examination. In real-time 2D-SWE systems, watching the liver motion is also helpful in confirming that the LS value is collected at the same point in respiration.

For most systems the ARFI pulse is maximized at 4.0 to 4.5 cm from the transducer. Therefore, the ROI for LS measurements ideally should be placed at least 1.5 to 2.0 cm from the liver capsule for pSWE and at 4.0 to 4.5 cm from the transducer. When using 2D-SWE the measurement box can be placed closer to the liver capsule as the reverberation artifact is identified and can be avoided in the ROI; this can be helpful in patients with increased BMI. Although most systems allow measurements to be taken as deep as 8 cm from the transducer, the strength of the ARFI pulse is usually attenuated significantly below 6 cm, especially in steatosis and cirrhotic livers, leading to less accurate measurements.[5] Most systems have a broad band transducer for ARFI imaging. As the ARFI pulse traverses the liver, it is attenuated with the higher frequencies affected more than the lower frequencies. Thus, the mean frequency of the ARFI pulse varies as it traverses the liver, particularly in steatotic and cirrhotic livers. The shear wave speed varies with the ARFI frequency so obtaining the measurements at the same depth for repeat examinations is important.

If the patient ate before the examination this increases portal flow and increases LS as noted previously. This can only increase the LS which may lead to overestimating the degree of LF. If the patient's LS values are not elevated (normal), there is no need to repeat the examination. If the values are increased, commenting that the LS value may be increased due to eating should be mentioned in the report. The clinician can then decide if a repeat examination (with fasting) is clinically indicated. If the patient ate adding a comment such as "The patient ate before the examination which can elevate the liver stiffness and overestimate the degree of liver fibrosis."

For patients receiving treatment for LF, non-invasive LS assessment can monitor if fibrosis is progressing or regression on treatment. With the advent of treatments for Hepatitis C it is clear that regression of the fibrosis or cirrhosis is possible over the time course of years.[74] However, even with sustained viral response and decrease in fibrosis, the risk of HCC is still present, and the patient needs continued monitoring for HCC.[75,76] It is important to note that the LS values will drop significantly after treatment due to the resolution of inflammation and NOT due to a change in fibrosis; therefore, cut-off values should not be used in post treatment patients. The change over time should be used.[6]

SUMMARY

CLD is a substantial world-wide problem. Any process that incites liver inflammation can lead to LF and progress to cirrhosis. It is now known that treating the inciting cause can lead stop the progression of the fibrosis or even reverse it. Therefore, a non-invasive method that can accurately stage the degree of LF is needed to assess the degree of fibrosis, determine when treatment should be initiated, monitor treatment, and evaluate for complications.

With a combination of B-mode, color Doppler and SWE, patients can be classified into the degree of fibrosis/inflammation for appropriate treatment and identify complications. SWE using ARFI technology has been shown to be an accurate method of assessing LS, but the technique requires a strict protocol. Most systems are now employing a quality measure assessing the displacement curves used to estimate the shear wave speed; this allows for more confidence in the LS measurement.

An early diagnosis of liver steatosis is critical because patients with MASLD have a risk for cardiovascular diseases, development of type 2 diabetes mellitus, and all-cause mortality higher than the general population. Moreover, MASLD may progress to MASH that may lead to severe fibrosis, liver-related events and risk of HCC.

Currently, for the quantification of liver steatosis, several noninvasive techniques are available.

MR techniques (such as MRI-PDFF) are the most accurate and are used as validated substitutes of liver biopsy for diagnosing and grading liver steatosis and for monitoring changes over time in clinical trials. Indeed, they can appreciate even small changes in liver fat content, but the significant threshold change used for clinical trials is 30%. Newer quantitative US techniques are becoming available and will provide a quick, non-invasive, accurate method for assessing the degree of liver fat and allow for serial follow-up to monitor treatment.

CLINICS CARE POINTS

- Elastography can accurately stage the degree of LF allowing for appropriate treatment and surveillance.
- For accurate assessment of LS, adherence to a strict protocol is required.
- The combination of the conventional US examination and elastography is a powerful tool in the assessment of CID.
- At LS values of 2.6–2.9 m/s (20–25 kPa), there is a high probability of clinically significant PHT.

DISCLOSURE

R.G. Barr has received a speaker honorarium from Canon Medical systems, Philips Ultrasound, Siemen Healthineers, Mindray, Samsung Ultrasound, Hologic Ultrasound. He has received research grants from Philips Ultrasound, Canon Ultrasound, Canon MRI, Samsung, South Korea, Siemens Healthineers, Germany, Hologic, United States, Mindray and equipment grants from Canon Medical Systems, United States, Philips Ultrasound, and Siemens Healthineers. He receives royalties from Thieme Publishers and Elsevier Publisher. He is on the advisory panels of Bracco Diagnostics and Lantheus.

REFERENCES

1. World Health Organization. Viral hepatitis. Report from the secretariat. Geneva, Switzerland: World Health Organization; 2010.
2. Angulo P. Nonalcoholic fatty liver disease. N Engl J Med 2002;346:1221–31.
3. Poynard T, Munteanu M, Deckmyn O, et al. Validation of liver fibrosis biomarker (FibroTest) for assessing liver fibrosis progression: proof of concept and first application in a large population. J Hepatol 2012;57:541–8.
4. Anthony PP, Ishak KG, Nayak NC, et al. The morphology of cirrhosis: definition, nomenclature, and classification. Bull World Health Organ 1977;55:521–40.
5. Barr RG, Ferraioli G, Palmeri ML, et al. Elastography Assessment of Liver Fibrosis: Society of Radiologists in Ultrasound Consensus Conference Statement. Ultrasound Q 2016;32:94–107.
6. Barr RG, Wilson SR, Rubens D, et al. Update to the Society of Radiologists in Ultrasound Liver Elastography Consensus Statement. Radiology 2020;296:263–74.
7. Riazi K, Azhari H, Charette JH, et al. The prevalence and incidence of NAFLD worldwide: a systematic review and meta-analysis. Lancet Gastroenterol Hepatol 2022;7:851–61.
8. Rinella ME. Nonalcoholic fatty liver disease: a systematic review. JAMA 2015;313:2263–73.
9. Simon TG, Roelstraete B, Khalili H, et al. Mortality in biopsy-confirmed nonalcoholic fatty liver disease: results from a nationwide cohort. Gut 2021;70:1375–82.
10. Rinella ME, Neuschwander-Tetri BA, Siddiqui MS, et al. AASLD Practice Guidance on the clinical assessment and management of nonalcoholic fatty liver disease. Hepatology 2023;77:1797–835.
11. Nasr P, Fredrikson M, Ekstedt M, et al. The amount of liver fat predicts mortality and development of type 2 diabetes in non-alcoholic fatty liver disease. Liver Int 2020;40:1069–78.
12. Ratziu V, Charlotte F, Heurtier A, et al. Sampling variability of liver biopsy in nonalcoholic fatty liver disease. Gastroenterology 2005;128:1898–906.
13. El-Badry AM, Breitenstein S, Jochum W, et al. Assessment of hepatic steatosis by expert pathologists: the end of a gold standard. Ann Surg 2009;250:691–7.
14. Wilson SR, Withers CE. Chapter 4 : "The Liver". In: Rumack CM, Wilson SR, Charboneau JW, editors. Diagnsotic Ultrasound. 3rd edition. St. Louis, MO: Elsevier Mosby; 2005. p. 77–145.
15. Elsayes KM, Shaaban AM, Rothan SM, et al. A Comprehensive Approach to Hepatic Vascular Disease. Radiographics 2017;37:813–36.
16. Fasel JH, Schenk A. Concepts for liver segment classification: neither old ones nor new ones, but a comprehensive one. J Clin Imaging Sci 2013;3:48.
17. Ferraioli G, Soares Monteiro LB. Ultrasound-based techniques for the diagnosis of liver steatosis. World J Gastroenterol 2019;25:6053–62.
18. Barr RG. "Conventional ultrasound findings in chronic liver disease". In: Barr RG, Ferraioli G, editors. Chapter 2 in Multiparametric Ultrasound for the Assessment of Diffuse Liver Disease. Philadelphia, PA: Elsevier; 2024. p. 7–24.
19. Gerstenmaier JF, Gibson RN. Ultrasound in chronic liver disease. Insights Imaging 2014;5:441–55.
20. Marshall RH, Eissa M, Bluth EI, et al. Hepatorenal index as an accurate, simple, and effective tool in

screening for steatosis. AJR Am J Roentgenol 2012; 199:997–1002.
21. Ferraioli G, Barr RG, Berzigotti A, et al. WFUMB Guidelines/Guidance on Liver Multiparametric Ultrasound. PArt 2: Guidance on Liver Fat Quantification. Ultrasound Med Biol 2024;50(8):1088–98.
22. Ferraioli G, Berzigotti A, Barr RG, et al. Quantification of liver fat content with ultrasound: A WFUMB position paper. Ultrasound Med Biol 2021;47:2803–20.
23. Shen F, Zheng RD, Shi JP, et al. Impact of skin capsular distance on the performance of controlled attenuation parameter in patients with chronic liver disease. Liver Int 2015;35:2392–400.
24. Ferraioli G, Tinelli C, Lissandrin R, et al. Controlled attenuation parameter for evaluating liver steatosis in chronic viral hepatitis. World J Gastroenterol 2014;20:6626–31.
25. Petroff D, Blank V, Newsome PN, et al. Assessment of hepatic steatosis by controlled attenuation parameter using the M and XL probes: an individual patient data meta-analysis. Lancet Gastroenterol Hepatol 2021;6:185–98.
26. Karlas T, Petroff D, Sasso M, et al. Individual patient data meta-analysis of controlled attenuation parameter (CAP) technology for assessing steatosis. J Hepatol 2017;66:1022–30.
27. Ferraioli G, Barr RG, Berzigotti A, et al. WFUMB Guidelines/Guidance on Liver Multiparametric Ultrasound. Part 2: Guidance on Liver Fat Quantification. Ultrasound Med Biol 2024. https://doi.org/10.1016/j.ultrasmedbio.2024.03.014.
28. Labyed Y, Milkowski A. Novel Method for Ultrasound-Derived Fat Fraction Using an Integrated Phantom. J Ultrasound Med 2020;39:2427–38.
29. Jeon SK, Lee JM, Joo I, et al. Two-dimensional Convolutional Neural Network Using Quantitative US for Noninvasive Assessment of Hepatic Steatosis n NAFLD. Radiology 2023;307:e221510.
30. Bao J, Lv Y, Wang K, et al. A comparative study of ultrasound attenuation imaging, controlled attenuation parameters, and magnetic resonance spectroscopy for the detection of hepatic steatosis. J Ultrasound Med 2023;42:1481–9.
31. Cassinotto C, Jacq T, Anselme S, et al. Diagnostic performance of attenuation to stage liver steatosis with MRI proton density fat fraction as reference: a prospective comparison of three US Machines. Radiology 2022;305:353–61.
32. Dioguardi Burgio M, Castera L, Oufighou M, et al. Prospective comparison of attenuation imaging and controlled attenuation parameter for liver steatosis diagnosis in patients with nonalcoholic fatty liver disease and type 2 diabetes. Clin Gastroenterol Hepatol 2023. https://doi.org/10.1016/j.cgh.2023.11.034.
33. Ferraioli G, Maiocchi L, Raciti MV, et al. Detection of liver steatosis with a novel ultrasound-based technique: a pilot study using MRI-derived proton density fat fraction as the gold standard. Clin Transl Gastroenterol 2019;10:e00081.
34. Lee DH, Cho EJ, Bae JS, et al. Accuracy of two-dimensional shear wave elastography and attenuation imaging for evaluation of patients with nonalcoholic steatohepatitis. Clin Gastroenterol Hepatol 2021;19: 797–805 e797.
35. Sugimoto K, Moriyasu F, Oshiro H, et al. The role of multiparametric us of the liver for the evaluation of nonalcoholic steatohepatitis. Radiology 2020;296:532–40.
36. Bae JS, Lee DH, Suh KS, et al. Noninvasive assessment of hepatic steatosis using a pathologic reference standard: comparison of CT, MRI, and US-based techniques. Ultrasonography 2022;41:344–54.
37. Fujiwara Y, Kuroda H, Abe T, et al. The b-mode image-guided ultrasound attenuation parameter accurately detects hepatic steatosis in chronic liver disease. Ultrasound Med Biol 2018;44:2223–32.
38. Imajo K, Toyoda H, Yasuda S, et al. Utility of ultrasound-guided attenuation parameter for grading steatosis with reference to MRI-PDFF in a large cohort. Clin Gastroenterol Hepatol 2022;20:2533–2541 e2537.
39. Kuroda H, Oguri T, Kamiyama N, et al. Multivariable Quantitative US Parameters for Assessing Hepatic Steatosis. Radiology 2023;309:e230341.
40. Tada T, Kumada T, Toyoda H, et al. Utility of attenuation coefficient measurement using an ultrasound-guided attenuation parameter for evaluation of hepatic steatosis: comparison With MRI-determined proton density fat fraction. AJR Am J Roentgenol 2019;212:332–41.
41. Jang JK, Choi SH, Lee JS, et al. Accuracy of the ultrasound attenuation coefficient for the evaluation of hepatic steatosis: a systematic review and meta-analysis of prospective studies. Ultrasonography 2022;41:83–92.
42. Ferraioli G, Kumar V, Ozturk A, et al. US Attenuation for Liver Fat Quantification: An AIUM-RSNA QIBA Pulse-Echo Quantitative Ultrasound Initiative. Radiology 2022;302:495–506.
43. Ferraioli G, Raimondi A, Maiocchi L, et al. Liver Fat Quantification With Ultrasound: Depth Dependence of Attenuation Coefficient. J Ultrasound Med 2023; 42:2247–55.
44. Ferraioli G, Raimondi A, De Silvestri A, et al. Toward acquisition protocol standardization for estimating liver fat content using ultrasound attenuation coefficient imaging. Ultrasonography 2023;42:446–56.
45. Dillman JR, Thapaliya S, Tkach JA, et al. Quantification of Hepatic Steatosis by Ultrasound: Prospective Comparison With MRI Proton Density Fat Fraction as Reference Standard. AJR Am J Roentgenol 2022; 219:784–91.
46. Freeman MP, Vick CW, Taylor KJ, et al. Regenerating nodules in cirrhosis: sonographic appearance with anatomic correlation. AJR Am J Roentgenol 1986; 146:533–6.

47. Di Lelio A, Cestari C, Lomazzi A, et al. Cirrhosis: diagnosis with sonographic study of the liver surface. Radiology 1989;172:389–92.
48. Simonovsky V. The diagnosis of cirrhosis by high resolution ultrasound of the liver surface. Br J Radiol 1999;72:29–34.
49. Giorgio A, Amoroso P, Lettieri G, et al. Cirrhosis: value of caudate to right lobe ratio in diagnosis with US. Radiology 1986;161:443–5.
50. Harbin WP, Robert NJ, Ferrucci JT Jr. Diagnosis of cirrhosis based on regional changes in hepatic morphology: a radiological and pathological analysis. Radiology 1980;135:273–83.
51. Tchelepi H, Ralls PW, Radin R, et al. Sonography of diffuse liver disease. J Ultrasound Med 2002;21: 1023–32 [quiz 1033-1024].
52. Hosey RG, Mattacola CG, Kriss V, et al. Ultrasound assessment of spleen size in collegiate athletes. Br J Sports Med 2006;40:251–4 [discussion 251-254].
53. Bolognesi M, Merkel C, Sacerdoti D, et al. Role of spleen enlargement in cirrhosis with portal hypertension. Dig Liver Dis 2002;34:144–50.
54. Shiina T, Nightingale KR, Palmeri ML, et al. WFUMB guidelines and recommendations for clinical use of ultrasound elastography: Part 1: basic principles and terminology. Ultrasound Med Biol 2015;41:1126–47.
55. Ferraioli G, Filice C, Castera L, et al. WFUMB guidelines and recommendations for clinical use of ultrasound elastography: Part 3: liver. Ultrasound Med Biol 2015;41:1161–79.
56. Guglielmo FF, Barr RG, Yokoo T, et al. Liver Fibrosis, Fat, and Iron Evaluation with MRI and Fibrosis and Fat Evaluation with US: A Practical Guide for Radiologists. Radiographics 2023;43:e220181.
57. Palmeri MNK, Fielding S, et al. RSNA QIBA ultrasound shear wave speed Phase II phantom study in viscoeastic media. IEEE Ultrason Symosium International 2015;397–400.
58. Ferraioli G, De Silvestri A, Lissandrin R, et al. Evaluation of Inter-System Variability in Liver Stiffness Measurements. Ultraschall der Med 2018. https://doi.org/10.1055/s-0043-124184.
59. Zeng J, Zheng J, Jin JY, et al. Shear wave elastography for liver fibrosis in chronic hepatitis B: Adapting the cut-offs to alanine aminotransferase levels improves accuracy. Eur Radiol 2018. https://doi.org/10.1007/s00330-018-5621-x.
60. Ferraioli G, Barr RG. Ultrasound liver elastography beyond liver fibrosis assessment. World J Gastroenterol 2020;26(24):3413–20.
61. Cosgrove D, Piscaglia F, Bamber J, et al. EFSUMB guidelines and recommendations on the clinical use of ultrasound elastography. Part 2: Clinical applications. Ultraschall der Med 2013;34:238–53.
62. Giovanna Ferraioli MD VW-SWM, Laurent Castera MD, PhD, Annalisa Berzigotti MD, Ioan Sporea MD, PhD , Christoph F Dietrich MD, PhD, MBA , Byung Ihn Choi MD, Stephanie R Wilson MD, Masatoshi Kudo MD, Richard G. Barr MD, PhD. Liver Ultrasound Elastography: An Update to the WFUMB GUIDELINES AND RECOMMENDATIONS Ultrasound in Medicine and Biology 2018.
63. Berzigotti A. Advances and challenges in cirrhosis and portal hypertension. BMC Med 2017;15:200.
64. van Leeuwen DJ, Howe SC, Scheuer PJ, et al. Portal hypertension in chronic hepatitis: relationship to morphological changes. Gut 1990;31:339–43.
65. Nagula S, Jain D, Groszmann RJ, et al. Histological-hemodynamic correlation in cirrhosis-a histological classification of the severity of cirrhosis. J Hepatol 2006;44:111–7.
66. Ripoll C, Groszmann R, Garcia-Tsao G, et al. Hepatic venous pressure gradient predicts clinical decompensation in patients with compensated cirrhosis. Gastroenterology 2007;133:481–8.
67. Groszmann RJ, Garcia-Tsao G, Bosch J, et al. Beta-blockers to prevent gastroesophageal varices in patients with cirrhosis. N Engl J Med 2005;353: 2254–61.
68. Sharma M, Rameshbabu CS. Collateral pathways in portal hypertension. J Clin Exp Hepatol 2012;2: 338–52.
69. Mallet M, Rudler M, Thabut D. Variceal bleeding in cirrhotic patients. Gastroenterol Rep (Oxf) 2017;5: 185–92.
70. Colecchia A, Montrone L, Scaioli E, et al. Measurement of spleen stiffness to evaluate portal hypertension and the presence of esophageal varices in patients with HCV-related cirrhosis. Gastroenterology 2012;143:646–54.
71. Takuma Y, Nouso K, Morimoto Y, et al. Measurement of spleen stiffness by acoustic radiation force impulse imaging identifies cirrhotic patients with esophageal varices. Gastroenterology 2013;144:92–101 e102.
72. Takuma Y, Nouso K, Morimoto Y, et al. Portal hypertension in patients with liver cirrhosis: diagnostic accuracy of spleen stiffness. Radiology 2016;279: 609–19.
73. de Franchis R, Baveno VIF. Expanding consensus in portal hypertension: Report of the Baveno VI Consensus Workshop: Stratifying risk and individualizing care for portal hypertension. J Hepatol 2015;63:743–52.
74. Marcellin P, Gane E, Buti M, et al. Regression of cirrhosis during treatment with tenofovir disoproxil fumarate for chronic hepatitis B: a 5-year open-label follow-up study. Lancet 2013;381:468–75.
75. Fattovich G, Stroffolini T, Zagni I, et al. Hepatocellular carcinoma in cirrhosis: incidence and risk factors. Gastroenterology 2004;127:S35–50.
76. Maan R, Feld JJ. Risk for hepatocellular carcinoma after hepatitis C virus antiviral therapy with direct-acting antivirals: case closed? Gastroenterology 2017;153:890–2.

Ovarian-Adnexal Reporting and Data System Ultrasound v2022
From Origin to Everyday Use

Catherine H. Phillips, MD[a],*, Krupa Patel-Lippmann, MD[a],
Jennifer Huang, MD[b], Lori M. Strachowski, MD[c],
Katherine E. Maturen, MD, MS[d]

KEYWORDS

- O-RADS • Ultrasound • Ovarian/adnexal lesions • Ovarian cancer • Ovarian neoplasm

KEY POINTS

- Ovarian-Adnexal Reporting and Data System (O-RADS) is an evidence-based clinical support system that helps to accurately characterize adnexal and ovarian lesions and predict the risk of malignancy. There are separate versions for ultrasound (US) and magnetic resonance imaging (MRI).
- O-RADS US provides suggested follow-up imaging and clinical management, which vary by assessment category.
- The O-RADS US v2022 update improves accuracy of the risk stratification and management system and allows the system to be incorporated into all pelvic US reports.
- Familiarization with the system, technical components of US examinations, and O-RADS US reporting practices will enable the reader to incorporate the system into their clinical practice.

INTRODUCTION

Ultrasound (US) is the imaging test of choice for initial evaluation of ovarian and adnexal pathology. In 2018, the American College of Radiology (ACR) Ovarian-Adnexal Reporting and Data System (O-RADS) US committee published a lexicon with the goal of providing an evidence-based consensus recognized vocabulary for describing normal and abnormal ovarian and adnexal findings.[1] This vocabulary included morphologic descriptors and definitions that help stratify ovarian and adnexal findings based on their sonographic features and assign an associated risk of malignancy (ROM). A subsequent article from the group in 2020 built on this lexicon foundation and outlined risk stratification categories with corresponding ROM based on existing data, as well as management recommendations.[2,3] Based on additional information from validation studies and feedback from users, the O-RADS US system was updated (O-RADS US v2022; Box 1) to clarify recommendations, incorporate new data, and address clinical challenges.[4] These updates were also incorporated into a smart phone app, which allows O-RADS US to be easily integrated into every day clinical practice.[5]

The O-RADS US v2022 system includes three main components: Governing concepts, O-RADS score with risk assessment, and suggested

---

[a] Department of Radiology and Radiological Sciences, Vanderbilt University Medical Center, 1211 Medical Center Drive, Nashville, TN, USA; [b] Department of Radiology, Abdominal Imaging and Intervention, Brigham and Women's Hospital, 75 Francis Street, Boston, MA, USA; [c] Department of Radiology and Biomedical Imaging & Obstetrics, Gynecology and Reproductive Sciences, University of California San Francisco, 1001 Potrero Avenue 1X57, San Francisco, CA 94110, USA; [d] Department of Radiology and Ob/Gyn, Michigan Medicine, 1500 East Medical Center Dr, B1 D530G, Ann Arbor, MI, USA
* Corresponding author.
E-mail address: catherine.phillips@vumc.org

> **Box 1**
> **Outline of major updates from O-RADS US v2022. For complete list of updates please see original reference[4]**
>
> **Major O-RADS US v2022 updates**
>
> *Governing concepts updates*
>
> Expanded applicability criteria to include normal ovaries
>
> Clarified management in patients of uncertain menopausal status and when uterus is absent. Added early and late menopause for management of hemorrhagic cysts
>
> US specialist definition expanded to include importance of experience
>
> Outlined that transabdominal images alone are enough to provide O-RADS US score; transvaginal not required
>
> Interval change assessed with average linear dimension (L + W + H)/3
>
> Clarifies that O-RADS US system can be applied to most lesions regardless of patient symptoms or risk, but that management can be modified. Recommendations are not requirements
>
> *Lexicon terms updates*
>
> "Bilocular" for cystic lesions
>
> "Shadowing" for solid lesions
>
> Number of locules and lack of internal vascularity added for dermoid cysts, endometriomas, and hemorrhagic cysts
>
> Hyperechoic component of dermoid cysts clarified as to be "diffuse" or "regional"
>
> "Punctate echogenic foci" added as a possible descriptor for endometriomas
>
> "Hydrosalpinx" definition updated to include anechoic fluid-filled tubular structure
>
> *Management recommendation updates*
>
> Clinical management added for all categories
>
> O-RADS US 0: Repeat US or MRI
>
> O-RADS US 1: No follow-up or additional management
>
> O-RADS US 2: Less follow-up of simple cysts. Surveillance limited to 24 months, previously 5 years; for classic benign lesions, option to follow-up within 3 months if features are suggestive only and overall assessment is uncertain
>
> O-RADS US 3: Follow-up ultrasound within 6 months is now an option; MRI remains an option for solid lesions
>
> O-RADS US 4: Gyn-oncologist imaging protocol now an option
>
> O-RADS US 5: Gyn-oncologist imaging protocol clarified as an option

management. Governing concepts provide insight into how and when to use O-RADS US v2022, clarify definitions, and outline technical considerations (**Fig. 1**).[6] Users should become familiar with governing concepts before implementing the system into their practice, as they provide rules for system use. The O-RADS US v2022 score is a numeric risk assessment based on lexicon terms, presence and morphology of solid and cystic components, and additional features including lesion size and color Doppler characteristics (**Figs. 2** and **3**).[7] There are 6 O-RADS US v2022 risk assessment categories (0–5) with increasing associated ROM from 1 to 5 (**Table 1**). Suggested management is specific for each risk category and has both clinical and imaging components. These recommendations are based on retrospective studies, better align with published expert consensus on adnexal cysts,[8] and represent a unified approach to management best practices based on multidisciplinary panel consensus.[4]

With this background and framework, the goal of this article is to outline the O-RADS US v2022 system and introduce methods to incorporate it into daily clinical practice.

IMAGING TECHNIQUES

Optimized images are key to both detecting and appropriately diagnosing ovarian or adnexal lesions. Unlike most other imaging modalities, the dynamic nature of US acquisition allows the interpreting physician to have real-time influence on diagnostic quality, and radiologists have a variety of potential methods to improve visualization. Due to this dynamic nature, US also allows for harmonization of imaging and physical examination. Interpretation of US findings should be done in context of patient symptoms, laboratory values, and prior imaging, when available. Complete technical guidance for US examinations has been provided for O-RADS US v2022[9] and key components will be highlighted here.

Equipment and Documentation

It is recommended that US equipment with transabdominal and transvaginal probes, color Doppler, and cine clip capabilities be used to image the ovaries and adnexa. As a general rule, transvaginal scanning is preferred to transabdominal scanning

O-RADS™ Ultrasound v2022 — Governing Concepts

Release Date: November 2022

1. O-RADS Ultrasound (US) applies to the ovaries, lesions involving (or suspected to involve) the ovaries and/or fallopian tubes, and paraovarian cysts, when the intent is to stratify risk of malignancy. Scenarios when O-RADS does not apply include (but are not limited to): pelvic inflammatory disease, ectopic pregnancy, torsion of a normal ovary, and those lesions clearly identified as non-ovarian/non-tubal in origin (eg, an exophytic or broad ligament myoma). If the origin of a lesion is indeterminate, options include CT and MRI.

2. Most nonvisualized and all absent ovaries are classified as "O-RADS: not applicable". When only one ovary is visualized, it may be assessed per lexicon descriptors to obtain an O-RADS score. An exam may be considered "O-RADS 0: technically inadequate" when ovarian visualization is expected based on the indication for the exam but is not seen.

3. In cases of multiple or bilateral lesions, each lesion should be separately characterized, and management driven by the lesion with the highest O-RADS score. Separate recommendations should be provided when management of one lesion is independent of the other.

4. When menopausal status is relevant for risk stratification or management, patient should be categorized as pre– or postmenopausal. The postmenopausal category is defined as amenorrhea ≥1 year; (early = postmenopausal for <5 years, late = postmenopausal for ≥5 years). If uncertain or the uterus is absent, manage as per the postmenopausal status if age is >50; (early = >50 but <55, late = ≥55).

5. Some O-RADS US management recommendations include the involvement of a physician whose practice includes a focus on ultrasound assessment of adnexal lesions, denoted as an "ultrasound specialist". While there are no mandated requirements or guidelines that define such a specialist, potential qualifications include sufficient experience with the appearance of adnexal pathology on US to improve the likelihood of correct diagnoses and participation in quality assurance activities related to adnexal imaging.

6. Imaging assessment of a lesion is generally based on transvaginal technique. Transabdominal imaging may add characterization and may suffice when transvaginal technique is not feasible or limited. When possible, orthogonal cine clips are strongly encouraged.

7. Single largest diameter of a lesion is used for risk stratification (scoring) and management. Reporting three dimensions is helpful to assess interval change, for which average linear dimension ([L+W+H]/3) should be used.

8. Lexicon terminology and lesion characterization apply to most lesions regardless of risk or symptoms. When uncertain about feature selection, (eg, smooth versus irregular, color score, etc.) use the higher risk category to score the lesion.

9. Management recommendations should serve as guidance rather than requirements and are based on average risk and no acute symptoms. Individual case management may be modified by risk (eg, personal or family history of ovarian cancer, BRCA mutation, etc.), symptoms, other clinical factors, and professional judgement, regardless of the O-RADS score.

© 2023 American College of Radiology® | All rights reserved

Fig. 1. American College of Radiology Ovarian-Adnexal Reporting and Data System Ultrasound v2022 (O-RADS US v2022) governing concepts. (O-RADS™ Ultrasound v2022 — Governing Concepts. Release Date: November 2022. © 2023 American College of Radiology.)

alone. Equipment maintenance and monitoring should be consistent with the American College of Radiology (ACR)-American Association of Physicists in Medicine (AAPM) Technical Standard for Diagnostic Medical Physics Performance Monitoring of Real Time Ultrasound Equipment.[10] Image acquisition and documentation should follow the established practice parameters for performance of female pelvic US.[11]

Technique

Grayscale and color or power Doppler images of any ovarian or adnexal lesion in orthogonal planes are required. Whenever possible, orthogonal cine clips of a lesion in its entirety are strongly encouraged to ensure that the interpreting radiologist has completely visualized the lesion and can accurately detect its features. Cine clips with color or power Doppler can also be helpful, but are not required, for troubleshooting and confirming findings of internal vascularity identified on static images. The gain, field of view, and focal zone settings should be optimized, and the highest frequency transducer that allows adequate penetration should be used. The size of a detected lesion should be measured in 3 orthogonal planes.

American College of Radiology

O-RADS™ US v2022 — Assessment Categories

Release Date: November 2022

O-RADS Score	Risk Category [IOTA Model]	Lexicon Descriptors		Management: Pre-menopausal	Management: Post-Menopausal
0	Incomplete Evaluation [N/A]	Lesion features relevant for risk stratification cannot be accurately characterized due to technical factors		Repeat US study or MRI	
1	Normal Ovary [N/A]	No ovarian lesion		None	
		Physiologic cyst: follicle (≤3 cm) or corpus luteum (typically ≤3 cm)			
2	Almost Certainly Benign [<1%]	Simple cyst	≤3 cm	N/A (see follicle)	None
			>3 cm to 5 cm	None	Follow-up US in 12 months[a]
			>5 cm but <10 cm	Follow-up US in 12 months[a]	
		Unilocular, smooth, non–simple cyst (internal echoes and/or incomplete septations)	≤3 cm	None	Follow-up US in 12 months[a]
		Unilocular, smooth, non–simple cyst (internal echoes and/or incomplete septations) / Bilocular, smooth cyst	>3 cm but <10 cm	Follow-up US in 6 months[a]	
		Typical benign ovarian lesion (see "Classic Benign Lesions" table)	<10 cm	See "Classic Benign Lesions" table for descriptors and management	
		Typical benign extraovarian lesion (see "Classic Benign Lesions" table)	Any size		
3	Low Risk [1 – <10%]	Typical benign ovarian lesion (see "Classic Benign Lesions" table), ≥10 cm		Imaging: • If not surgically excised, consider follow-up US within 6 months[b] • If solid, may consider US specialist (if available) *or* MRI (with O-RADS MRI score)[c] Clinical: Gynecologist	
		Uni- or bilocular cyst, smooth, ≥10 cm			
		Unilocular cyst, irregular, any size			
		Multilocular cyst, smooth, <10 cm, CS <4			
		Solid lesion, ± shadowing, smooth, any size, CS = 1			
		Solid lesion, shadowing, smooth, any size, CS 2–3			
4	Intermediate Risk [10 – <50%]	Bilocular cyst without solid component(s)	Irregular, any size, any CS	Imaging: Options include: • US specialist (if available) *or* • MRI (with O–RADS MRI score)[c] *or* • Per gyn–oncologist protocol Clinical: Gynecologist with gyn–oncologist consultation *or* solely by gyn–oncologist	
		Multilocular cyst without solid component(s)	Smooth, ≥10 cm, CS <4		
			Smooth, any size, CS 4		
			Irregular, any size, any CS		
		Unilocular cyst with solid component(s)	<4 pps or solid component(s) not considered a pp; any size		
		Bi- or multilocular cyst with solid component(s)	Any size, CS 1–2		
		Solid lesion, non-shadowing	Smooth, any size, CS 2–3		
5	High Risk [≥50%]	Unilocular cyst, ≥4 pps, any size, any CS		Imaging: Per gyn-oncologist protocol Clinical: Gyn-oncologist	
		Bi- or multilocular cyst with solid component(s), any size, CS 3–4			
		Solid lesion, ± shadowing, smooth, any size, CS 4			
		Solid lesion, irregular, any size, any CS			
		Ascites and/or peritoneal nodules[d]			

GLOSSARY

Smooth and irregular: refer to **inner** walls/septation(s) for **cystic** lesions, and **outer** contour for **solid** lesions; irregular inner wall for cysts = <3 mm in height	Solid: excludes blood products and dermoid contents; solid lesion = ≥80% solid; solid component = protrudes ≥3 mm (height) into cyst lumen off wall or septation
Shadowing: must be diffuse or broad to qualify; excludes refractive artifact	pp = papillary projection; subtype of solid component surrounded by fluid on 3 sides
CS = color score; degree of intralesional vascularity; 1 = none, 2 = minimal flow, 3 = moderate flow, 4 = very strong flow	Bilocular = 2 locules; multilocular = ≥3 locules; bilocular smooth cysts have a lower risk of malignancy, regardless of size or CS
Postmenopausal = ≥1 year amenorrhea (early: <5 yrs; late: ≥5 yrs); if uncertain or uterus surgically absent, use age >50 years (early = >50 yrs but <55 yrs, late = ≥55 yrs)	

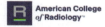

Fig. 2. American College of Radiology Ovarian-Adnexal Reporting and Data System Ultrasound v2022 (O-RADS US v2022) assessment categories with corresponding nomenclature and numeric risk of malignancy. *Shorter imaging follow-up may be considered in some scenarios (eg, clinical factors). If smaller (≥10%–15% decreases in average linear dimension), no further surveillance. If stable, follow-up US at 24 months from initial examination. If enlarging (≥10%–15% increase in average linear dimension), consider follow-up US at 12 and 24 months from initial examination, then management per gynecology. For changing morphology, reassess using lexicon descriptors. *Clinical management with gynecology as needed.* **There is a paucity of evidence for defining the optimal duration or interval for imaging surveillance. Shorter follow-up may be considered in some scenarios (eg, Clinical factors). If stable, follow-up at 12 and 24 months from initial examination, then as clinically indicated. For changing morphology, reassess using lexicon descriptors. †MRI with contrast has higher specificity for solid lesions, and cystic lesions with solid component(s). ††Not due to other malignant or nonmalignant etiologies; must consider other etiologies of ascites in categories 1 to 2. O-RADS™ US v2022 — Assessment Categories. Release Date: November 2022 © 2023 American College of Radiology.

O-RADS™ US v2022 — Classic Benign Lesions

Release Date: November 2022

Lesion	Descriptors and Definitions For any atypical features on initial or follow-up exam, use other lexicon descriptors (eg, unilocular, multilocular, solid, etc.)	Management If sonographic features are only suggestive, and overall assessment is uncertain, consider follow-up US within 3 months

Typical Hemorrhagic Cyst	Unilocular cyst, **no internal vascularity**[a], <u>and at least one</u> of the following:
	• Reticular pattern (fine, thin intersecting lines representing fibrin strands)
	• Retractile clot (intracystic component with straight, concave, or angular margins)
		Imaging:
		○ Premenopausal:
		  • ≤5 cm: None
		  • >5 cm but <10 cm: Follow-up US in 2–3 months
		○ Early postmenopausal (<5 years):
		  • <10 cm, options to confirm include:
		    ▪ Follow-up US in 2–3 months <u>or</u>
		    ▪ US specialist (if available) <u>or</u>
		    ▪ MRI (with O-RADS MRI score)
		○ Late postmenopausal (≥5 years):
		  • Should not occur; recategorize using other lexicon descriptors.
		Clinical: Gynecologist[b]

Typical Dermoid Cyst	Cystic lesion with ≤3 locules, **no internal vascularity***, <u>and at least one</u> of the following: • Hyperechoic component(s) (diffuse or regional) with shadowing • Hyperechoic lines and dots • Floating echogenic spherical structures	Imaging: ○ ≤3 cm: May consider follow-up US in 12 months[c] ○ >3 cm but <10 cm: If not surgically excised, follow-up US in 12 months[c] Clinical: Gynecologist[b]

Typical Endometrioma	Cystic lesion with ≤3 locules, **no internal vascularity**[a], homogeneous low–level/ground glass echoes, and smooth inner walls/septation(s)
	• ± Peripheral punctate echogenic foci in wall
		Imaging:
		○ Premenopausal:
		  • <10 cm: If not surgically excised, follow-up US in 12 months[c]
		○ Postmenopausal:
		  • <10 cm <u>and initial exam</u>, options to confirm include
		    ▪ Follow-up US in 2–3 months <u>or</u>
		    ▪ US specialist (if available) <u>or</u>
		    ▪ MRI (with O-RADS MRI score)
		Then, if not surgically excised, recommend follow-up US in 12 months[c]
		Clinical: Gynecologist[b]

Typical Paraovarian Cyst	Simple cyst separate from the ovary	Imaging: None Clinical: Gynecologist[b]
Typical Peritoneal Inclusion Cyst	Fluid collection with ovary at margin or suspended within that conforms to adjacent pelvic organs • ± Septations (representing adhesions)	Imaging: None Clinical: Gynecologist[b]
Typical Hydrosalpinx	Anechoic, fluid–filled tubular structure • ± Incomplete septation(s) (representing folds) • ± Endosalpingeal folds (short, round projections around inner walls)	

Fig. 3. American College of Radiology Ovarian-Adnexal Reporting and Data System Ultrasound v2022 (O-RADS US v2022) classic benign lesions with associated lexicon descriptors and definitions in the second column and management recommendations in the third column. *Excludes vascularity in walls or intervening septation(s). **As needed for management of clinical issues. †There is a paucity of evidence for defining the need, optimal duration or interval of timing for surveillance. If stable, consider US follow-up at 24 months from initial examination, then as clinically indicated. Specifically, evidence does support an increased risk of malignancy in endometriomas following menopause and those present greater than 10 years. (O-RADS™ US v2022 — Classic Benign Lesions. Release Date: November 2022. © 2023 American College of Radiology.)

Additionally, to differentiate solid components (≥3 mm) from wall irregularity (<3 mm) in cystic lesions, the height of the projection into the cavity should be measured. Images with and without calipers are suggested if calipers could obscure lesion assessment.

Ultrasound Artifacts and Scanning Tips

Acoustic shadowing is a US artifact that results from an increased attenuation of the US beam by a lesion compared to adjacent structures, creating a hypoechoic zone posterior/deep to the lesion.

Table 1
O-RADS US v2022 risk assessment categories and associated risk of malignancy

O-RADS Score	Risk Category	Risk of Malignancy (%)
0	Technically inadequate	N/A
1	Normal ovary	0
2	Almost certainly benign	<1
3	Low risk	1 to <10
4	Intermediate risk	10 to <50
5	High risk	≥50

Shadowing is associated with benign dermoid cysts and fibromatous lesions and can be a useful feature to downgrade solid lesions when the outer margins are smooth. It is important to note that shadowing should be broad or diffuse in shape due to attenuation of sound through the structure. Shadowing should not be confused with refractive artifact, which results from sound traveling through adjacent tissues with different acoustic impedances, appearing as linear or focal areas of hypoechogenicity within or posterior to the lesion at the site of the apposed tissue types[4] or reflection of the beam striking the edge of a curved structure.

Spatial compounding is a technique used to optimize the appearance of sonographic images by enhancing resolution of tissue planes and reducing noise, but compounding can mask the appearance of posterior acoustic shadowing typically seen with conventional sonography. Turning off spatial compounding, when feasible, may be needed to identify shadowing artifacts. Furthermore, it is important to adjust color Doppler scale to assess for low velocity flow within solid components or septations. This can be accomplished by optimizing the color box to fit the region of interest and decreasing the color scale until a "flash" is achieved and then increasing the scale by one. By optimizing the color scale, it is possible to accurately assess the color score (CS). When flow is equivocal, spectral Doppler can demonstrate a waveform and distinguish flow signal from noise. When flow is minimal, power Doppler can augment sensitivity for slow flow. O-RADS US CS is a subjective assessment of the degree of internal blood flow within a lesion and includes 4 levels: CS 1 (no flow), CS 2 (minimal flow), CS 3 (moderate flow), and CS 4 (very strong flow).[1]

The use of sliding maneuvers, documented with clips, is helpful to confirm lesion location as intraovarian (lesion moves with the ovary when pressure is applied with the transducer) or extraovarian (lesion moves separately from the ovary). These maneuvers can also be helpful for assessing for underlying deep penetrating endometriosis or adhesions. Rapid, gentle probe pressure or "jiggling" can be used to characterize internal cyst contents and determine if internal echoes are mobile or fixed.

HOW TO APPROACH A LESION ON ULTRASOUND

The majority of incidentally detected adnexal observations are either physiologic or benign.[12] Thus, the first and most important distinction in O-RADS US is to differentiate physiologic and classic benign findings from cystic or solid lesions, which require further morphologic evaluation and scoring. The O-RADS US system applies an algorithmic approach to assessing lesions with the ultimate goal of increasing the likelihood of correct diagnoses (**Fig. 4**).[13]

Normal Ovary and Physiologic Cysts

The first major category of observations to consider are physiologic cysts that occur in premenopausal patients, including the follicle and corpus luteum (CL). A follicle is a unilocular, anechoic, cyst with smooth inner walls 3 cm or less; this appearance is considered a simple cyst when greater than 3 cm and in postmenopausal patients. A CL may appear as a thick-walled cyst with smooth or crenulated inner walls. Internally, a CL may be anechoic, have internal echoes (representing blood products) or no apparent cystic center and apposed walls resulting in a solid appearance. Color Doppler is helpful in the diagnosis of a CL, particularly when solid in appearance, by demonstrating peripheral vascularity. While most corpora lutea are 3 cm or less, morphologic features play a greater role in accurate characterization than a discriminatory size cutoff. Physiologic findings are not considered "lesions."

Classic Benign Lesions

The next major category is the classic benign lesion (CBL) with 6 subtypes (3 intraovarian and 3 extraovarian). These demonstrate typical features, well described in prior literature, without more suspicious characteristics, that allow one to make a specific diagnosis. The most common to arise from the ovary is a hemorrhagic cyst, which is an avascular, unilocular cyst with an internal reticular pattern or retractile clot. Because hemorrhagic cysts generally arise from follicles,

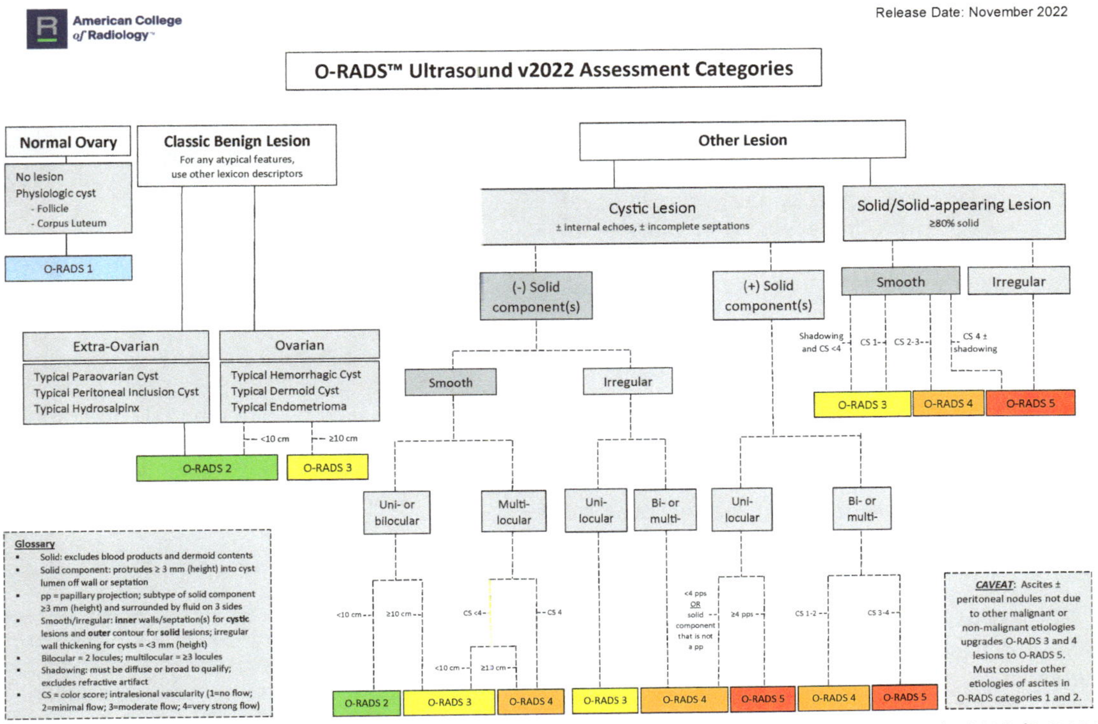

Fig. 4. American College of Radiology Ovarian-Adnexal Reporting and Data System Ultrasound v2022 (O-RADS US v2022) assessment categories algorithm. (O-RADS™ Ultrasound v2022 Assessment Categories. Release Date: November 2022. © 2023 American College of Radiology.)

they should never occur in late postmenopause (≥5 years of menopause); in this setting, other lexicon terms should be used for cystic or solid lesions. A typical ovarian dermoid cyst has 3 locules or less, no internal vascularity and at least 1 of the following: hyperechoic lines and dots, a diffuse or regional hyperechoic component with shadowing, or floating echogenic spherical structures. A typical endometrioma is an avascular cyst with 3 locules or less and homogenous low-level or ground glass echoes, commonly ovarian in location. An optional feature for endometriomas is the presence of peripheral punctate echogenic foci, which are specific for the diagnosis, though uncommon. Hemorrhagic cysts, dermoid cysts, and endometriomas under 10 cm are O-RADS US 2; if 10 cm or greater, they are O-RADS US 3 (see **Fig. 3**).

The remaining CBLs are adnexal, but extraovarian. First is a paraovarian cyst, which is a simple cyst adjacent to but separate from the ovary and includes paratubal cysts. Second is a peritoneal inclusion cyst, where a loculated fluid collection with or without septations surrounds the ovary. These result from prior surgery or inflammatory process, with scarring and adhesions leading to this accumulation of benign serous peritoneal fluid. The collection should conform to adjacent pelvic organs, and the presence of follicles may help distinguish the ovary from a solid component. Third, a hydrosalpinx is an anechoic, fluid-filled tubular structure separate from the ovary. When seen, incomplete septations (representing folding of the tube) and endosalpingeal folds, which present as equidistantly spaced nodular excrescences along the inner walls, assist in the diagnosis. These 3 classic benign extraovarian lesions receive O-RADS US score 2, and overall size is not relevant for scoring.

While many CBLs will have the typical features described earlier, overall assessment may be uncertain; in this setting, short interval follow-up US may be obtained in 2 to 3 months to allow another opportunity at characterization.

Other Lesions

When an observation does not fulfill criteria for a typical physiologic cyst or CBL, it is placed within the remaining third category, which includes 5 subtypes as follows:

- Unilocular cyst without solid components
- Unilocular cyst with solid components
- Bilocular or multilocular cyst without solid components

- Bilocular or multilocular cyst with solid components
- Solid lesion

A unilocular cyst has no complete septations, a bilocular cyst has a single smooth, thin, complete septation, and a multilocular cyst has 2 or more septations. Purely cystic lesions are almost never malignant, but risk increases with number of locules and irregular or nodular inner walls and septations. Irregularity of inner walls and/or septations when not a true solid component is defined as focal thickening less than 3 mm in height and is worrisome enough to increase the ROM and the O-RADS US score. If the inner wall is smooth, risk stratification will further depend on maximum size of the lesion (<10 cm vs $\geq$10 cm), as well as the CS (1–3 vs 4) if multilocular. Management of unilocular and bilocular smooth cysts depends on specified size ranges when less than 10 cm. For unilocular smooth cysts, management will also differ based on the assessment of internal contents as simple or non-simple defined as internal echoes or incomplete septations.

A solid component may be seen in cystic lesions and is defined as focal wall thickening or solid tissue arising from a cyst wall or septation and protruding into the cyst cavity 3 mm or greater in height, but the largest size of the component is immaterial beyond the 3 mm threshold.[14] Notably, blood products and dermoid contents are not considered solid components in the O-RADS US schema, and denoting them as such will incorrectly upgrade a lesion. Given the most predictive feature for malignancy is solid components followed by complete septations, these two features are the primary focus of the assessment for cystic lesions. A subtype of solid component is the papillary projection that is surrounded by fluid on 3 sides. If a solid component is present, the locularity determines the next step in stratification. For unilocular cysts with solid components, the number of papillary projections (<4 vs $\geq$4) is relevant for scoring, whereas the degree of internal vascularity (CS 1–2 vs 3–4) is relevant for stratifying bilocular and multilocular cystic lesions with solid components. Overall lesion size is not used for scoring cystic lesions with solid components.

A solid lesion consists of 80% or greater solid component. Assessing the outer contour of a solid lesion is the first step in risk stratification. An irregular or lobular outer contour is worrisome enough to stratify the lesion as an O-RADS US 5 (high risk) lesion without need for further US feature assessment. A smooth outer contour warrants interrogation with color Doppler to determine the CS. When very strong flow (CS 4) is seen, assessment is complete. With less than very strong flow, the presence of broad or diffuse shadowing, commonly seen with fibromatous lesions, is sought. The size of a solid lesion is not relevant for risk assessment.

O-RADS US V2022 ASSESSMENT CATEGORIES AND MANAGEMENT

Using the aforementioned morphologic descriptors, O-RADS US v2022 can be used to stratify ovarian and adnexal lesions into risk assessment categories to help predict the likelihood of malignancy. The following section delineates each O-RADS US category with examples and associated management.

O-RADS US 0: Incomplete due to Technical Factors

O-RADS US 0 is used when an evaluation is incomplete due to technical factors, such as large lesion size, incomplete or nonvisualization, or absence of color or power Doppler images of the lesion (**Fig. 5**). Repeat US or MRI are both options for additional management based on the clinical scenario and patient factors.

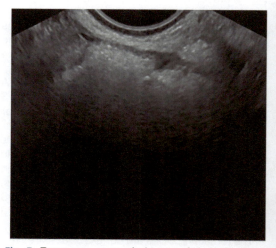

Fig. 5. Transverse grayscale image of the left adnexa in a 48 year old BRCA carrier who presented for annual screening ultrasound. The left ovary was not visualized due to bowel gas. In this case, ovarian visualization is required and expected, so an O-RADS US score of 0 (technically inadequate) is appropriate. Repeat US could be considered if the technical limitations are expected to improve, status after bowel movement, for example. Alternatively, MRI is also an option based on clinical factors and patient scenario.

O-RADS US 1: Normal Ovary

O-RADS US 1 is used for the classification of a normal ovary with no focal observations, or a physiologic cyst (follicle or CL). This category is associated with 0% ROM (**Figs. 6** and **7**). No imaging follow-up or additional management is needed for O-RADS US 1. Reporting with O-RADS US is optional in this setting, and its use will depend on the clinical setting and individual practice preferences.

O-RADS US 2: Almost Certainly Benign

O-RADS US 2 lesions are almost certainly benign, with less than 1% ROM. This risk category includes simple cysts less than 10 cm, unilocular nonsimple cysts with smooth inner walls less than 10 cm, bilocular cysts with smooth inner walls less than 10 cm, as well as lesions less than 10 cm that can be classified as "classic benign lesions" (**Figs. 8** and **9**). Given the spectrum of lesions in this category, various imaging management options are available based on menopausal status, lesion size, and imaging features (see **Figs. 2** and **3**). Clinical management of O-RADS US 2 lesions is by a gynecologist, as needed.

O-RADS US 3: Low Risk

O-RADS US 3 lesions have a low ROM (1% to <10%).[3,15–18] These include unilocular and bilocular cysts greater than 10 cm, unilocular cysts with irregular inner walls, smooth solid lesions without shadowing or internal flow, solid lesions with shadowing and less than very strong internal flow (CS <4), and multilocular cysts with smooth inner walls less than 10 cm and with less than very strong internal flow (CS <4). CBLs measuring 10 cm or greater are also included in this category (**Figs. 10** and **11**). Imaging management options for O-RADS US 3 lesions includes follow-up US within 6 months, if not excised. Alternatively, if solid, an evaluation by a US specialist or MRI (with O-RADS MRI score) is suggested. Clinically, O-RADS US 3 lesions may be managed by a gynecologist.

O-RADS US 4: Intermediate Risk

O-RADS US 4 lesions are intermediate risk, with a 10% to less than 50% ROM.[15,16,18–20] This category includes a large spectrum of lesions (see **Fig. 2**) including cystic lesions with solid components or irregular walls, as well as nonshadowing smooth solid lesions with minimal-to-moderate internal flow (CS 2–3; **Fig. 12** and **13**). Imaging management for O-RADS US 4 lesions includes a US specialist (if available), MRI (with O-RADS MRI score) or per gyn-oncologist. Clinical management of O-RADS US 4 lesions is the lowest O-RADS US score to include a gyn-oncologist, either in conjunction with a gynecologist or through direct management by a gyn-oncologist.

O-RADS US 5: High Risk

O-RADS US 5 lesions are the most suspicious for malignancy, with 50% or greater ROM.[15,16,18–20] The malignancy can be either primary adnexal or from metastatic lesions. O-RADS US 5 lesions include unilocular cysts with 4 or greater papillary

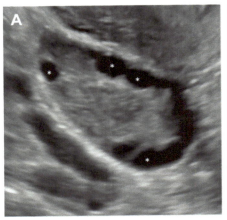 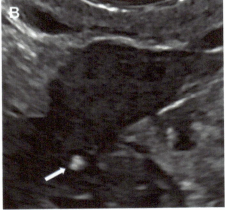

Fig. 6. Normal sonographic appearance of the ovary in a premenopausal (*A*) and postmenopausal (*B*) patient. Note the presence of small anechoic follicles (*asterisk*) in the premenopausal ovary and punctate echogenic foci (*white arrow*) in the postmenopausal ovary. O-RADS US score is 1. No further imaging or clinical management is needed.

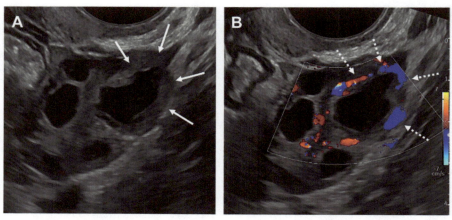

Fig. 7. Physiologic corpus luteum on grayscale (*A*) and color Doppler (*B*) images. This is the typical appearance of a corpus luteum, which is a unilocular thick-walled ovarian cyst (*white arrows*) typically 3 cm or less ± internal echoes and crenulated inner walls. Note the peripheral vascularity on color Doppler (dashed *arrow*). O-RADS US score is 1. No follow-up imaging or clinical management is needed.

projections, bilocular or multilocular cysts with solid components and moderate-to-strong internal vascularity (CS 3–4), and solid lesions with strong internal flow or irregular margins. Additionally, an adnexal O-RADS 3 or 4 lesion with ascites and/or peritoneal nodularity is always scored O-RADS US 5 regardless of lesion morphology (**Figs. 14–16**). Imaging and clinical management is per gyn-oncology.

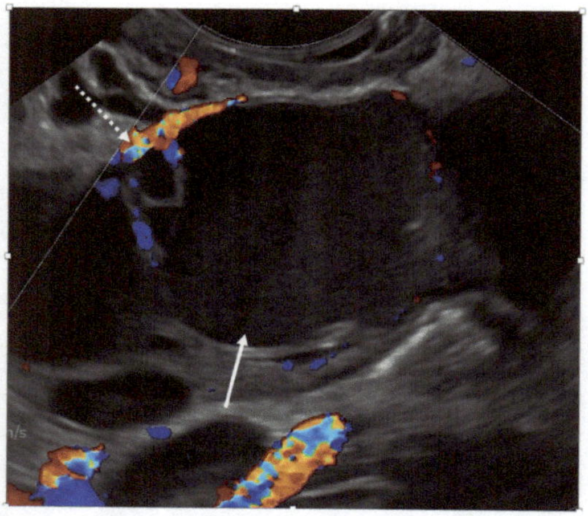

HOW TO REPORT

A comprehensive guide to utilizing O-RADS US v2022 in a pelvic US report and structured reporting templates are available through the ACR Web site.[21,22] The purpose of this section is to highlight the key components and approaches to reporting O-RADS US v2022.

When approaching an examination where O-RADS US utilization would be appropriate, relevant clinical history should be included in the report indication, including age and menopausal status as well as any relevant clinical context: for example, symptoms, physical examination findings, laboratory values, high-risk status, oncologic history, prior gynecologic surgeries, and so forth. As delineated in the Governing Concepts, clinical presentation will often help guide the user to decide if O-RADS US is applicable. For example, O-RADS US would not apply to patients presenting with acute clinical scenarios unrelated to malignancy such as ovarian hyperstimulation syndrome, pelvic inflammatory disease, torsion of an otherwise normal ovary, potential ectopic pregnancy, or tubo-ovarian abscess. Similarly, if a lesion seen on pelvic US is clearly nonovarian/adnexal in origin such as an exophytic uterine myoma, O-RADS US would not apply.

If the origin of a pelvic mass cannot be determined with US, O-RADS US should not be utilized

Fig. 8. Classic benign lesion—Endometrioma less than 10 cm. Sagittal color Doppler image of the right ovary in a 34 year old patient demonstrating a 2.8 cm unilocular cystic structure filled with internal homogeneous low-level echoes and an internal fluid–fluid level (straight *arrow*); while fluid–fluid levels are nonspecific and not included in the O-RADS lexicon, they are not uncommon in endometriomas. There is no internal color Doppler flow, but flow is noted in the adjacent ovary (dashed *arrow*). The O-RADS US score is 2. In this premenopausal patient, follow-up ultrasound in 12 months is suggested unless the finding is surgically excised. Management of clinical issues is per gynecology.

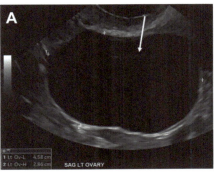 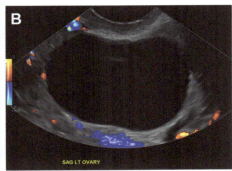

Fig. 9. Sagittal grayscale (*A*) and color Doppler (*B*) images of the left ovary in a 69 year old woman presenting with a history of ovarian cysts. Note the small amount of reverberation artifact in the near field (*arrow*, A), a commonly seen artifact. The finding is a unilocular, anechoic cyst with smooth inner walls, measuring up to 4.6 cm and meets criteria of a simple cyst, O-RADS US 2. In a postmenopausal woman, follow-up ultrasound in 12 months is suggested. Management of clinical issues is per gynecology.

(or a score 0 could be considered), and further imaging with either computed tomography (CT) or MRI could be appropriate for problem solving. If an ovarian lesion is seen, but lesion features cannot be adequately assessed sonographically, the score is O-RADS US 0 and further evaluation with either repeat US or MR would be appropriate. When the ovary is surgically absent or not visualized and visualization is not expected such as in a postmenopausal patient, O-RADS US is not applicable in most cases and can be reported as "O-RADS US N/A." However, certain clinical scenarios may call for utilization of O-RADS US 0 in the setting of ovarian nonvisualization. For example, O-RADS US 0 could be used for follow-up of a previously seen lesion on US or other modality as well as in the setting of expected visualization such as ovarian cancer screening in a high-risk patient.

Once a lesion is identified and adequately assessed, the findings section of the report should include lesion laterality and location (ovarian, adnexal, or extraovarian), and the lesion should be described using lexicon descriptors. Adnexal observations can be divided into 3 general categories: physiologic findings, classic benign lesions, and nonphysiologic cystic or solid lesions. Single largest diameter of the lesion should be reported at a minimum, with documentation of all 3 dimensions encouraged, especially if management includes imaging follow-up. When assessing interval change, report the average linear dimension (length + height + width)/3. Ascites or peritoneal nodules should be mentioned, if present.

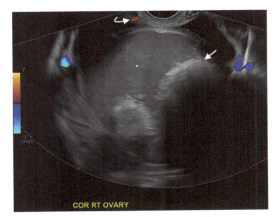

Fig. 10. Classic benign lesions—Dermoid cyst greater than 10 cm. Transvaginal color Doppler image of the right ovary containing a 11.6 cm unilocular cyst with regional hyperechoic components with shadowing (*straight arrow*). Additional internal echoes are noted within the lesion (*asterisk*). No internal flow is seen on color Doppler (*curved arrow*). Finding is consistent with a dermoid cyst, which would be scored O-RADS US 2 when less than 10 cm. However, given size 10 cm or greater, score is O-RADS US 3. If not surgically excised, follow-up ultrasound within 6 months is recommended. Management of clinical issues is per gynecology.

The report impression should include a brief summary of the lesion or lesions if multiple, listed from most to least concerning with the corresponding assessment category and management recommendations. The assessment category should include both the score and the associated terminology/risk category (eg, O-RADS US 2, almost certainly benign). Alternatively, the score can be listed in the impression, and the terminology can be in a legend or glossary form at the end of the report for clinician reference (such as in **Table 1**). Providing the associated ROM with the risk score and reference link to the ACR O-RADS Web site are optional. In the era of immediate patient access to reports, a reasonable

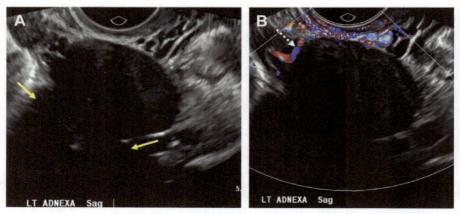

Fig. 11. Transvaginal grayscale (*A*) and color Doppler (*B*) image of the left ovary in a 44 year old woman presenting with pain. In the left ovary, there is a 4.1 cm solid hypoechoic mass with smooth outer margins, broad posterior shadowing (*yellow arrows*). No internal color Doppler flow is seen (color score 1) but peripheral flow is noted (*dashed white arrow*). The O-RADS US score is 3. Follow-up imaging options of this solid lesion include MRI with O-RADS MRI score or follow-up ultrasound in 6 months, if not surgically excised. This patient opted for MRI where the lesion was found to have markedly T2 hypointense signal consistent with a benign fibromatous lesion and was downscored to O-RADS MRI 2. Management of clinical issues is per gynecology.

approach to this may be inclusion of ROM for reassurance in normal, almost certainly benign, and low-risk lesions. Alternatively, omitting ROM in intermediate and high-risk lesions would allow the clinician to communicate the implications of these findings directly with the patient and address expected questions/concerns at that time.

There are many clinical tools and resources available on the ACR Web site to help with seamless integration of O-RADS into clinical practice.[22] These tools are designed both for seasoned users to confirm scoring in challenging cases and for new and novice users trying to learn the system. Documents including technical guidance, sample report, and templates are provided to help integrate O-RADS into the workflow as well as clinical tools such as an algorithm and a link to the smartphone app, which can be used when actively assessing lesions.

FUTURE DIRECTIONS

The RADS are living documents, to be refined and improved over time based on user feedback and

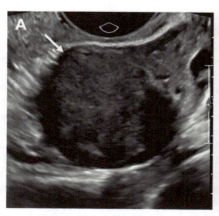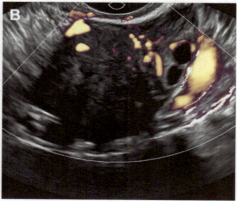

Fig. 12. Transvaginal grayscale (*A*) and color Doppler (*B*) images of the left ovary in a 19 year old patient presenting with abdominal pain. In the left ovary, there is a solid mass with smooth outer margins (*white arrow*) and no posterior shadowing. There is minimal-to-moderate internal flow on color Doppler (CS 2–3). The O-RADS US score is 4. Further imaging evaluation with MRI or per gyn-oncologist would be suggested with clinical follow-up with a gynecologist with gyn-oncologist or solely gyn-oncologist.

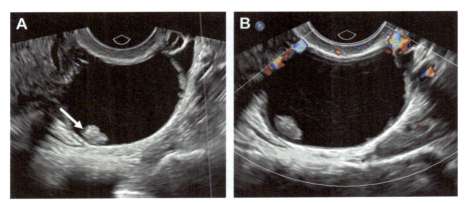

Fig. 13. Transvaginal grayscale (*A*) and color Doppler (*B*) images of the left ovary in a 31 year old patient presenting with a history of right ovarian borderline tumor. In the left ovary, there is a unilocular cyst with smooth inner margins, few internal echoes and single papillary projection (*white arrow*). There is no internal flow on color Doppler (CS 1). The O-RADS US score is 4. Further evaluation with MRI or per gyn-oncologist would be suggested with clinical follow-up with a gynecologist with gyn-oncologist or solely gyn-oncologist. Patient opted for resection with pathology demonstrating a serous borderline tumor.

emerging evidence. The Breast Imaging Reporting and Data System, now in its fifth edition, is entering its fourth decade in clinical practice and continues to evolve.[23] Similarly, O-RADS will be revised as needed, to incorporate new evidence and improve usability.

Although the original evidence basis supporting both O-RADS US and MRI was robust, knowledge gaps persist (**Box 2**). O-RADS US is driven by morphologic descriptors, and perceptions may vary among individuals. Several existing articles have briefly evaluated interreader concordance as part of a diagnostic performance evaluation, demonstrating good or better kappa statistics (0.7–0.8).[19,20] The ACR has supported a comprehensive prospective evaluation of reproducibility for individual US features and overall O-RADS US score, which is currently underway.

Other knowledge gaps pertain to specific features and populations. For example, the vascularity score is subjective lacking quantitative thresholds, and its reproducibility is unknown. It is possible

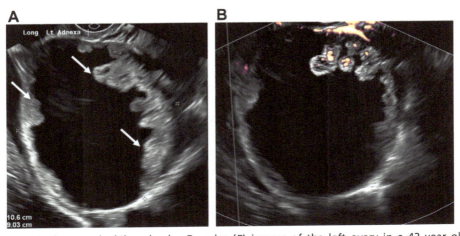

Fig. 14. Transvaginal grayscale (*A*) and color Doppler (*B*) images of the left ovary in a 42 year old patient presenting with abnormal uterine bleeding. In the left ovary, there is a 10.6 cm unilocular cyst with greater than 4 papillary projections. There is moderate internal flow on color Doppler (CS 3). Finding is consistent with an O-RADS US 5 lesion. Unfortunately, this patient was lost to follow-up as she was visiting from another country; however, imaging per gyn-oncologist was recommended with clinical follow-up with gyn-oncologist.

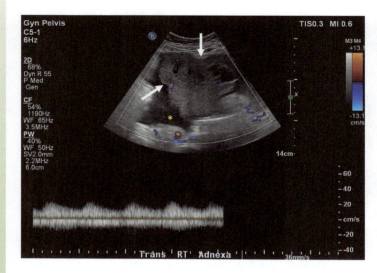

Fig. 15. A 68 year old female patient presenting with abdominal pain and pelvic mass seen on same day CT. Transabdominal spectral color Doppler image demonstrated a solid 11.9 cm right adnexal mass with irregular outer margin (*white arrows*). Minimal internal color Doppler flow was noted (CS 2). Ascites was also noted (*yellow asterisk*). The O-RADS US score is 5. Further imaging per gyn-oncologist was suggested with clinical follow-up with gyn-oncologist. This mass was surgically removed, and pathology returned high-grade serous carcinoma.

that emerging techniques for flow quantification could improve diagnostic performance,[24] or it may be that O-RADS can perform adequately with a more simplified or even binary vascularity score. The potential contribution of contrast-enhanced ultrasound (CEUS) for risk stratification is incompletely understood,[25] and the role of CEUS requires evaluation before it can be incorporated into O-RADS US. Diagnostic performance in children and adolescents,[26] as well as management in high-risk groups, such as patients with deleterious gene mutations (eg, BReast Cancer (BRCA) gene mutations, Lynch Syndrome, and so forth), has not been fully evaluated.

Finally, the relationship between US and MRI and their complementary roles for adnexal mass characterization are an area of ongoing research. US is the primary imaging modality for adnexal mass assessment, and a recent meta-analysis shows pooled O-RADS US 4 and 5 scores with 95.6% sensitivity and 76.6% specificity for the detection of malignancy.[27] However, as the confirmatory modality, MRI can provide additional specificity[28] and potentially decrease surgical intervention for benign lesions.[29] Currently, MRI is cited as a management option for O-RADS US 3 lesions that are solid or exhibit solid components, and also for O-RADS 4 lesions. Future research may expand or refine these recommendations, potentially incorporating additional test attributes such as patient preference, cost, and even environmental impact.

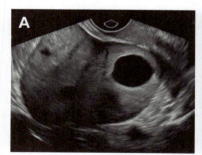
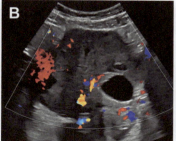
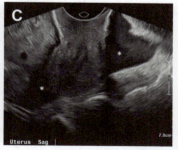

Fig. 16. A 29 year old patient presenting for evaluation of incidentally noted pelvic mass on CT. Transvaginal (*A, C*) and transabdominal (*B*) images demonstrate a 9.4 cm solid lesion with smooth outer contour and no associated shadowing. Moderate internal flow is seen on Doppler (CS 3). Ascites with low-level internal echoes is noted (*asterisk*). The O-RADS US score is 5. Clinical follow-up with gyn-oncologist was recommended. Patient expired shortly after this exam due to sepsis and heart failure. Pathology returned adenocarcinoma with signet ring features, likely metastatic from GI source.

> **Box 2**
> **Ovarian-Adnexal Reporting and Data System knowledge gaps and opportunities.**
>
> Intrareader and interreader concordance of feature descriptions and O-RADS US risk score
>
> Reproducibility of 4 point vascularity score and potential to simplify
>
> Capacity to incorporate CEUS features or quantitative flow metrics
>
> Management in high-risk population (BRCA, Lynch, other gene mutations)
>
> Diagnostic performance and management in children and adolescents
>
> Optimal utility of MRI after US
>
> Cost-effectiveness analysis of O-RADS approach

- context of patient symptoms, laboratory values, and prior imaging, when available.
- Optimal sonographic technique is needed to accurately assess an adnexal lesion. Optimization of color Doppler settings is important and helps differentiate solid components from internal debris, which can have similar grayscale sonographic appearance.
- Imaging and clinical management recommendations are also now available for each of the 6 O-RADS US risk categories.
- The size of a CBL is important for risk stratification. A CBL with maximum diameter less than 10 cm will be assigned an O-RADS US 2 (almost certainly benign) score while those 10 cm or greater will be assigned O-RADS US 3 (low risk) score.

SUMMARY

O-RADS US v2022 is an evidence-based and structured method for reporting and assessing ROM in ovarian and adnexal lesions. It can be applied to normal ovaries as well as ovarian/adnexal lesions, allowing it to be incorporated into everyday clinical practice. Risk assessment tables and the smart phone app are useful tools for assigning the appropriate O-RADS scores and management recommendations. Familiarization with the governing concepts, risk assessment categories and tables, technical requirements, and "how to report" documents ensure correct use of the system. Ongoing research will help refine and streamline the system, intending to standardize and enhance sensitivity, specificity, and management with the ultimate goal of optimal care for patients with ovarian and adnexal lesions.

CLINICS CARE POINTS

- O-RADS US v2022 is an evidence-based clinical support system that helps to accurately characterize adnexal and ovarian findings, assigning lesions an estimated ROM.
- O-RADS US should be used when the intent is to stratify the ROM of adnexal finding and thus should not be used in certain clinical scenarios including ectopic pregnancy, pelvic inflammatory disease, or for lesions that are not adnexal (ie, pedunculated myoma).
- Familiarization with US techniques and expected artifacts will help ensure optimized imaging and lesion characterization. Interpretation of US findings should be done in

ACKNOWLEDGMENTS

The authors would like to thank Rochelle Andreotti, MD, for her tremendous contributions to O-RADS and for her feedback on this article.

DISCLOSURE

The authors have nothing to disclose.

REFERENCES

1. Andreotti RF, Timmerman D, Benacerraf BR, et al. Ovarian-adnexal reporting lexicon for ultrasound: a white paper of the ACR ovarian-adnexal reporting and data system committee. J Am Coll Radiol 2018;15(10):1415–29.
2. Andreotti RF, Timmerman D, Strachowski LM, et al. O-RADS US risk stratification and management system: a consensus guideline from the ACR Ovarian-Adnexal Reporting and Data System Committee. Radiology 2020;294(1):168–85.
3. Timmerman S, Valentin L, Ceusters J, et al. External Validation of the Ovarian-Adnexal Reporting and Data System (O-RADS) Lexicon and the International Ovarian Tumor Analysis 2-Step Strategy to Stratify Ovarian Tumors Into O-RADS Risk Groups. JAMA Oncol 2023;9(2):225–33.
4. Strachowski LM, Jha P, Phillips CH, et al. O-RADS US v2022: An Update from the American College of Radiology's Ovarian-Adnexal Reporting and Data System US Committee. Radiology 2023; 308(3):e230685.
5. Zhan J, Diao XH, Jin JM, et al. Superb Microvascular Imaging-A new vascular detecting ultrasonographic technique for avascular breast masses: A preliminary study. Eur J Radiol 2016;85(5):915–21.

6. O-RADS Ultrasound 2022- Govering Concepts. 2022. Available at: https://www.acr.org/-/media/ACR/Files/RADS/O-RADS/O-RADS–US-v2022-Governing-Concepts-only.pdf.
7. ACR ORADS v2022 Assessment categories- Tables 2022. Available at: https://www.acr.org/-/media/ACR/Files/RADS/O-RADS/US-v2022/O-RADS–US-v2022-Assessment-Categories.pdf.
8. Levine D, Patel MD, Suh-Burgmann EJ, et al. Simple adnexal cysts: SRU consensus conference update on follow-up and reporting. Radiology 2019;293(2):359–71.
9. Phillips C, Strachowski L. O-RADS US v2022 technical guidance. 2023. Available at: https://www.acr.org/-/media/ACR/Files/RADS/O-RADS/O-RADS-US-Technical-Guidance.pdf. [Accessed 22 February 2024].
10. ACR–AAPM standard for diagnostic medical physics performance monitoring of real time ultrasound equipment. 2021. Available at: https://www.acr.org/-/media/ACR/Files/Practice-Parameters/US-Equip.pdf.
11. ACR–ACOG–AIUM–SPR–SRU Practice parameter for the performance of ultrasound of the female pelvis Revised 2019 (cited 2023 December 8).
12. Smith-Bindman R, Poder L, Johnson E, et al. Risk of malignant ovarian cancer based on ultrasonography findings in a large unselected population. JAMA Intern Med 2019;179(1):71–7.
13. O-RADS Ultrasound v222. Assessment categories algorithm. 2022. Available at: https://www.acr.org/-/media/ACR/Files/RADS/O-RADS/US-v2022/O-RADS-US-v2022-Assessment-Categories-Algorithm.pdf. [Accessed 16 February 2024].
14. O-RADS Ultrasound. v2022 Lexicon Categories, Terms, and Definitions 2023. Available at: https://www.acr.org/-/media/ACR/Files/RADS/O-RADS/O-RADS-US-v2022-Lexicon-Terms-Table-2023.pdf. [Accessed 29 February 2024].
15. Hack K, Gandhi N, Bouchard-Fortier G, et al. External validation of O-RADS US Risk Stratification and Management System. Radiology 2022;304(1):114–20.
16. Jha P, Gupta A, Baran TM, et al. Diagnostic performance of the ovarian-adnexal reporting and data system (O-RADS) ultrasound risk score in women in the United States. JAMA Netw Open 2022;5(6):e2216370.
17. Guo Y, Phillips CH, Suarez-Weiss K, et al. Inter-reader agreement and intermodality concordance of O-RADS US and MRI for assessing large, complex ovarian-adnexal cysts. Radiol Imaging Cancer. 2022;4(5):e220064.
18. Phillips CH, Guo Y, Strachowski LM, et al. The ovarian/adnexal reporting and data system for ultrasound: from standardized terminology to optimal risk assessment and management. Can Assoc Radiol J 2023;74(1):44–57.
19. Basha MAA, Metwally MI, Gamil SA, et al. Comparison of O-RADS, GI-RADS, and IOTA simple rules regarding malignancy rate, validity, and reliability for diagnosis of adnexal masses. Eur Radiol 2021;31(2):674–84.
20. Cao L, Wei M, Liu Y, et al. Validation of American College of Radiology Ovarian-Adnexal Reporting and Data System Ultrasound (O-RADS US): Analysis on 1054 adnexal masses. Gynecol Oncol 2021;162(1):107–12.
21. Stachowski L, Phillips C, O-RADS US v2022. How to report: Essential components and lexicon descriptors. 2023. Available at: https://www.acr.org/-/media/ACR/Files/RADS/O-RADS/O-RADS-US-v2022-Sample-reports-FINAL.pdf. [Accessed 22 February 2024].
22. Strachowski L, Frederick-Dyer K. O-RADS US v2022: Report Template Sample. 2023. Available at: https://www.acr.org/-/media/ACR/Files/RADS/O-RADS/O-RADS-US-v2022-report-template-sample-FINAL.pdf. [Accessed 22 February 2024].
23. Burnside ES, Sickles EA, Bassett LW, et al. The ACR BI-RADS experience: learning from history. J Am Coll Radiol 2009;6(12):851–60.
24. Ruan L, Liu H, Xiang H, et al. Application of O-RADS US combined with MV-Flow to diagnose ovarian-adnexal tumors. Ultrasonography 2024;43(1):15–24.
25. Shi Y, Li H, Wu X, et al. O-RADS combined with contrast-enhanced ultrasound in risk stratification of adnexal masses. J Ovarian Res 2023;16(1):153.
26. Wang H, Wang L, An S, et al. American college of radiology ovarian-adnexal reporting and data system ultrasound (O-RADS): Diagnostic performance and inter-reviewer agreement for ovarian masses in children. Front Pediatr 2023;11:1091735.
27. Lee S, Lee JE, Hwang JA, et al. O-RADS US: a systematic review and meta-analysis of category-specific malignancy rates. Radiology 2023;308(2):e223269.
28. Campos A, Villermain-Lecolier C, Sadowski EA, et al. O-RADS scoring system for adnexal lesions: Diagnostic performance on TVUS performed by an expert sonographer and MRI. Eur J Radiol 2023;169:111172.
29. Dabi Y, Rockall A, Razakamanantsoa L, et al. O-RADS MRI scoring system has the potential to reduce the frequency of avoidable adnexal surgery. Eur J Obstet Gynecol Reprod Biol 2024;294:135–42.

Challenges in Ultrasound of the Gallbladder and Bile Ducts: A Focused Review and Update

Benjamin S. Strnad, MD, Katerina S. Konstantinoff, MD, Daniel R. Ludwig, MD*

KEYWORDS

- Acute cholecystitis • Cystic artery velocity • Gallbladder polyps • Contrast-enhanced US
- Biliary duct dilatation

KEY POINTS

- While ultrasound (US) is fundamental for assessment of acute cholecystitis, its measured performance has declined and would benefit from standardization in interpretation and reporting.
- Cystic artery velocity is a promising technique in diagnosis of acute cholecystitis but lacks supporting data and requires further study to define its clinical role and utility.
- Recent Society of Radiologists in Ultrasound consensus management guidelines for commonly identified, incidental gallbladder polyps aim to reduce unnecessary follow-up and surgery, but still require prospective and systematic evaluation.
- Lack of enhancement on contrast-enhanced US has high negative predictive value for excluding blood flow and is more useful than color Doppler evaluation for differentiating tumefactive sludge from gallbladder neoplasm.
- Incidental biliary duct dilatation is common in clinical practice. A recently presented algorithmic approach incorporating liver chemistries can help determine which patients need further evaluation.

INTRODUCTION

Ultrasound (US) is generally considered the initial imaging modality of choice in patients with right upper quadrant pain or suspected biliary obstruction.[1–4] It uses no ionizing radiation, is cost-effective, and can be performed portably in patients who are unstable. Real-time imaging allows for assessment of the mobility of intraluminal structures and presence of a sonographic Murphy sign (SMS).[5] Furthermore, it has the highest sensitivity of any modality for the diagnosis of cholelithiasis.[6] Important limitations of US include its operator dependence and potential for image degradation by larger patient body habitus or intervening bowel gas.

Despite the ubiquitous role of US in the evaluation of the gallbladder and biliary system, a number of challenges in clinical practice limit its utility as a stand-alone imaging modality. Accordingly, US is considered a highly effective screening test, but the presence of positive or indeterminate findings on US frequently prompt further evaluation with computed tomography (CT), magnetic resonance imaging with cholangiopancreatography (MRI/MRCP), or hepatobiliary scintigraphy. In the current article, the authors provide a focused review of the literature, highlighting current knowledge gaps and future directions for US of the gallbladder and bile ducts. Selected topics include routine evaluation of acute cholecystitis (AC),

---

Mallinckrodt Institute of Radiology, Washington University School of Medicine, 510 S. Kingshighway Boulevard, Campus Box 8131, Saint Louis, MO 63110, USA
* Corresponding author.
E-mail address: ludwigd@wustl.edu

cystic artery velocity (CAv) for the diagnosis of AC, incidental gallbladder polyps, contrast-enhanced US (CEUS), and incidental biliary duct dilatation.

Ultrasound of Acute Cholecystitis

The clinical diagnosis of AC relies on physical examination signs localizing inflammation to the right upper quadrant, systemic signs of inflammation and confirmatory imaging findings. The imaging findings of AC include confirmation of gallstones in appropriate patients and various secondary findings of gallbladder inflammation or obstruction.[7] Multiple imaging modalities are used to confirm AC including US, hepatobiliary scintigraphy, CT and MRI/MRCP. US is widely considered the most appropriate initial test because of its high accuracy, low cost, and broad availability.[3] Although early studies found US to have positive and negative predictive values for AC exceeding 90%, its reported performance has declined substantially in more recent large meta-analyses, with pooled sensitivity and specificity of 81% and 83%, respectively, in 2012, and 69% and 79%, respectively, in 2023.[8–10] Meanwhile, recent data suggest that CT and MRI have comparable or superior performance to US in the diagnosis of AC.[10] The explanations for and implications of these evolving performance metrics are not yet understood.

Detection of gallstones with US is a well-established and usually straightforward component of the US diagnosis of AC.[6] The role of secondary findings–how they are defined, their relative significance, and how many are necessary or sufficient to make a confident diagnosis–remains surprisingly ambiguous, however. The best-established secondary US findings are the "SMS" and thickening of the gallbladder wall. Additional secondary findings include gallbladder distension and identification of an impacted stone within the gallbladder neck (**Fig. 1**).

The SMS, first reported in the late 1970s as an elaboration on the widely accepted SMS, was arguably the first reported secondary US finding of AC. Early studies reported a positive predictive value of 92% in association with stones and a negative predictive value, absent stones, of 95%.[8] It was later recognized that the SMS may be absent in gangrenous cholecystitis due to ischemic denervation of the gallbladder.[11] The first definitions of the SMS were "the point of maximal abdominal tenderness over the sonographically localized gallbladder," noting "…if there was no tenderness over the gallbladder, or if tenderness was the same over the gallbladder as in adjacent regions, [the SMS] was negative."[12,13] Key features of the SMS were therefore "tenderness," an objective sign assessed by the examiner (as opposed to "pain," a symptom reported by the patient) and a deliberate comparison of tenderness at multiple sites on the abdomen. However, descriptions of the SMS have varied widely in terms of how tenderness or pain is defined and assessed.[14,15] This variation and the evolution of radiology practice since the late 1970s toward near-universal scanning by sonographer technologists with remote image interpretation by radiologists may account for decreased performance of this feature. Assessment of the SMS in the setting of opioid analgesia also presents an increasingly common ambiguity. When a sonographer is unfamiliar with the patient's baseline prior to medication, or if the sonographer is not trained or experienced in assessment of objective signs of abdominal tenderness, the SMS may be less reliable. A prospective study of emergency room patients randomized to receive placebo or meperidine reported that the performance of the SMS was unaffected by meperidine when assessed by emergency providers trained in bedside US, but that sensitivity of the SMS was as low as 17% when obtained by sonographers after medication was given, with many sonographers noting that the SMS could not be assessed. The same authors noted an increasing trend among emergency providers toward early prescription of analgesics to patients with suspected AC.[16]

After the SMS, gallbladder wall thickening is the other major, longest established secondary US finding of AC. Defining abnormal thickness as greater than 2 mm, a widely cited early study showed a high positive predictive value of 95% in association with gallstones.[8] A thickness greater than 3 mm is now widely considered to be the threshold for abnormal,[6,17] although proposed thresholds have varied from 2 to 5 mm. As with the SMS, there is a lack of consistency in the literature regarding where and how the gallbladder wall should be measured, or how to deal with partial or focal wall thickening. Gallbladder wall edema has also been described variably in the literature, but its distinction as a feature from wall thickening is not clear, with some authors describing a distinct, "hypoechoic layer" in the gallbladder wall and others describing a "striated appearance" of the wall in association with gangrenous cholecystitis.[15,18] There are also a wide variety of conditions other than cholecystitis that can cause gallbladder wall thickening, limiting the specificity of this finding in patients with chronic liver disease, acute hepatitis, heart failure, and many other conditions.[6] Notably, early studies

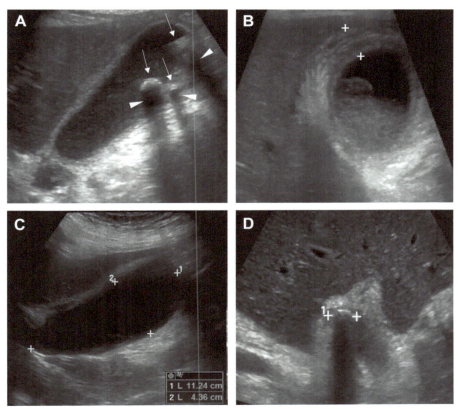

Fig. 1. Findings of acute cholecystitis on US in different patients. (A) Gallstones appear as echogenic intraluminal structures (arrows) with posterior acoustic shadowing (arrowheads). (B) Transverse view of the gallbladder with marked gallbladder wall thickening (calipers, 11 mm). (C) Gallbladder distention, most commonly described as luminal width greater than 4 cm. (D) Transverse view of impacted stone in gallbladder neck (calipers), which could not be dislodged with changes in patient positioning.

of this finding excluded patients with ascites and only included positive patients referred specifically for evaluation of suspected biliary disease, likely a very different population than those undergoing evaluation of abdominal pain in the emergency department today.

Several other secondary findings of AC have been described but are generally less supported by data and are variably applied in practice. Distension of the gallbladder lumen, for example, often defined as a luminal width greater than 4 cm, is a common secondary finding of AC. However, the gallbladder may also be distended in the fasting state, a typical scenario in patients with abdominal pain. Gallbladder size at baseline can also vary substantially from person to person. Due to these factors, defining gallbladder distension by a specific diameter or size threshold has limited positive predictive value, as low as 65%.[15] The tense gallbladder fundus sign has also been described as a marker of gallbladder distension and/or obstruction on CT[19]; however, no equivalent findings have been described on US. Notably, the absence of gallbladder distension using a luminal diameter threshold of less than 2.2 cm is likely to exclude AC.[20]

Direct visualization of an obstructing stone in the gallbladder neck or cystic duct and demonstration of its non-mobility has been proposed as another secondary finding, but has not been studied extensively. An impacted stone in the neck is identified by absence of anechoic bile between the stone and the walls of the gallbladder neck, and does not displace from the neck when moving the patient from supine to left lateral decubitus to nearly prone position.[21] In patients with a gallbladder-oriented steeply in the cranio-caudal axis, moving the patient to an upright or even standing position may be necessary to displace the stone.

Despite the emergence of these and other secondary findings omitted from this discussion, there is no consensus as to their relative significance in making the diagnosis. The only available meta-analyses of US performance for AC describe extensive heterogeneity among studies regarding how many findings were considered diagnostic, representing a significant limitation. As illustrated earlier, there is and has always been considerable ambiguity in assignment of even the most fundamental secondary features of AC. In combination with evolving practice in radiology and emergency departments, this ambiguity has likely contributed to the declining performance of US in diagnosis of AC. Focused training for sonographers in assessment of the SMS, especially in the setting of prior analgesia, as well as direct involvement by the radiologist whenever possible in ambiguous cases, will likely improve the utility of this important secondary finding. A comprehensive guidance system, akin to the Liver Reporting & Data System, to establish universal standards for interpretation and reporting, would also likely improve the performance of US in practice and facilitate clinical research and data collection. Finally, incorporation of novel techniques like CAv, as detailed in the subsequent section, provides further potential for improvement.

Cystic Artery Velocity

Pericholecystic inflammatory changes that occur in AC are commonly visualized on hepatobiliary scintigraphy as the "hot rim" sign, and on contrast-enhanced CT or CEUS as hyperemia of the hepatic parenchyma adjacent to the gallbladder fossa.[22,23] Correlations have been similarly described between increased color or power Doppler signal within the gallbladder wall and AC in the older US literature.[24–28] With routine use of spectral Doppler, quantitative parameters of pericholecystic hyperemia have essentially replaced qualitative assessment, which is notoriously dependent on the color Doppler settings which are utilized (eg, gain, frequency, range).[7]

Both peak hepatic artery velocity (HAv) and CAv have been associated with AC in various reports in the literature and with variable performance.[29–32] In a series of patients, 21 with AC and 14 with chronic cholecystitis (CC), peak HAv 100 cm/s or greater had an accuracy of 69% for the diagnosis of AC.[30] In a larger recent study which included 119 patients with AC and 117 with CC, a simple model incorporating peak HAv 96 cm/s or greater, gallbladder distention, and wall abnormalities had an area under the operating curve of 0.75, and sensitivity and specificity of only 60% and 83%, respectively, for differentiating AC from CC.[32] Increased peak HAv is not specific for AC, nor is it necessarily specific to primary hepatobiliary disease. Accordingly, an evaluation of a series of patients with peak HAv 200 cm/s or greater found that elevations could be attributed to a variety of causes including generalized infection and sepsis.[33]

Peak CAv, on the other hand, is likely more specific than peak HAv in the evaluation for pericholecystic inflammation (**Fig. 2**). An older study found that a peak CAv of greater than 40 cm/s was indicative of AC in patients with cirrhosis and a thickened gallbladder wall, though only 6 patients with AC were included.[29] In a recent study performed by Perez and colleagues, peak CAv was evaluated in 43 patients who presented to the emergency department with right upper quadrant pain, 25 with AC and 18 with CC, as well as in 30 control patients.[31] The authors found that a peak CAv 40 cm/s or greater was highly associated with AC, with positive predictive value of 95% and an overall accuracy 81% when used alone. However, this study was performed retrospectively, and the majority of patients screened for inclusion were excluded either because CAv was not measured, or they did not undergo definitive treatment within 6 days after imaging.

In our practice, we have encountered a number of patients with elevated peak CAv but who do not have AC, which may occur from variety of factors including hyperdynamic state, shock, hepatitis, and pancreatitis (**Fig. 3**A, B). Spuriously normal peak CAv, on the other hand, may occur in early AC or low cardiac output states (**Fig. 3**C, D). Further study is needed to determine the true performance CAv in practice and define its utility in combination with other more established features of AC. CAv will likely serve as a tiebreaking feature if grayscale findings are equivocal and/or SMS cannot be elicited.

Gallbladder Polyps

Gallbladder polypoid lesions are relatively common incidental imaging findings, and while the vast majority represent benign etiologies such as pseudotumors (eg, cholesterol polyps, inflammatory polyps), epithelial tumors (eg, adenomas), or mesenchymal tumors (eg, fibromas, lipomas, hemangiomas), a small percentage are or may become malignant.[34] Gallbladder cancer often presents at late stage and thus identifying high risk or precursor lesions would be of benefit; however, only 6% of gallbladder malignancies are associated with polyps.[35] In an attempt to address the frequent and prolonged imaging follow-up of many gallbladder polyps as well as potentially unnecessary surgical resections, the Society of Radiologists in Ultrasound (SRU) published updated consensus follow-up and management guidelines

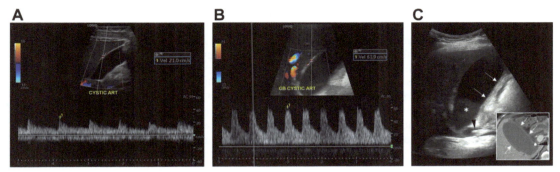

Fig. 2. Angle-corrected peak systolic velocity (PSV) of the cystic artery in two different patients (*A* and *B-C*, respectively). Color Doppler is used to identify the cystic artery branch along the gallbladder–liver interface and the angle-corrected PSV is measured using spectral Doppler. Normal PSV is less than 40 cm/s. (*A*) Normal cystic artery velocity (21 cm/s) and grayscale sonographic appearance of the gallbladder in a 26 year old man with 2 weeks of vague right upper quadrant pain. (*B*) Elevated cystic artery velocity (62 cm/s) in a 50 year old woman with cholelithiasis and 2 days of acute right upper quadrant pain. Corresponding grayscale imaging of the gallbladder (*C*) and contemporaneous axial contrast-enhanced CT image (*C*, inset) show gallbladder distention, wall thickening (*arrows*), sludge (*asterisk*), and an impacted stone in the gallbladder neck (*arrowhead*), consistent with acute cholecystitis.

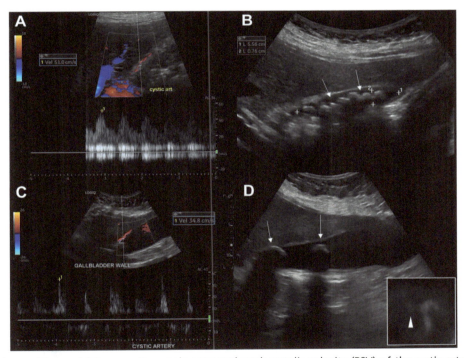

Fig. 3. False positive and false negative angle-corrected peak systolic velocity (PSV) of the cystic artery in two different patients (*A–B* and *C–D*, respectively). (*A, B*) Elevated cystic artery velocity (51 cm/s) in a 20 year old pregnant woman undergoing evaluation for epigastric abdominal pain. The gallbladder was collapsed around numerous shadowing gallstones (*arrows, B*). Sonographic Murphy sign was negative. Symptoms improved after antacid therapy. (*C, D*) Normal cystic artery velocity (35 cm/s) in a 46-year-old woman presenting with severe right upper quadrant pain, nausea, vomiting, and leukocytosis. There were two large shadowing stones in the gallbladder (*arrows, B*), one of which was impacted in the gallbladder neck. There was mild gallbladder distention but no significant wall thickening. Sonographic murphy sign was reported negative though the patient had received intravenous analgesic medication. Subsequent hepatobiliary scintigraphy study (inset) showed no filling of the gallbladder during initial 60 minutes of imaging or within 30 minutes after administration of morphine (*arrowhead*). Acute cholecystitis with significant pericholecystic inflammation was found at the time of surgery.

in 2021.[36] Previous guidelines did not take polyp morphology into account and were based predominantly on polyp size, symptoms, and patient risk factors.[37,38] The updated SRU guidelines risk-stratify polyps based on morphology, followed by more nuanced recommendations based on size. In applying the new guidelines, substantially fewer polyps meet criteria for long-term follow up and surgical management. A flowchart summarizing the updated guidance is shown in **Fig. 4**.

These recommendations apply only to high-quality US examinations where polyps are confidently differentiated from mimics such as sludge or adenomyomatosis. Additionally, the algorithm should not be applied if there is an obviously invasive or suspicious lesion, or in patients with primary sclerosing cholangitis (PSC). Patients with PSC are at increased risk for biliary malignancy and separate imaging surveillance recommendations exist for this population.[23] Once an eligible gallbladder polyp is identified on US, the first step is to risk-stratify based on morphology. The shape of the polyp is assessed and placed into one of three categories: pedunculated polyps which have a "ball-on-the-wall" appearance, or a thin stalk are considered "extremely low risk"; pedunculated polyps with a thick or wide stalk, or sessile morphology polyps are "low risk"; and polyps with adjacent focal wall thickening 4 mm or greater are "indeterminate risk". Within each category, follow-up and management recommendations are then made based on size of the polyp (see **Fig. 4**). For polyps that meet criteria for follow-up, an additional change in the updated guidelines was made regarding the cutoff for interval annual threshold growth. This was raised from 2 mm/year to 4 mm/year based on recent data from a very large 20-year cohort, which suggested the natural history of many benign polyps can involve small fluctuations in size, whether it be slight growth, or decrease in size.[39]

Of note, these new guidelines were created based on expert consensus rather than prospective data or meta-analysis and have not yet undergone systematic evaluation or validation. Further study is essential in this regard. Additionally, the new recommendations hinge upon morphology of the polyp for risk stratification, which has a significantly higher potential for inter-reader variability than polyp size. Fortunately, a recent inter-reader study found substantial agreement among abdominal radiologists for SRU consensus risk category assignment.[40]

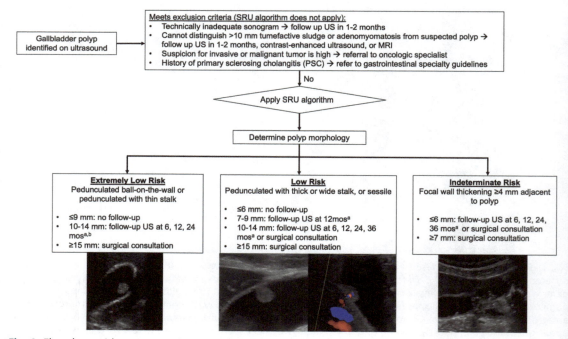

Fig. 4. Flowchart with representative examples adapted from the updated SRU follow-up and management recommendations for gallbladder polyps. If there is uncertainty between the categories, select the low-risk category.
[a]If size increases by 4 mm or more in 12 months or less or the polyp reaches threshold size for its category, surgical consultation is recommended. If the polyp decreases in size by 4 mm or more, additional follow-up is unnecessary.
[b]Surgical consultation may be appropriate for polyps 10 to 14 mm in the extremely low-risk category.

Contrast-Enhanced Ultrasound

CEUS is an US technique with expanding applications in abdominal imaging.[41,42] The contrast consists of microbubbles of inert gas stabilized by a phospholipid or albumin shell. Insonating these microbubbles at low power after intravenous injection creates harmonics that can be isolated and imaged selectively while suppressing the echoes from surrounding tissues. This creates very high contrast resolution and reproduces the effect of MRI digital subtraction techniques while allowing the operator to observe tissue perfusion continuously in real time. US contrast agents are also safe for use in patients with renal failure or in those with severe allergies to iodinated or gadolinium-based contrast agents. Allergic type or cardiopulmonary adverse reactions to US contrast have been reported but are thought to be extremely rare.[42]

Differentiation of gallbladder malignancy from gallbladder wall inflammation or tumefactive sludge are areas in which CEUS shows most promise as a problem-solving tool (**Fig. 5**). In the setting of chronic, complicated, or xanthogranulomatous cholecystitis, all of which can mimic gallbladder malignancy when they produce mass-like thickening of the gallbladder wall or when inflammation involves adjacent liver or other organs, CEUS can help by demonstrating a benign (progressive and delayed or absent) or a malignant (washout) pattern of enhancement. Tumefactive sludge in the gallbladder lumen, which can simulate a mass, can usually be identified by demonstrating its mobility on repositioning the patient. When patients cannot be repositioned, or when sludge fills most of the gallbladder lumen, CEUS can exclude malignancy by showing absence of enhancement within the sludge.[23,43,44] The lack of enhancement on CEUS has exceptionally high negative predictive value

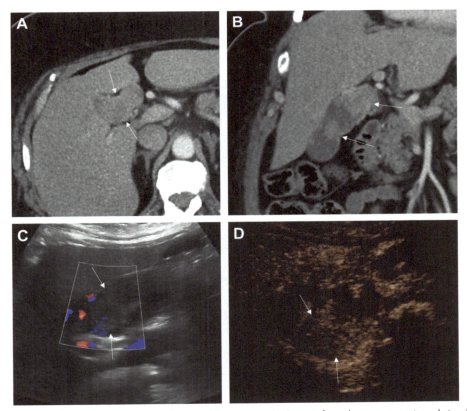

Fig. 5. Incidental gallbladder mass in a 66 year old woman which was found to represent an intracholecystic papillary neoplasm (ICPN). Axial and coronal contrast-enhanced CT images (*A* and *B*, respectively) show multiple endoluminal polypoid lesions with soft tissue attenuation involving the gallbladder neck and body (*arrows*). Color Doppler US image (*C*) shows echogenic intraluminal material in the gallbladder lumen without internal color flow (*arrows*), suggestive of tumefactive sludge. However, subsequently obtained contrast-enhanced US image (*D*) confirms the presence of internal enhancement, most consistent with a gallbladder neoplasm. Cholecystectomy and central hepatectomy was performed, which found IPCN without invasive carcinoma.

(98%) for excluding blood flow in a solid-appearing mass and is unequivocally superior to color Doppler in this regard.[45]

CEUS may serve as useful adjunct in the initial workup of AC by demonstrating reactive hepatic parenchymal enhancement adjacent to the gallbladder fossa when other secondary findings are equivocal,[23] or may facilitate early detection of complicated or ruptured cholecystitis by showing subtle ulceration or small defects in the gallbladder wall which would otherwise be missed on B-mode imaging.[23,46] Studies of CEUS for the evaluation of complicated cholecystitis remain limited to single institutional series. Larger, prospective evaluations of CEUS in this context, and comparisons of its performance with CT or MRI, are still lacking.

Biliary Duct Dilatation

In patients with jaundice or a cholestatic pattern of liver injury, US is commonly performed to evaluate for biliary duct dilatation in order to differentiate biliary obstruction from intrahepatic cholestasis.[2,4] Biliary duct dilatation in this context is commonly indicative of biliary obstruction, whereas normal caliber bile ducts have a very high negative predictive value.[47] However, biliary duct dilatation is unlikely to indicate biliary obstruction in the absence of clinical symptoms or elevated liver chemistries. Indeed, biliary duct enlargement is an exceedingly common incidental finding in clinical practice and the majority of asymptomatic cases are attributable to advanced age or prior cholecystectomy (**Fig. 6**).[48,49] We recently presented an algorithmic approach for the management of biliary duct dilatation in an AJR Expert Panel review[50] and will briefly summarize the relevant recommendations.

The initial step is to assess whether an enlarged bile duct meets size criteria for biliary duct dilatation, which is defined as greater than 6 mm in the general population, greater than 8 mm in patients aged 60 years and older, and greater than 10 mm in patients with prior cholecystectomy. On US, the extrahepatic bile duct is often measured at its proximal, mid, and distal segments. Rather than relying on different thresholds depending on the location where the duct is measured, a simpler and more reliable approach

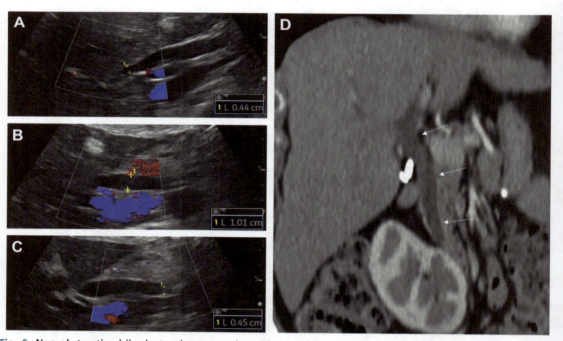

Fig. 6. Non-obstructive bile duct enlargement in a 57 year old woman with prior cholecystectomy presenting with left-sided abdominal pain and normal liver chemistries. Serial longitudinal ultrasound images of the extrahepatic bile duct (*A–C*) show enlargement of the extrahepatic bile duct measuring 4, 10, and 5 mm in the proximal (*A*, calipers), mid (*B*, calipers), and distal segments (*C*, calipers), respectively. Contemporaneous oblique coronal contrast-enhanced CT image (*D*) shows mild central and diffuse extrahepatic bile duct enlargement to the level of the ampulla with a gradual distal taper (*arrows*). Findings are most consistent with reservoir effect is the setting of prior cholecystectomy and the degree of duct enlargement does not meet criteria for biliary duct dilation (ie, >10 mm after prior cholecystectomy).

is to use the greatest diameter of the extrahepatic duct at any location along its course. Measurements should be performed perpendicular to the long axis of the bile duct, and the duct measured from inner-wall to inner-wall (see **Fig. 6**A–C).

Once it is determined that the bile duct is dilated, the next step is to correlate with clinical factors, the most important of which is liver chemistries. There are multiple patterns of liver chemistry elevations, though alkaline phosphatase, gamma-glutamyl transpeptidase (GGT), and conjugated bilirubin are considered biliary-associated enzymes and are invariably elevated in a cholestatic pattern of liver injury. Elevated biliary-associated enzymes in the setting of biliary duct dilation should prompt further evaluation with MRI/MRCP with IV contrast (when feasible) to evaluate for an obstructing lesion or less common etiologies of biliary duct dilatation including a peri-ampullary duodenal diverticulum, intraductal papillary neoplasm of the bile duct (IPN-B), or choledochal cyst. Any suspicious findings on MRI/MRCP should be further evaluated using endoscopic ultrasound (EUS) with endoscopic retrograde cholangiopancreatography (ERCP) if intervention is required. Notably, if a bile duct stone is identified on the initial US, ERCP is performed for stone extraction; additional imaging with MRI/MRCP is considered unnecessary according to clinical society guidelines.[51]

SUMMARY

US is well established as the initial imaging modality of choice in patients with right upper quadrant pain because of its low cost, good performance, portability, and accessibility. Despite its stability as a preferred imaging modality in this setting, US of the gallbladder and bile ducts faces a number of emerging challenges in contemporary practice and also continues to evolve. A particular challenge discussed at length in this review is the persisting lack of consensus and standardization in the US diagnosis of AC, which has likely contributed to a decline in diagnostic performance. We hope this can be addressed through development of a standardized reporting and data system that can more clearly define and integrate the various US findings of AC and their correlates on complementary imaging modalities. New US techniques reviewed here, including CAv measurement for suspected AC and CEUS for distinction of benign and malignant gallbladder processes, are promising but require further study. New guidance summarized here on US in management of incidentally detected gallbladder polyps and biliary dilation will likely clarify reporting and reduce the need for unnecessary follow-up imaging and surgical management.

CLINICS CARE POINTS

- Ultrasound is an established imaging technique for the diagnosis of acute cholecystitis, though a lack standardization in interpretation and reporting has likely contributed to a measurable decline in its diagnostic performance.
- Cystic artery velocity has potential value for the diagnosis of acute cholecystitis, especially in patients with equivocal grayscale findings, but further study is needed define its clinical role and utility.
- Application of recent SRU consensus management guidelines for gallbladder polyps will likely reduce unnecessary follow-up and surgery, but validation studies are needed.
- Contrast-enhanced ultrasound has high negative predictive value for excluding blood flow and better performance than color Doppler for differentiating tumefactive sludge from gallbladder neoplasm.
- Implementation of a recently presented algorithmic approach to incidental biliary duct dilation can help determine which patients need further evaluation.

DISCLOSURE

The authors have nothing to disclose.

REFERENCES

1. Kwo PY, Cohen SM, Lim JK. ACG Clinical Guideline: Evaluation of Abnormal Liver Chemistries. Off J Am Coll Gastroenterol ACG 2017;112(1):18–35.
2. Hindman NM, Arif-Tiwari H, Kamel IR, et al. ACR Appropriateness Criteria® Jaundice. J Am Coll Radiol 2019;16(5):S126–40. Elsevier.
3. Peterson CM, McNamara MM, Kamel IR, et al. ACR appropriateness criteria® right upper quadrant pain. J Am Coll Radiol 2019;16(5):S235–43. Elsevier.
4. Arif-Tiwari H, Porter K, Kamel I. Abnormal Liver Function Tests, ACR Appropriateness Criteria® American College of Radiology. J Am Coll Radiol 2023.
5. Foley WD, Quiroz FA. The Role of Sonography in Imaging of the Biliary Tract. Ultrasound Q 2007;23(2):123–35.
6. Middleton WD, Morgan T. Ultrasound: the requisites. Amsterdam, Netherlands: Elsevier Health Sciences; 2015.

7. Yokoe M, Hata J, Takada T, et al. Tokyo Guidelines 2018: diagnostic criteria and severity grading of acute cholecystitis (with videos). J Hepato-Biliary-Pancreat Sci 2018;25(1):41–54.
8. Ralls PW, Colletti PM, Lapin SA, et al. Real-time sonography in suspected acute cholecystitis. Prospective evaluation of primary and secondary signs. Radiology 1985;155(3):767–71.
9. Kiewiet JJS, Leeuwenburgh MMN, Bipat S, et al. A Systematic Review and Meta-Analysis of Diagnostic Performance of Imaging in Acute Cholecystitis. Radiology 2012;264(3):708–20. Radiological Society of North America.
10. Childs DD, Lalwani N, Craven T, et al. A meta-analysis of the performance of ultrasound, hepatobiliary scintigraphy, CT and MRI in the diagnosis of acute cholecystitis. Abdom Radiol 2024;49(2):384–98.
11. Simeone JF, Brink JA, Mueller PR, et al. The sonographic diagnosis of acute gangrenous cholecystitis: importance of the Murphy sign. AJR Am J Roentgenol 1989;152(2):289–90.
12. Ralls PW, Halls J, Lapin SA, et al. Prospective evaluation of the sonographic murphy sign in suspected acute cholecystitis. J Clin Ultrasound 1982;10(3):113–5.
13. Sherman M, Ralls P, Quinn M, et al. Intravenous cholangiography and sonography in acute cholecystitis: prospective evaluation. Am J Roentgenol 1980;135(2):311–3. American Roentgen Ray Society.
14. Finberg HJ, Birnholz JC. Ultrasound evaluation of the gallbladder wall. Radiology 1979;133(3 Pt 1):693–8.
15. Borzellino G, Massimiliano Motton A, Minniti F, et al. Sonographic diagnosis of acute cholecystitis in patients with symptomatic gallstones. J Clin Ultrasound 2016;44(3):152–8.
16. Noble VE, Liteplo AS, Nelson BP, et al. The impact of analgesia on the diagnostic accuracy of the sonographic Murphy's sign. Eur J Emerg Med 2010;17(2):80.
17. Engel J, Deitch E, Sikkema W. Gallbladder wall thickness: sonographic accuracy and relation to disease. Am J Roentgenol 1980;134(5):907–9.
18. Teefey SA, Baron RL, Bigler SA. Sonography of the gallbladder: significance of striated (layered) thickening of the gallbladder wall. Am J Roentgenol 1991;156(5):945–7. American Roentgen Ray Society.
19. An C, Park S, Ko S, et al. Usefulness of the tensile gallbladder fundus sign in the diagnosis of early acute cholecystitis. AJR Am J Roentgenol 2013;201(2):340–6.
20. Shaish H, Ma HY, Ahmed FS. The utility of an underdistended gallbladder on ultrasound in ruling out acute cholecystitis. Abdom Radiol N Y 2021;46(6):2498–504.
21. Nelson M, Ash A, Raio C, et al. Stone-In-Neck phenomenon: a new sign of cholecystitis. Crit Ultrasound J. SpringerOpen 2011;3(2):115–7.
22. Zhang P, Dyer RB. The hot rim sign. Abdom Radiol 2018;43(12):3530–1.
23. Lyshchik A, Dietrich CF, Sidhu PS, et al. Fundamentals of CEUS. Amsterdam, Netherlands: Elsevier; 2019.
24. Jeffrey RB, Nino-Murcia M, Ralls PW, et al. Color Doppler sonography of the cystic artery: comparison of normal controls and patients with acute cholecystitis. J Ultrasound Med 1995;14(1):33–6.
25. Schiller VL, Turner RR, Sarti DA. Color doppler imaging of the gallbladder wall in acute cholecystitis: sonographic-pathologic correlation. Abdom Imaging 1996;21(3):233–7.
26. Uggowitzer M, Kugler C, Schramayer G, et al. Sonography of acute cholecystitis: comparison of color and power Doppler sonography in detecting a hypervascularized gallbladder wall. Am J Roentgenol 1997;168(3):707–12.
27. Soyer P, Brouland JP, Boudiaf M, et al. Color velocity imaging and power Doppler sonography of the gallbladder wall: a new look at sonographic diagnosis of acute cholecystitis. AJR Am J Roentgenol 1998;171(1):183–8. American Public Health Association.
28. Draghi F, Ferrozzi G, Calliada F, et al. Power Doppler ultrasound of gallbladder wall vascularization in inflammation: clinical implications. Eur Radiol 2000;10(10):1587–90.
29. Tochio H, Nishiuma S, Okabe Y, et al. Diagnosis of acute cholecystitis in patients with liver cirrhosis: waveform analysis of the cystic artery by color Doppler imaging. J Med Ultrason 2004;31(1):21–8.
30. Loehfelm TW, Tse JR, Jeffrey RB, et al. The utility of hepatic artery velocity in diagnosing patients with acute cholecystitis. Abdom Radiol N Y 2018;43(5):1159–67.
31. Perez MG, Tse JR, Bird KN, et al. Cystic artery velocity as a predictor of acute cholecystitis. Abdom Radiol N Y 2021;46(10):4720–8.
32. Navarro SM, Chen S, Situ X, et al. Sonographic Assessment of Acute Versus Chronic Cholecystitis. J Ultrasound Med 2023;42(6):1257–65.
33. Ramirez MV, McGahan JP, Loehfelm TW, et al. Markedly elevated hepatic arterial velocity-HAV greater than 200 cm/s-is not specific to hepatobiliary disease. J Clin Ultrasound JCU 2020;48(9):532–7.
34. Andrén-Sandberg A. Diagnosis and management of gallbladder polyps. North Am J Med Sci 2012;4(5):203–11.
35. Okamoto M, Okamoto H, Kitahara F, et al. Ultrasonographic evidence of association of polyps and stones with gallbladder cancer. Am J Gastroenterol 1999;94(2):446–50.
36. Kamaya A, Fung C, Szpakowski J-L, et al. Management of Incidentally Detected Gallbladder Polyps:

Society of Radiologists in Ultrasound Consensus Conference Recommendations. Radiology 2022;305(2): 277–89. Radiological Society of North America.
37. Sebastian S, Araujo C, Neitlich JD, et al. Managing incidental findings on abdominal and pelvic CT and MRI, Part 4: white paper of the ACR Incidental Findings Committee II on gallbladder and biliary findings. J Am Coll Radiol JACR 2013;10(12):953–6.
38. Wiles R, Thoeni RF, Barbu ST, et al. Management and follow-up of gallbladder polyps. Eur Radiol 2017;27(9):3856–66.
39. Szpakowski J-L, Tucker L-Y. Outcomes of Gallbladder Polyps and Their Association With Gallbladder Cancer in a 20-Year Cohort. JAMA Netw Open 2020;3(5):e205143.
40. Anderson MA, Mercaldo S, Cao J, et al. Society of Radiologists in Ultrasound Consensus Conference Recommendations for Incidental Gallbladder Polyp Management: Interreader Agreement Among Ten Radiologists. AJR Am J Roentgenol 2024. https://doi.org/10.2214/AJR.23.30720.
41. Russell G, Strnad BS, Ludwig DR, et al. Contrast-Enhanced Ultrasound for Image-Guided Procedures. Tech Vasc Intervent Radiol 2023;100913. https://doi.org/10.1016/j.tvir.2023.100913.
42. Chung YE, Kim KW. Contrast-enhanced ultrasonography: advance and current status in abdominal imaging. Ultrasonography 2015;34(1):3–18.
43. Liu L-N, Xu H-X, Lu M-D, et al. Contrast-Enhanced Ultrasound in the Diagnosis of Gallbladder Diseases: A Multi-Center Experience. PLoS One 2012; 7(10):e48371.
44. Kumar I, Yadav YK, Kumar S, et al. Utility of Contrast-Enhanced Ultrasound in Differentiation between Benign Mural Lesions and Adenocarcinoma of Gallbladder. J Med Ultrasound 2020;28(3):143.
45. Alrashed A, Ahmad H, Khalili K, et al. Negative Predictive Value of Contrast-Enhanced Ultrasound in Differentiating Avascular Solid-Appearing From Vascularized Masses: A Retrospective Consecutive Study. J Ultrasound Med 2018;37(12):2935–42.
46. Sagrini E, Pecorelli A, Pettinari I, et al. Contrast-enhanced ultrasonography to diagnose complicated acute cholecystitis. Intern Emerg Med 2016;11(1):19–30.
47. Cooperberg PL, Li D, Wong P, et al. Accuracy of common hapatic duct size in the evaluation of extrahepatic biliary obstruction. Radiology 1980;135(1): 141–4. Radiological Society of North America.
48. McArthur TA, Planz V, Fineberg NS, et al. The common duct dilates after cholecystectomy and with advancing age: reality or myth? J Ultrasound Med 2013;32(8):1385–91.
49. McArthur TA, Planz V, Fineberg NS, et al. CT evaluation of common duct dilation after cholecystectomy and with advancing age. Abdom Imaging 2015; 40(6):1581–6.
50. Ludwig DR, Itani M, Childs DD, et al. Biliary Duct Dilatation: AJR Expert Panel Narrative Review. AJR Am J Roentgenol 2023. https://doi.org/10.2214/AJR.23.29671.
51. Buxbaum JL, Abbas Fehmi SM, Sultan S, et al. ASGE guideline on the role of endoscopy in the evaluation and management of choledocholithiasis. Gastrointest Endosc 2019;89(6):1075–105.e15.

Ultrasound of the Upper Urinary Tract

Margarita V. Revzin, MD, MS, FAIUM, FSRU, FSAR, FACR[a],*, Benjamin Srivastava[b], John S. Pellerito, MD, FSRU, FAIUM[c]

KEYWORDS

- Sonography • Doppler ultrasound • Renal contrast-enhanced ultrasound • Renal elastography
- Renal cyst • Upper genitourinary infection • Renal mass • Chronic renal disease

KEY POINTS

- Conventional and advanced ultrasound (US) plays a primary role in the assessment and diagnosis of the kidneys and bladder pathologies and their management.
- US is the first-line imaging modality for the evaluation of urinary obstruction, nephrolithiasis, renal vascular pathologies, and genitourinary infection with advanced techniques such as contrast-enhanced US gaining popularity in the diagnosis of renal malignancies; and shear wave elastography emerging as a technique for evaluation of the degree of chronic renal fibrosis.
- Conventional US is the modality of choice in evaluation of urinary bladder masses, causes of bladder outlet obstruction, and post treatment follow-up of urinary retention.

INTRODUCTION

Conventional and advanced ultrasound (US) techniques are essential in evaluation of a number of renal and ureteral pathologies (**Table 1**).[1] Kidney diseases can result from a wide range of genetic, hemodynamic, toxic, infectious, and autoimmune factors. Although the diagnosis of kidney disease usually involves analysis of clinical presentation, serum blood, and urine, these parameters are often insufficient to make a definitive diagnosis. US imaging as a first look can narrow down the diagnosis and guide choices regarding additional imaging and overall patient management.

US is non-invasive, portable, and safe; it does not utilize ionizing radiation or intravenous iodinated contrast material, and can detect structural, functional, and hemodynamic changes within the kidney.[1] New methods, such as contrast-enhanced US (CEUS) and elastography can allow more accurate assessment of renal masses and chronic renal disease.[2,3] Microbubbles can also help assess renal vascular patency and cortical perfusion in native and transplanted kidneys. When utilized, these methods greatly advance the diagnosis of renal and bladder diseases and safe monitoring of patients with serial follow-up examinations.

This article reviews the role of US imaging in the evaluation of suspected renal and ureteral disorders with emphasis on key sonographic features, utility of Doppler, and advanced techniques such as microflow imaging and CEUS.

ANATOMY

Kidneys have a relatively complex anatomy. Depending on the patient size, gender, and age, the kidneys range in size from 9 to 13 cm. Atrophic kidneys usually measure less than 8 cm in length and demonstrates heterogeneous and echogenic renal parenchyma (see **Fig. 3**).[4] On US, the bean-shaped kidneys consist of fibrofatty echogenic renal sinus and relatively hypoechoic renal cortex. The renal cortex is slightly more hypoechoic than

---

[a] Department of Radiology and Biomedical Imaging, Yale School of Medicine, New Haven, CT, USA; [b] Wilton Public High School, Wilton, CT 06897, USA; [c] Department of Radiology, Division of US, CT and MRI, Peripheral Vascular Laboratory, North Shore - Long Island Jewish Health System
* Corresponding author. 156 Mather Street, Wilton, CT 06897.
E-mail address: Margarita.revzin@yale.edu
Twitter: @MargaritaRevzin (M.V.R.)

Table 1 Grades of hydronephrosis	
Grade of Hydronephrosis	Characteristic Appearance
Grade 0	No hydronephrosis
Grade 1	Dilatation of renal pelvis only
Grade 2	Dilatation of renal pelvis and dilatation of a few calyces
Grade 3	Dilatation of renal pelvis and dilatation of all calyces
Grade 4	Dilatation of renal pelvis, dilatation of all calyces, and thinning of the renal parenchyma.

the liver and substantially more hypoechoic than the spleen. Heart-shaped pyramids are either isoechoic or slightly hypoechoic relative to the renal cortex (**Figs. 1** and **2**).[5] In patients with medical renal disease, the echogenic renal cortex is easy to characterize relative to the adjacent liver parenchyma (**Fig. 3**A, B). Echogenic kidneys are considered a "nonspecific finding" and can occur with other renal conditions such as chronic renal failure, drug-induced toxicity, metabolic disease, and infection. The intrarenal collecting and vascular systems travel through the echogenic renal sinus and may be seen as tubular anechoic structures converging at the renal hilum if dilated.[5] Although the surface of the kidneys is generally smooth, a common variant, called the junctional parenchymal defect, can produce a wedge-shaped indentation on the surface of the kidney near the junction of the upper and middle thirds of the renal cortex. This incomplete embryologic fusion of the upper and lower poles can be confused for scarring, traumatic injury, or a mass. Triangular shape and location of the defect are the keys to differentiate it from pathologic processes. A central wall of cortical tissue (*Column of Bertin*) can protrude into the renal sinus simulating a mass (**Fig. 4**).[6,7] Location in the mid third of the kidney, identical echogenicity as the renal cortex, uninterrupted continuation of the vessels into the tissue, and occasionally presence of a small hypoechoic pyramid are features that aid in differentiation of the column from pathologies (see **Fig. 4**A–C). Another common variant is *duplication of the intrarenal collecting system*, characterized by central band of cortex between the upper and lower pole (**Fig. 5**A, B).[8]

CONGENITAL ANOMALIES

Kidney agenesis is a rare congenital anomaly of the kidneys, where one of the kidneys is not developed resulting in empty renal fossa, contralateral kidney hypertrophy and linear shape of the ipsilateral adrenal gland rather than V-shaped configuration. It is associated with anomalies of the Mullerian duct. In women it can be seen with morphologic anomalies of the uterus and in man it may present with seminal vesicle anomaly or anomaly of the vas deferens. *Ectopic kidney* can be positioned anywhere in the abdomen and even thorax and usually has a blood supply from the adjacent vessels (**Fig. 6**A, B).[8] In contrast, a *ptotic kidney* is located lower than expected but still maintains the vascular supply from the abdominal aorta with the main renal artery originating at the same level as the normally positioned kidney. Crossed fused ectopia can also occur and may present as a very large kidney in a renal fossa with empty contralateral renal fossa. The ectopic kidney is fused with its upper pole to the lower pole of normally positioned kidney (**Fig. 7**A–D). The ureters maintain 2 normal urinary bladder insertion sites, and vascular supply is

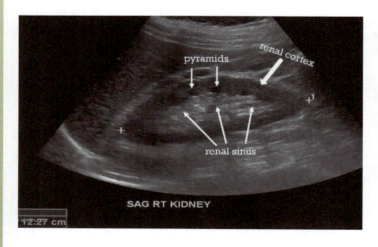

Fig. 1. Anatomy of the kidney on ultrasound (US). Grayscale US of the right kidney in sagittal plane demonstrates bean-shaped kidney with fibrofatty echogenic renal sinus (long thin *arrows*) and relatively hypoechoic renal cortex (short thick *arrow*). The renal cortex is slightly more hypoechoic than the adjacent liver echogenicity and substantially more hypoechoic than the spleen (not shown). Heart/roundish-shaped pyramids are hypoechoic relative to the renal cortex (short thin *arrows*).

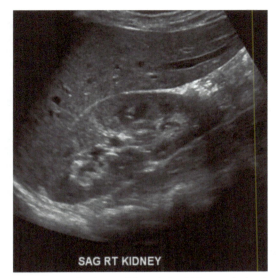

Fig. 2. Normal echogenicity of the kidney relative to the liver. Grayscale ultrasound (US) of the right kidney in sagittal plane demonstrates hypoechoic renal cortex relative to the hepatic parenchyma.

not altered. *Horseshoe kidney* is one of the most common fusion anomalies characterized by a variable thickness band of renal tissue (isthmus) extending from both lower poles to connect anterior to the aorta below the level of the inferior mesenteric artery (**Fig. 8**).[8]

PRINCIPLES OF EXAMINATION AND TECHNIQUE

There are several key elements to a successful renal examination. Although usually patients do not need to fast for general kidney assessment, adequate patient preparation can be essential when evaluating renal vasculature, for example, in the setting of suspected renal artery stenosis (RAS) or vascular thrombosis. Fasting can also decrease amount of bowel gas, improving visualization of the deeply positioned kidneys.

Curvilinear (2 – 5 MHz) transducers are used to maximize US beam penetration. Grayscale, color, spectral, and power Doppler are utilized for general assessment of the kidneys. Various parameters are optimized for better visualization of the examined structures, including but not limited to acoustic window, depth, brightness, focal zone, velocity scale, wall filter, and angle of insonation. When pathology is suspected, other more advanced US techniques and applications such as B-flow, microflow imaging, and CEUS can be helpful for more definitive diagnosis, especially for the assessment of vascular patency, mass vascularity, or kidney parenchymal perfusion in native kidney and renal transplants. Elastography can also improve confidence in the assessment of chronic and acute renal failure.

The US examination is performed with the patient in the supine position. The kidneys are examined in longitudinal and transverse scan planes with the transducer placed on the flanks using liver and spleen as acoustic windows. Supine and the lateral decubitus positions can be included when visualization of the kidney is obscured by bowel gas, with the transducer moved dorsally.

NONVASCULAR RENAL DISORDERS
Obstruction

One of the most common indications for renal US is renal insufficiency or suspected obstructive uropathy.[9] In most cases, bilateral obstruction is

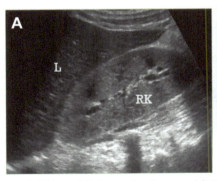
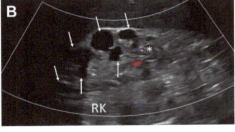

Fig. 3. Echogenic kidney. (*A*) Grayscale ultrasound (US) of the right kidney obtained in the sagittal plane demonstrates renal cortex (RK) substantially more echogenic than the hepatic parenchyma (L). The findings are nonspecifically associated with medical renal disease. (*B*) Acquired cystic renal disease in a patient with long-standing chronic renal disease. Color Doppler image of the right kidney obtained in a sagittal plane demonstrates atrophic (less than 8 cm in length) kidney (RK) with markedly echogenic and slightly heterogeneous renal cortex (*asterisk*) resulting in a loss of corticomedullary differentiation. Multiple renal cortical cysts of various size and complexity (*arrows*) are indicative of acquired cystic renal disease.

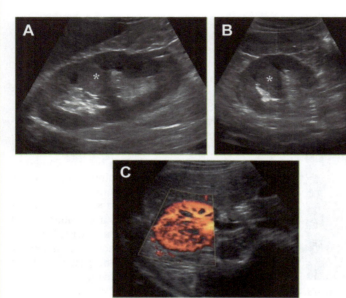

Fig. 4. Hypertrophied *column of Bertin*. (*A, B*) Grayscale ultrasound (US) of the right kidney obtained in sagittal (*A*) and transverse (*B*) planes demonstrates a rounded mass-like structure (*asterisks* in A, B) located in the mid third of the kidney and protruding into the renal sinus. The structure is isoechoic to renal cortex, indicative of column of Bertin. A small hypoechoic renal pyramid may be seen within column of Bertin (not shown). (*C*) Power Doppler image in the transverse plane shows uninterrupted continuation of the vessels into the column, which differentiates it from a neoplasm, which splays vessels around the mass and demonstrates disorganized neovascularity.

required for renal insufficiency to develop. Untreated obstruction may result in irreversible renal functional impairment, thus necessitating prompt diagnosis and management. Obstruction can be due to variable etiologies, including but not limited to obstructive stone, mass, external lymphadenopathy, abscess, pelvic mass/neoplasm, retroperitoneal fibrosis, among other etiologies. Hydronephrosis refers to dilatation of the intrarenal collecting system, including calyceal and pelvic dilatation. Hydroureteronephrosis describes dilation of the intrarenal and extrarenal collecting systems, including dilation of the ureters (≥ 5 mm in diameter) (**Fig. 9**A, B). It is important to note that 3 mm should be considered the upper limit of normal size for unobstructed ureters on unenhanced helical computed tomography (CT).[10] The overall reported diagnostic accuracy of US in detecting hydronephrosis is 85.2%, with a specificity of 84.4% and a sensitivity of 89.9%.[11] In addition to its ability to detect hydronephrosis, US also helps to differentiate acute obstructive hydronephrosis from non-obstructive hydronephrosis (for example physiologic hydronephrosis from gravid uterus, or persistently dilated collecting systems due to previous episodes of obstruction, or active physiologic diuresis, or overdistension of the urinary bladder and vesicoureteral reflux). All of these processes will show dilated collecting systems but without obstructive cause. The sensitivity of US in detecting urinary tract obstruction is 93%.[12] On US, hydronephrosis can be differentiated from peripelvic cysts by demonstrating convergence of the dilated calices to the level of the dilated renal pelvis, resembling a glove appearance with

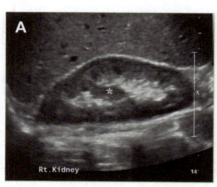 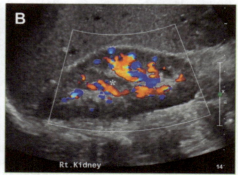

Fig. 5. Renal duplicated collecting system. (*A, B*) Grayscale (*A*) and color Doppler (*B*) ultrasound (US) images of the right kidney obtained in sagittal plane show a band of cortical tissue (*asterisks*) separating the renal sinus into superior and inferior segments.

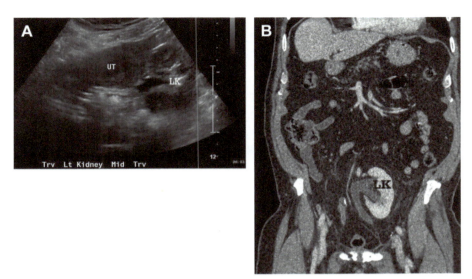

Fig. 6. Ectopic pelvic kidney. (*A*) Grayscale ultrasound (US) of the left kidney in sagittal plane demonstrates ectopic positioning of the left kidney in the pelvis (LK). Note that the ectopic kidney shows mild fullness of the collecting system and is adjacent to the uterus (UT). (*B*) Contrast-enhanced computed tomography (CECT) image in coronal plane demonstrates confirms pelvic located of the left kidney (LK) with mild hydronephrosis.

all the intrarenal segments communicating with the renal pelvis. Spectral Doppler can increase confidence in the diagnosis of obstructive hydronephrosis by demonstrating relatively elevated resistive index (RI), although this concept is still controversial as many processes may result in elevated RI.[13] There are 5 grades of obstruction recognized ranging from slight expansion of the intrarenal collecting system to end-stage hydronephrosis with cortical thinning (**Table 1**). In the setting of long-standing obstructive uropathy, the renal cortex becomes thin allowing differentiating chronic from acute obstruction (**Fig. 10**). Color Doppler can help distinguish prominent renal vessels from the collecting system (**Fig. 11**A–D). Due to bowel gas distension obscuring evaluation of the mid and lower pelvic organs, only the proximal and the most distal segments of the ureter are commonly visualized on US. Identification of an echogenic focus within the lumen with posterior shadowing and upstream ureteral dilatation can help to make accurate diagnosis (see

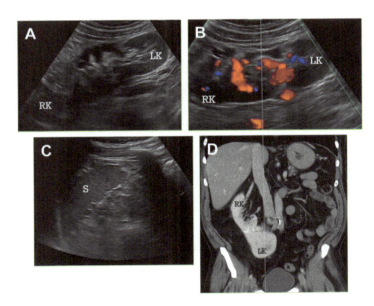

Fig. 7. Crossed fused renal ectopia. (*A–C*) Grayscale (*A, C*) and color Doppler (*B*) ultrasound (US) images of the upper abdomen obtained in the sagittal plane demonstrate fusion of upper pole of the left ectopic kidney (LK) to lower pole of the normally located right kidney (RK). Color Doppler demonstrates flow to the fused kidneys with the left main renal artery supplying the left ectopically positioned kidney and the right main renal artery supplying the right kidney. Note: empty left renal fossa with only spleen (S) present in the left upper abdomen. (*D*) Contrast-enhanced computed tomography (CECT) image depicting the positioning of the fused kidneys in the right abdomen and relationship of the right and left kidneys (RK, LK), as well as their corresponding vascular supply.

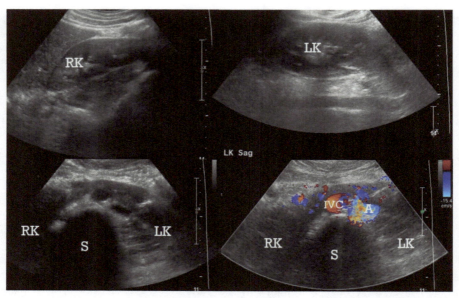

Fig. 8. Horseshoe kidney. Top row shows sagittal grayscale images of the right (RK) and left (LK) portions of the kidneys located in the corresponding right and left renal fossa. Bottom row grayscale (left) and color Doppler (right) images obtained in the transverse plane over the lower abdomen show the connecting isthmus crossing anterior to the retroperitoneal great vessels, aorta (A) and inferior vena cava (IVC) with the renal parenchyma of right (RK) and left (LK) limb of the horseshoe draping over the spine (S).

Fig. 11). The mid segment of the ureter is rarely seen on US unless it is severely dilated and tortuous. Doppler US can improve renal stone visualization and confidence by demonstrating a twinkling artifact.[14,15] Analysis of ureteral jets using Doppler can assist in the evaluation of potentially obstructed kidney and assess the degree of obstruction. Thus, in the presence of obstruction, ureteral jets usually are absent or in the case of partial obstruction, the jets can be markedly diminished.[16] In the setting of nonobstructive hydronephrosis, the ureteral jets are maintained. US is the most optimal imaging modality for serial follow-up of the patients with obstructive stones to monitor for relief of obstruction, which would be suggested by reappearance of the ureteral jets and resolution of hydronephrosis. Urolithiasis is the most common cause of hydronephrosis in the adult patient and has a prevalence of 10% – 15%.[17] In a study of 210 patients with hydronephrosis, B-mode US imaging determined the cause of hydronephrosis in 65.2% of cases with

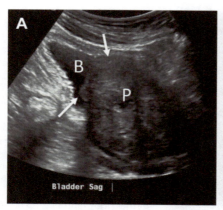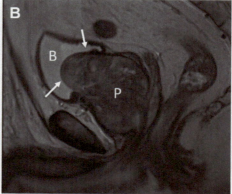

Fig. 9. Benign prostatic hypertrophy. (A) Grayscale image of the bladder in sagittal plane demonstrates a large slightly heterogeneous prostate gland (P) indenting the urinary bladder base (arrows). The bladder is partially decompressed (B) with mild wall trabeculation and thickening. (B) Sagittal T2 FS MR image of the prostate gland shows markedly enlarged heterogeneous prostate gland (P) indenting the bladder (B) base (arrows).

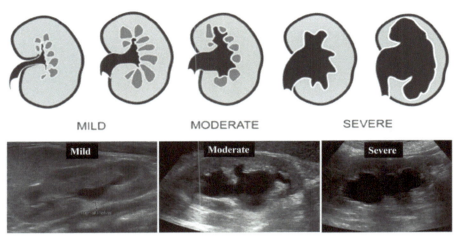

Fig. 10. Hydronephrosis grades. Schematic diagram and grayscale images of the right kidney in sagittal plane show mild (*left*), moderate (*mid*) and severe (*right*) hydronephrosis. Note that at grades 1, 2 there is only mild dilatation of the renal pelvis, and the calyces are not yet dilated. When hydronephrosis progresses to grade 3, 4, calyces become dilated, and the renal pelvis dilates to a higher degree. Blunting of fornices and flattening of papillae are also present. With severe hydronephrosis, the renal cortex becomes thinner with subsequent irreversible renal atrophy. There is also near complete loss of borders between the renal pelvis and calyces.

urolithiasis being the cause of obstruction in 60% of the patients. The detection rate of urinary stones was 50%, 61%, and 71.4% for grades 1, 2, and 3 hydronephrosis, respectively.[18] When an obstructive etiology is not identified on US, further imaging with CT urography is required. Presence of hematuria and obstruction without renal stones should raise concern for an underlying neoplasm and warrant further imaging assessment using CT or magnetic resonance (MR) urography, which allow evaluation of the entire upper and lower collecting systems (**Fig. 12**A–C). If the dilated calyces show internal debris, infection such as pyonephrosis is suspected, and correlation with urinalysis and clinical presentation should be made (**Fig. 13**A, B).[12] Pyonephrosis can cause rapid and permanent deterioration of renal function and should be decompressed as soon as it is detected.

Cystic Diseases

Renal cysts are the most frequently encountered renal lesions. They are seen in 50% of people over age of 50 y.[19] They may increase in size and become complex due to development of septations, precipitation of milk of calcium in the wall, and internal hemorrhage. The main US characteristics of a simple renal cyst include anechoic lumen, well-defined back wall, acoustic posterior enhancement, lack of internal flow, and imperceptible avascular wall (too thin to measure) (**Fig. 14**). Harmonic imaging and real-time compounding can aid in minimizing internal artifacts within the cysts, which can be encountered by imaging the cysts from different approaches.

By location, renal cysts can be divided into the cortical and parapelvic (originating in the renal sinus, commonly multiple) (see **Fig. 14**; **Fig. 15**A, B). Doppler US helps to differentiate the renal cysts from aneurysms, pseudoaneurysms (PSAs), arteriovenous fistulas, and vascular cystic neoplasms by demonstrating characteristic flow patterns and specific waveforms within these structures.

Complex cysts are those with variable-thickness septations or filled with echogenic material and/or solid components. Number and thickness of the septations and presence of nodular components determine complexity of the cysts. Hemorrhagic cysts may show either a retracted clot or low amplitude echogenic material, and on the serial follow-up examinations will show evolution of the hemorrhage often resulting in decreased size of the cyst. When large in size, hemorrhagic cysts rarely can rupture and become superinfected (**Fig. 16**A–C). Proteinaceous cysts may also show echogenic material within but do not morphologically change with time. Calcifications occur in 1% to 3% of cysts as a sequela of prior infection, hemorrhage, or ischemia.[20] Thick globular calcification should raise suspicion for malignancy. CEUS has emerged as an alternative imaging modality compared to CT angiography and MR angiography (MRA) for evaluation of suspected complex renal cystic lesions suspicious for neoplasms. Presence of enhancing components within the cystic renal lesions or septal

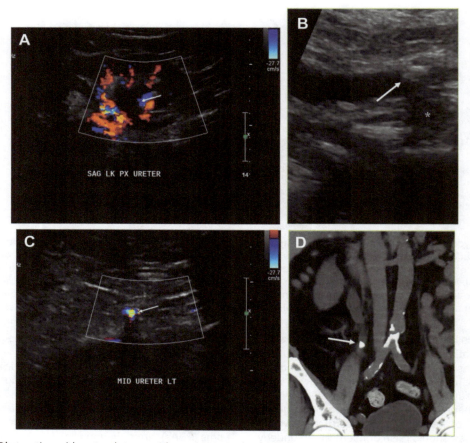

Fig. 11. Obstructive mid ureteral stone with resultant moderate hydroureteronephrosis. (A) Color Doppler image of the left kidney in sagittal plane demonstrates moderate hydroureteronephrosis. Note that the color Doppler helps differentiate vessels from the collecting system (arrow). (B) Grayscale images of the ureter shows dilated proximal right ureter, measuring 5 mm in diameter, to the level of an echogenic focus within its lumen with posterior shadowing seen in the proximal/mid ureter (arrow) indicative on an obstructing calculus. (C) Color Doppler image through the mid ureter shows twinkling artifact produced by the obstructive stone (arrow) (D) Nonenhanced coronal computed tomography (CT) confirms the findings demonstrating the obstructive calculus (arrow) and upstream hydroureteronephrosis.

enhancement should increase confidence in the diagnosis of a neoplasm.

Multiple cysts are usually seen in conditions such as autosomal dominant polycystic kidney disease (ADPKD), acquired cystic renal disease, von Hippel-Lindau disease (VHL), and tuberous sclerosis (TS).

In ADPKD, the various size and complexity cysts are seen in the bilateral enlarged kidneys occupying the renal cortex and medulla, and in more severe cases they may cause compression of the collecting systems.[21] Urine stasis resulting in solid appearance of the cysts due to formation of stones or hemorrhage are additional hallmarks of this condition (Fig. 17A–C).

VHL disease is another condition where presence of multiple cysts is one of its manifestations.

In fact, 30% – 70% of the patients with VHL have renal involvement in the form of multiple renal cysts.[21] The cysts may harbor malignancy developing within its walls; thus, their monitoring is a key for proper management of this patient population. The incidence of developing renal cell carcinoma (RCC) is 75% in a VHL patient with kidney involvement.[22] Over 90% of VHL patients will have more than 1 RCC, with earlier age of development when compared to sporadically developed RCC.[22,23] Bilateral RCC are seen in 75% of patients.[24] Other manifestations of VHL include pancreatic cysts, intracranial hemangioblastomas, pheochromocytomas, and scrotal papillary cystadenomas.

TS is a disorder characterized by a classic clinical triad consisted of mental retardation, seizures,

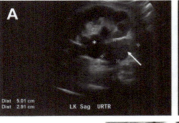
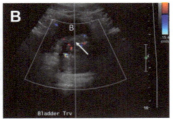
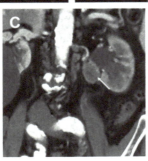

Fig. 12. Urothelial cancer resulting in hydronephrosis. (A) Grayscale ultrasound (US) image of the left kidney in sagittal plane demonstrates a hypoechoic infiltrating mass (arrow in A) in the proximal left ureter distending the ureter and resulting in the upstream moderate hydronephrosis (asterisk). (B) Color Doppler US image of the base of the urinary bladder in transverse plane shows a vascular mass (arrow in B) at the level of the left ureterovesicular junction (UVJ) indicative of a metastatic disease. (C) Coronal contrast-enhanced computed tomography (CECT) shows a hyperdense mass-like lesion in the left proximal ureter (arrow) with associated hydronephrosis. The findings are indicative of a multifocal urothelial cancer.

and cutaneous lesions. Renal cysts, seen in 95% of patients with TS, and neoplasms such as angiomyolipoma (AML), seen in 50% to 80% of patients, are also the hallmark of this multisystem disease. Cardiac, neural, pulmonary, and skeletal systems are usually affected.[25]

Benign Neoplasms

AMLs are the most common benign renal tumors and are composed of fat, muscle, and vessels. These asymptomatic tumors have no malignant potential but can increase in size and represent a source of bleeding due to ruptured microaneurysms. Due to high risk of bleeding, it is recommended to surgically excise AMLs when their size is greater than or equal to 4 cm in diameter.[26] On US, AMLs less than 2 cm are homogeneously echogenic (similar to the renal sinus), well-defined cortical renal lesions with posterior shadowing (**Fig. 18**A, B). It is essential to recognize that up to 20% of small RCC resemble AML.[27] Presence of cystic components in the RCC helps to distinguish them from AML. AMLs that are greater than 1 cm should be further evaluated with CT and MRI to evaluate for fat component.

Oncocytomas, a common type of renal neoplasm, comprise 5% of all renal neoplasms.[28] Their imaging appearance may be indistinguishable from other malignant lesions. Although central necrosis and hemorrhage are more often seen with oncocytomas, RCCs can also present with these features. Doppler image optimization may detect spoke-wheel pattern of vascular distribution with central scar that has been described in oncocytomas; however, the differentiation of oncocytoma from RCC is very difficult and can only be definitively done by assessment of

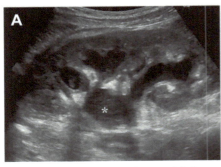
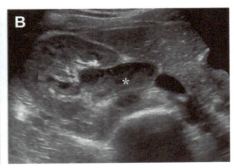

Fig. 13. Pyonephrosis in a 54-year-old man with fever and white count. (A, B) Grayscale images of the right kidney in sagittal (A) and transverse (B) planes show dilated intrarenal and extrarenal collecting system with echogenic intraluminal material resulting in moderate hydroureteronephrosis. Considering patient's clinical symptoms and urinalysis results, the findings are indicative of pyonephrosis, Urology consult was obtained, and patient was decompressed soon after the imaging was performed.

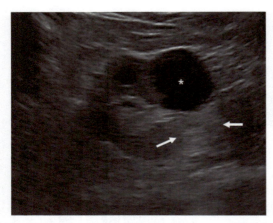

Fig. 14. Simple renal cyst. Grayscale ultrasound (US) in transverse plane shows a simple renal cyst with anechoic lumen (*asterisk*), well-defined back wall, acoustic posterior enhancement (*arrows*), and imperceptible avascular wall (too thin to measure). No flow was seen on color Doppler within the cyst or peripherally (not shown).

pathologic specimen.[29] Similar to RCC, these tumors are managed operatively with either nephrectomy, partial nephrectomy, or cryoablation.

Multilocular cystic nephroma is a benign neoplasm, which demonstrates indeterminate features on US, due to appearance of multiple septations. These tumors are characterized by multiple various size noncommunicating cysts and can affect either middle-aged women or young boys (**Fig. 19**A–D).[30] Because there is a significant overlap of multilocular cystic nephroma with RCC, they usually are managed with partial nephrectomy.

Malignant Neoplasms

RCC is the most common malignant renal parenchymal tumor accounting for 86% of all malignancies in the kidney.[31] Up to 60% of patients clinically present with hematuria; weight loss, fatigue, and anemia are less common presentations. RCC appearance on US varies significantly from iso- and hypoechoic masses to hyperechoic cortical masses, but they can also be located centrally in medulla or sinus (**Fig. 20**A, B). Multifocal presentation is common, especially in VHL or TS patients; the masses may be either entirely solid, have cystic and solid appearance, or contain nearly completely cystic components. Although conventional US cannot differentiate between the types of solid neoplasms and, more specifically, types of RCC, CEUS has proven to be capable of more definitive diagnosis based on the types of intensity curves that each type of tumor produces. Thus, papillary RCC subtype (which comprises 15% of all RCCs) demonstrates more weak and slow enhancement and clear cell RCC (ccRCC, which comprises 80% of all RCCs) shows rapid intense arterial enhancement (**Fig. 21**A–C). ccRCC more commonly shows cystic components (due to necrosis, hemorrhage, and cystic degeneration); calcifications; and presence of microscopic fat on MRI. Chromophobe RCC, which comprises 5% of all RCCs, has the most favorable prognosis and shows intermediate intensity curves.[32,33] Depending on patient age, comorbidities, and personal choice, RCCs can be managed by watchful waiting, surgically, or with minimally invasive procedures (cryoablation). Approximately 10% of RCC invade the renal veins (tumor-in-vein) and extend to the inferior vena cava and right atrium, necessitating multidisciplinary surgery (**Fig. 22**A, B).[34]

Renal medullary carcinoma—a very rare and highly aggressive type of RCC affecting younger patients with male predominance—is associated with sickle cell trait. Sonographically, the mass is centered in the renal medulla, usually

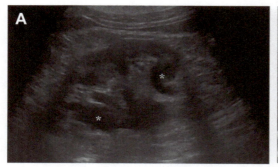
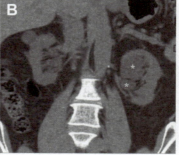

Fig. 15. (*A*, *B*) Parapelvic cyst. Grayscale ultrasound (US) image in sagittal plane shows 2 cystic structures in the renal sinus (*asterisks*) with resemblance of hydronephrosis. However, on real-time imaging and cine clips (not shown), these structures were not communicating compatible with parapelvic cysts. Correlative coronal nonenhanced CT (NECT) of the abdomen confirmed presence of parapelvic cysts (*asterisks*) and absence of hydronephrosis.

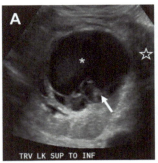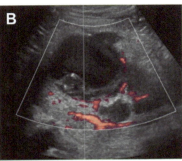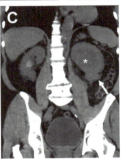

Fig. 16. Hemorrhagic superinfected cyst complicated by rupture. (A) Grayscale (A) and power Doppler (B) images of the left kidney in transverse plane demonstrate a complex cyst with a retracted clot (arrow) and low amplitude internal echoes (asterisk) compatible with a hemorrhagic cyst. Complex collection adjacent to the cyst (star) is compatible with spilled contents of the cyst after rupture. Peripheral flow is noted on the power Doppler but no internal vascularity. (C). Coronal NECT of the abdomen and pelvis demonstrates a hyperdense heterogeneous and poorly defined left renal cyst (asterisk) with evidence of rupture manifested as complex fluid in the perirenal fat adjacent to the kidney (arrow). On later examinations, the spilled fluid formed abscess requiring interventional radiology drainage.

demonstrates infiltrative nature, and may cause thrombus in the vein.[35]

Urothelial carcinomas (UTC) account for 10% of renal masses and can mimic centrally-located RCC.[36] They may show poorly defined borders and therefore, can be easily missed on US. The masses usually are isoechoic to the renal sinus and extend into the renal collecting system, resulting in either obliteration or irregular thick wall. Hydronephrosis may also be a presenting finding (see **Fig. 12**). If the primary UTC is in the urinary bladder, they present as a focal wall thickening of the bladder with or without detectable flow within on color Doppler, and can metastasize to

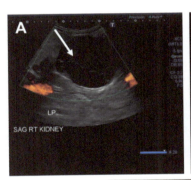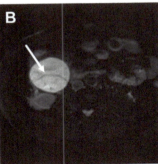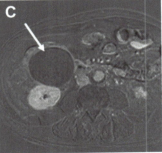

Fig. 17. Complex renal cyst. (A) Color Doppler US image in sagittal plane reveals a complex cyst with a thin septation in the lower pole of the right kidney (arrow). Note absence of flow in the septation and absence of nodular components. (B) Axial T2 weighted (T2WI) MRI of the abdomen shows a hypointense thin septation (arrow) within the renal cyst. (C) Axial fat suppressed (FS) T1WI subtraction MRI image after the administration of the gadolinium shows absence of the right renal cyst enhancement including absence of enhancement within the thin septation (arrow).

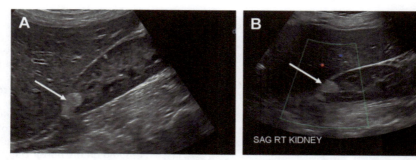

Fig. 18. Renal Angiomyolipoma (AML). (*A, B*) Grayscale (*A*) and color Doppler (*B*) ultrasound (US) images of the right kidney in sagittal plane show a small round echogenic homogeneous avascular mass in the upper renal cortex (*arrow*). The mass was also present on prior imaging 3 y ago and was unchanged in its size and morphologic appearance, indicative of AML.

1 or both kidneys. UTC often clinically presents with hematuria in the setting of absent obstructive stones.

Renal metastases are rare, accounting for only 0.9% of renal masses, most of which are solitary carcinomas.[37] Lung cancer is the most common primary site of renal metastases.

Renal lymphoma occurs in the setting of widespread nodal and extra-nodal lymphoma, and can present as a solitary, well- or ill-defined, or multifocal mass (**Fig. 23**A–C). Infiltrating type may result in the enlarged kidney(s) that on US will show preservation of corticomedullary differentiation.

Infections

Urinary tract infections are the most common urologic disease in the United States and annually account for over 7 million office visits and 1 million emergency department visits.[38]

When infection such as *Escherichia coli* migrates to the upper urinary tract or is seeded there hematogenously, both the renal pelvis and parenchyma become inflamed; thus, the condition is characterized as pyelonephritis. Classic symptoms of pyelonephritis include an abrupt onset of chills, fever (temperature of 100°F or greater), and unilateral or bilateral flank pain with costovertebral tenderness.[39] These "upper tract signs" are often accompanied by dysuria and urinary frequency and urgency. Acute pyelonephritis may also cause gastrointestinal symptoms, such as abdominal pain, nausea, vomiting, and diarrhea, which confuse the diagnosis. Laboratory findings include pyuria, leukocytosis, bacteriuria, and a positive urine culture. Blood tests may show leukocytosis

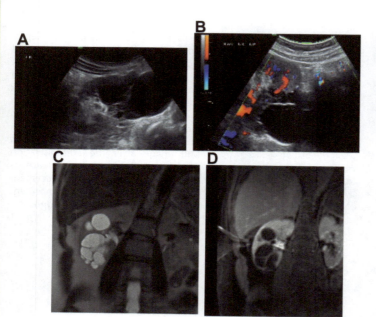

Fig. 19. Multilocular cystic nephroma. Grayscale (*A, B*) and color Doppler (*C, D*) ultrasound (US) images of the right kidney in sagittal plane show a cluster of various in size cysts in the lower pole. The cysts are not communicating, and normal parenchyma is present between the cysts. The findings are indicative of multilocular cystic nephroma.

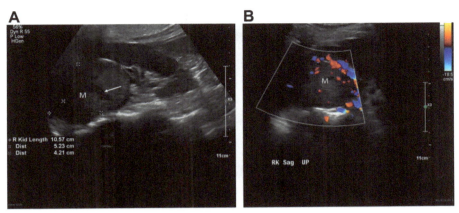

Fig. 20. Renal cell carcinoma (RCC). (*A, B*) Grayscale (*A*) and color Doppler (*B*) ultrasound (US) images of the right kidney obtained in sagittal plane show an upper pole solid mass (M) iso-to slightly hyperechoic to the renal cortex. Focal area of hypoechogenicity in the center of the mass (*arrow in A*) indicates focal necrosis. Disorganized flow is seen within the mass (M in *B*) on color Doppler.

with a neutrophilic shift, elevated erythrocyte sedimentation rate, elevated C-reactive protein levels, and occasionally positive blood cultures that grow the same organism as cultured from the urine.[39]

On US, early noncomplicated pyelonephritis may not be readily detectable. In more advanced forms, the kidneys may enlarge and show patchy heterogenous appearance with isolated or

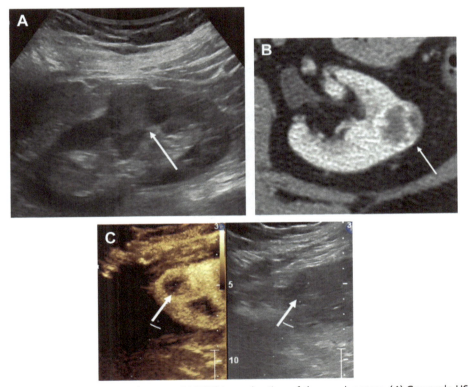

Fig. 21. Role of contrast-enhanced ultrasound (CEUS) in evaluation of the renal masses. (*A*) Grayscale US image in sagittal plane through the left kidney shows a solid slightly hyperechoic mass (*arrow*) in the mid portion of the kidney. (*B*) Coronal CECT image of the left kidney demonstrates heterogenous enhancement of a well-defined renal cortical partially exophytic mass (*arrow*). (*C*) CEUS image of the mass shows enhancing solid components (*arrow*), aiding with the biopsy of the enhancing solid component. Pathologic specimen showed clear cell subtype of renal cell carcinoma (RCC) (not shown).

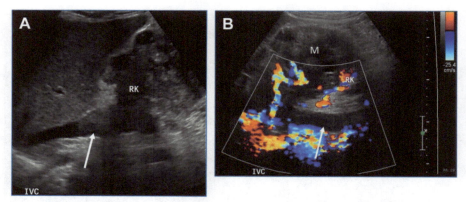

Fig. 22. RCC with inferior vena cava (IVC) invasion. Grayscale (A) and color Doppler (B) US images of the right kidney (RK) and IVC in sagittal plane show a large infiltrating solid vascular mass (M in B) with irregular borders infiltrating into the suprarenal (*arrows* in A) and infrarenal (*arrows* in B) IVC, indicative of tumor-in-vein extension of the renal cell carcinoma (RCC) (*arrows* in A, B).

multifocal areas of increased or decreased echogenicity resulting in striated appearance, similar to the findings on CT (**Fig. 24**A–C). Although nonspecific, in the correct clinical settings, urothelial thickening of the intrarenal collecting system should raise concern for infection. Color Doppler may also demonstrate diminished perfusion of the renal cortex due to vasoconstriction as a response to inflammation and parenchymal vascular congestion. Focal inflammation may present as a mass-like lesion (pseudotumor). US is helpful not only for evaluation of renal

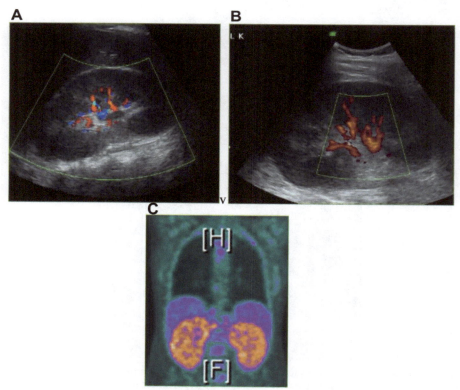

Fig. 23. Renal lymphoma. (A, B) Color Doppler of the right (A) and power Doppler of the left (B) kidney show bilateral renomegaly but with preservation of the differentiation between renal sinus and cortex. The right kidney measured 15.4 cm and the left kidney measured 16 cm (not shown). (C) PET CT in coronal plane demonstrates marked fludeoxyglucose (FDG) avidity of both kidneys compatible with diffuse lymphoma infiltration.

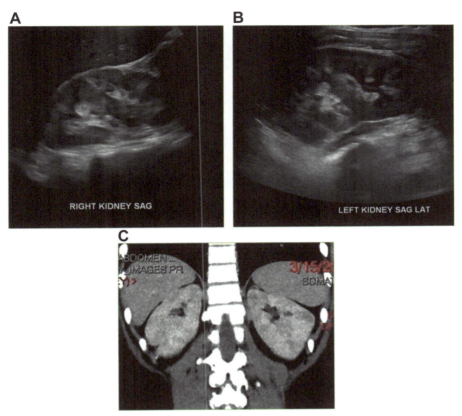

Fig. 24. Pyelonephritis. (*A, B*) Grayscale US images of the bilateral kidneys in sagittal plane show striated appearance of the renal cortex with alternating areas of hyper and hypoechogenicity. (*C*) Coronal CECT confirms striated appearance of the kidney parenchyma indicative of bilateral pyelonephritis.

parenchyma but also for identifying obstruction, cause of infection, or complication such as renal or perirenal abscess formation. An abscess may be seen either as a new simple cystic lesion or complex echogenic cyst, which was not seen on prior imaging (**Fig. 25**). Echogenic debris within the cyst is a representative of pus on US. Flow usually is observed peripherally and diminished in the renal parenchyma associated with the abscess due to inflammation and congestion (see **Fig. 25**A–D).[13] Infectious processes are often bilateral; therefore, assessment of both kidneys should be performed when pyelonephritis is suspected. Gas-producing bacteria may result in *emphysematous pyelonephritis* with echogenic foci representative of a gas seen in the renal parenchyma (**Fig. 26**A, B). This process predominately affects women suffering from diabetes and is considered a true emergency necessitating surgical consultation for nephrectomy as a treatment management. When gas is only confined to the collecting system and does not extend to the renal parenchyma, the process is called *emphysematous pyelitis*, and can be treated with medical management.[13] CT may be a helpful alternative cross-sectional modality for more definitive diagnosis and differentiation of involvement of the kidneys.

Other more chronic infectious processes such as xanthogranulomatous pyelonephritis (XGP) and tuberculosis may result in more complex appearance of the kidneys with a large conglomerate of stones (staghorn calculus) casting the renal calyces (in the case of XGP), or as an atrophic calcified kidney, also known as "putty kidney" (in the setting of genitourinary TB) (**Fig. 27**A–C). It is important to recognize that indwelling stones and stents may be a cause of persistent infection and should be managed with lithotripsy and stent removal and/or replacement.

Renal Calculi

Urolithiasis is a common entity affecting up to 12% of the United States of America (USA) population.[40,41] Overall, the prevalence is increasing and is higher in developed countries with males affected 3

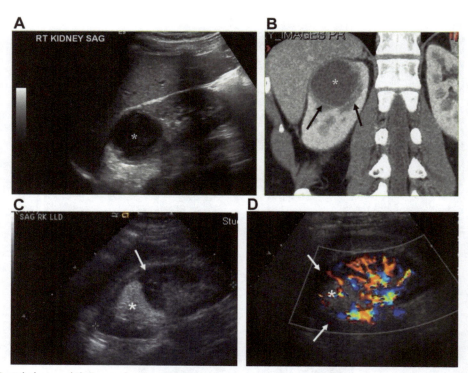

Fig. 25. Renal abscess. (*A*) Grayscale ultrasound (US) image of the right kidney in sagittal plane shows a complex renal cyst filled with echogenic internal debris manifested by low amplitude echoes (*asterisk*). Flow was seen in the periphery of the cyst. The cyst was not present on prior images (not shown). (*B*) Coronal contrast-enhanced computed tomography (CECT) image demonstrates the complex cyst (*asterisk*) with wall enhancement and surrounding hypodensity (*arrows*) consistent with vascular congestion; the findings are indicative of an abscess. (*C, D*) Grayscale and color Doppler (*D*) US images through the right kidney in sagittal plane in a different patient demonstrate new cystic change in the mid renal sinus (*arrow* in C) with associated edema of the renal sinus (*asterisks* in C, D) and diminished flow to the inflamed area on color Doppler (*arrows* in D) indicative of inflammation and congestion.

times more than females.[42] Urolithiasis presents a significant cost to USA, approaching 2.1 billion in USA in 2000. It is projected to be substantially higher in the future years.[43]

Major risk factors for the development of urolithiasis include low fluid intake, diets high in animal protein content; ureteropelvic junction obstruction, ADPKD; calyceal diverticula, and other

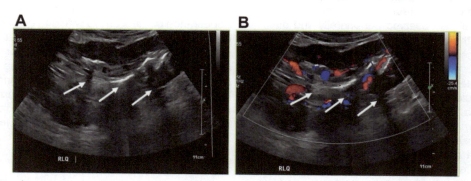

Fig. 26. Emphysematous pyelitis and pyelonephritis. (*A, B*) Grayscale (*A*) and color Doppler (*B*) ultrasound (US) images of the right lower quadrant renal transplant in sagittal plane show multiple linear echogenicities (*arrows*) with dirty posterior shadowing located predominately in the renal calyces indicative of emphysematous pyelitis. A few droplets of gas were also seen in the renal cortex (not shown) compatible with emphysematous pyelonephritis-a true emergency. Transplant team was consulted, and the patient underwent emergent transplant extraction.

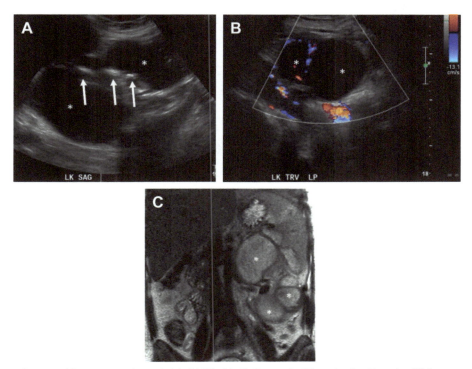

Fig. 27. Xanthogranulomatous pyelonephritis (XGP). (*A, B*) Grayscale (*A*) and color Doppler (*B*) images of the left kidney in sagittal plane show a large obstructive calculi in the renal sinus (*arrows* in A) and associated dilated renal calyces (*asterisks* in B) with vascular flow between the calyces. (*C*) Coronal T2 weighted image (T2WI) MR image of the left kidney demonstrates distorted architecture of the left kidney with dilated calyces and complex cysts indicative of XGP.

conditions resulting in urine stasis. Most stones are in the form of calcium oxalate or calcium phosphate, comprising over 80% of all stones.[44] Uric acid stone accounts for 5% to 10% of all calculi and are predisposed by the conditions such as Crohn's disease, chemotherapy, and gout.[44] Uric acid stones are radiolucent; therefore, they are best detected on US or CT. Staghorn calculi are usually formed by struvite or apatite stones and are associated with bacteria such as *Proteus, Pseudomonas, Staph aureus,* and *Klebsiella* bacteria. Staghorn stones are also defined as "partial" or "complete." A "partial" staghorn stone would include at least 2 calyces, while "complete" would indicate that at least 80% of the renal collecting system was involved.[45]

On US, stones usually are echogenic structures with posterior acoustic shadowing (**Fig. 28**A–D). Small size stones may not mount posterior shadowing and can represent a diagnostic challenge because their echogenicity is similar to the renal sinus. High frequency transducers and optimization of focal zone at the level of the presumable stone are the techniques that are used to improve visualization of the shadowing. Twinkling artifact is another hallmark of stones on color Doppler.

Arterial calcifications/atherosclerotic plaques, renal sinus echogenicity, and gas are well-recognized mimicker for the stones on US.

Although US has a high sensitivity to the stones, it is lower than CT. Location, for example, mid ureter stones and size of the stones less than 5 mm are conditions that may negatively impact sensitivity of stone detection by US. Patients should be always scanned while they have a full bladder to increase visibility of distal ureters and assess for a lodged stone at the ureterovesical junction. US can also assess for indirect findings of urolithiasis. Hydronephrosis, perinephric collections, increased resistive indices, presence of twinkling artifact, and absent ureteral jets are all helpful secondary signs of urolithiasis. Extracorporeal shock wave lithotripsy may be performed for stones larger than 4 mm.[46]

Medullary Nephrocalcinosis

Medullary nephrocalcinosis is the diffuse calcification of the renal medulla due to deposition of calcium salts within the parenchyma, specifically the calcium is deposited in the renal pyramids rather than collecting systems.[47] The echogenic

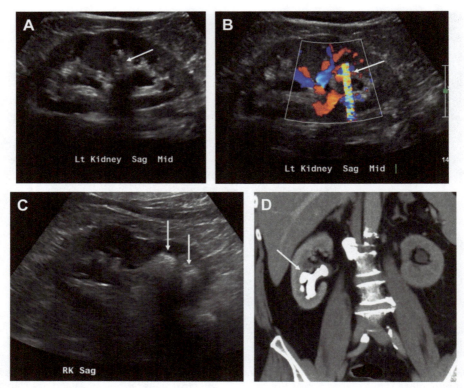

Fig. 28. Nonobstructive small and large staghorn renal calculi. (*A, B*) Grayscale (*A*) and color Doppler (*B*) images of the left kidney in sagittal plane show a small echogenic focus with posterior shadowing (*arrow* in A) and corresponding twinkling artifact (*arrow* in B) indicative of a nonobstructive renal stone. (*C*) Grayscale image in sagittal plane shows a large conglomerate of stones representing staghorn calculus with posterior shadowing, with the stones casting the lower calyces and extending in the renal sinus (*arrows* in C). (*D*) Correlative coronal NECT confirms presence of the right renal staghorn calculus without urinary obstruction (*arrow* in D).

renal pyramids are visible on US (**Fig. 29**). Three main conditions are responsible for this disease: hyperparathyroidism, renal tubular acidosis, and tubular ectasia. Progression of calcification in the pyramids is centripetal from the periphery to the center.[47]

Renal Parenchymal Disease

There are many causes of renal parenchymal disease. Renal insufficiency may develop acutely as a result of a systemic metabolic imbalance, obstructive uropathy, inflammatory/infectious cause, or chemical insult in the setting of oncologic treatment. Acute kidney failure often develops as a result of obstructive process, and one of the imaging findings would be a demonstration of hydronephrosis. If left untreated, acute renal failure may progress to chronic renal disease.

Chronic kidney disease (CKD) affects approximately 15% of adults in the United States or nearly 37 million people.[48] The Kidney Disease Improving Global Outcomes practice guidelines define CKD as abnormalities in kidney structure or function that are present for greater than 3 mo with health implications, which can be classified on the basis of cause, albuminuria category, or estimated glomerular filtration rate.[49] A characteristic sonographic appearance of the CKD is echogenic renal cortices, with or without perinephric small amount of fluid commonly seen (not related to an abscess, or infection or trauma) (see **Fig. 3**). It is important to note that medical renal disease is a commonly utilized term where the kidneys are echogenic. It is nonspecific term and may be seen with various conditions. There has been growing popularity of the use of US shear wave elastography in the assessment of the degree of CKD by the estimation of tissue stiffness and determination of risk stratification for the development of intra-renal fibrosis.[50–53] It has been shown that because intra-renal fibrosis is a final common pathway in a patient with CKD, it can be correlated with disease severity. Although this technique has a great amount of potential, it is still largely under the investigation.

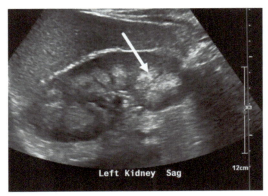

Fig. 29. Medullary nephrocalcinosis. Grayscale ultrasound (US) image of the left kidney shows hyperechoic renal pyramids (*arrow*) indicative of nephrocalcinosis.

Acquired cystic disease is one of the manifestations of chronic renal disease and is characterized by increased number and size of the cysts with time in the setting of atrophic, echogenic kidneys. Patients with long-term dialysis are prone for the development of this disease, with ACKD reported in 10% – 20% of patients after 1 to 3 y and more than 90% of patients after 5 to 10 y of dialysis.[54] Imaging findings include normally sized or atrophic kidneys with multiple small cysts of varying complexity, regardless of the initial cause of renal failure or the method of dialysis (see **Fig. 3**).[55] The incidence of RCC is 3-fold to 24-fold higher in patients with kidney failure than it is in the general population,[56] and patients with ACKD have more than a 100-fold increased risk[57] of RCC. Therefore, each lesion warrants careful evaluation to distinguish among simple cysts, cystic renal masses, and solid masses. Noncontrast CT is frequently performed in patients with renal disease and any indeterminate cystic lesion measuring between 20 and 70 HU.[58,59] CEUS is an excellent alternative to gadolinium-based contrast media or iodinated contrast media in this patient population.[33] One of the most serious complications of this disease is a retroperitoneal hemorrhage arising from the hemorrhagic cysts.

Renal Trauma

Although US is not the first-line imaging modality for evaluation of renal trauma, it can be used for the assessment of progression or resolution of the hematomas on serial follow-up US studies. Perinephric, intraparenchymal, and subcapsular hematomas can all be recognized. Similar to other locations of hematomas, depending on their stage/acuity, hematomas may range in echogenicity as anechoic, hypoechoic, hyperechoic, or heterogeneous. Subcapsular hematomas have a characteristic crescent shape located along the surface of the kidney(s). If the size of subcapsular hematoma is large, they may exert a mass effect on the renal parenchyma and result in vascular congestion, manifested as either high resistance arterial waveforms or reversal of diastolic flow in the main renal artery (**Fig. 30**A–C). Clinically, a patient may develop hypertension resistant to medical treatment, and increased serum creatinine level. Management in this setting is surgical with evacuation of the hematoma. CEUS is very helpful in identification of renal trauma such as acute extravasation in the case of shattered kidney or kidney laceration with hematoma formation, subcapsular hematoma, PSA, or arterio-venous fistula (AVF) formation.[60,61]

VASCULAR DISEASE

Doppler US is the most optimal imaging modality for evaluation of vascular abnormalities such as RAS, renal vein thrombosis (RVT), renal artery thrombosis (RAT), PSA, and AVF formation (**Figs. 31**A–D, **32**A–C and **33**).

RAS is one of the most common vascular pathologies. In 90% of cases, RAS is attributable to atherosclerotic disease, which usually causes stenosis of the origin of the main renal artery (see **Fig. 32**); this is in contrast to fibromuscular dysplasia, which is known for the involvement of the mid or distal segments of the main renal artery (see **Fig. 31**).[62] Most widely accepted criteria of RAS include threshold of peak systolic velocity (PSV) of 180 to 200 cm/sec; renal artery-to-aortic PSV ratio greater than or equal to 3.5, spectral broadening, and presence of tardus-parvus waveforms in the segmental vessels (see **Fig. 32**).[63] Secondary signs of RAS include tissue vibration at the site of stenosis, bruit artifact on spectral Doppler, and color aliasing.[63]

AVMs are characterized by high-amplitude low-resistance waveforms at the site of anastomosis. If the efferent venous branch is identified, arterialized waveform may be observed within this vein (see **Fig. 33**).

A PSA usually is located either within the renal parenchyma or anywhere along the course of the main renal artery. It may show peripheral thick rim of calcification with posterior shadowing limiting evaluation for the intraluminal flow. Careful waveform analysis should be performed for the definitive diagnosis. "Yin-yang" flow pattern is recognized in a large patent PSA sac. If PSA neck is identified, it demonstrates "to-and -fro" flow pattern on spectral Doppler. Congenital

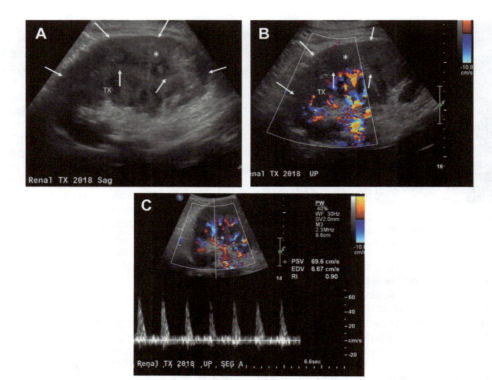

Fig. 30. Subcapsular hematoma. (*A–C*) Grayscale, color (*B*) and spectral Doppler (*C*) US images of renal transplant show a heterogeneous avascular hyperechoic collection (*asterisks* in *A, B*) surrounding the transplant kidney with smooth borders (*arrows*) and mass effect on the renal transplant parenchyma. Note that preservation of renal cortical perfusion aids in distinguishing the subcapsular hematoma from the renal cortex. High-resistance waveforms (resistive index [RI] 0.9) are seen in the segmental arteries indicative of renal congestion and development of Page kidney.

variants such as circumferential left renal vein or retro-aortic left renal vein can also be readily identified on US. Detection of a vessel posterior to the abdominal aorta should raise suspicion for this anatomic variant (**Fig. 34**A–C).

RENAL TRANSPLANT

Conventional and advanced renal US applications are invaluable in the evaluation of renal transplantation complications, especially in evaluation of potentially life-threatening vascular complications such as RAT, RAS, RVT, PSA, and AVF. Conventional US is the first-line imaging modality in the evaluation of renal transplant obstruction, infection, complications of transplant biopsy, pseudotumor, and assessment of malignancy (see **Figs. 26** and **30**). The sonographic characteristics are similar to those seen in native kidneys. Unfortunately, conventional US use in evaluation of transplant rejection is limited, with nonspecific secondary signs such as elevated resistive indices and renal cortical echogenicity being often observed with rejection.

Advanced techniques such as CEUS and shear wave elastography can be very helpful in the assessment of transplant rejection or development of renal fibrosis and scarring.[52,64–66] CEUS is a safe minimally invasive modality for initial imaging in patients with acute *rejection of a renal allograft* and vascular complications. In addition to superb assessment of tissue perfusion, CEUS offers quantitative estimation of renal blood flow, when used in conjunction with serum creatinine levels, can improve the diagnostic capability of US in the assessment of transplant organ rejection.[67,68] Quantitative analysis using time-intensity curve-derived analysis and abnormal quantitative indices have shown good potential in detection of rejection. Acute rejection shows an increase in time-to-peak, while non-rejection-related acute tubular necrosis (ATN) in grafts will show an increased mean transit time and regional blood volume.[69]

US-based elastography is another tool that may aid in the noninvasive assessment of renal transplant rejection. The parenchymal stiffness measured by the transient elastography technique

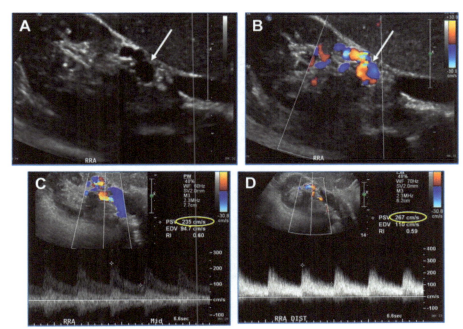

Fig. 31. Fibromuscular dysplasia (FMD) in a 25-year-old female presenting with high blood pressure resistant to the medical treatment. (*A–D*) Grayscale (*A*), color (*B*), and spectral Doppler (*C, D*) ultrasound (US) images of the right kidney demonstrate several areas of arterial lumen dilation and narrowing (*arrow* in A) with evidence of aliasing at the narrower areas (*arrow* in B) corresponding to elevated peak systolic velocities up to 235 and 267 cm/s (yellow ovals) seen on spectral Doppler in C, D. Note that areas of narrowing are located distal to the main renal artery origin/proximal segments. Given the patient's age and location of the renal artery stenotic areas, as well as aneurysmal dilatations, the findings are indicative of FMD.

correlates with underlying histologic interstitial fibrosis. Unfortunately, kidney stiffness is not solely related to the degree of fibrosis but is also related to functional and mechanical parameters. Although this new tool has promise, further validation is needed in clinical practice.[66]

CEUS is a valuable tool for the evaluation of vascular transplant complications with a sensitivity of 100%, a specificity of 66.7%, a positive predictive value of 71.4%, and a negative predictive value of 100%, which is comparative to other cross-sectional imaging modalities.[70]

Both Doppler and CEUS can be used to accurately diagnose *transplant* RAS.

It is the most common vascular complication of renal transplantation with incidence rate ranging from 3% to 23%.[71,72] Similar to the native kidneys, transplant RAS clinically presents with hypertension refractory to treatment occurring in 93% of cases, often as a single event (53%) or combined with a decline in renal function (44%).[73] Direct signs of transplant RAS are seen at the site of narrowing and include elevated PSV, abnormal ratio of PSV in the main renal artery with respect to the external iliac artery, and presence of aliasing due to turbulence.[74] The most accepted criteria for transplant RAS is detection of main renal artery PSV greater than or equal to 250 cm/sec and greater than or equal to 1.8 ratio of the main renal artery PSV to the PSV of the ipsilateral external iliac artery, and presence tardus-parvus waveform distal to the stenosis.[74] When transplant RAS is hemodynamically significant, endovascular techniques including percutaneous transluminal angioplasty and stent placement are first-line treatments, followed by surgery in refractory cases or in the setting of complex arterial anatomy.[71]

Transplant RAT is a rare but devastating complication with an incidence of less than 1%, which may result in graft loss and thus require accurate and quick diagnosis.[75,76] Risk factors include hyperacute rejection, anastomotic occlusion, kinking of the renal artery, or presence of an intimal flap. Clinically, patients with RAT present with tenderness over the graft, hypertension, and acute anuria. Depending on the degree of vascular involvement, a part of entire allograft infarction may occur. On Doppler US, a segmental infarct appears as a hypoechoic mass-like or wedge-shaped avascular region. Absent arterial and

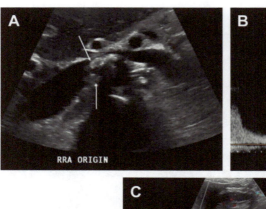
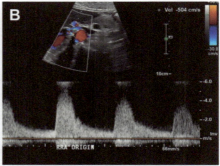
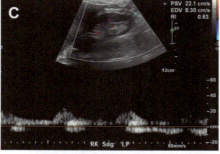

Fig. 32. Renal artery stenosis (RAS) in 86-year-old woman with uncontrolled hypertension. (A) Grayscale US image at the level of the main right renal artery origin shows a large circumferential calcified plaque (arrow in A). (B) Spectral Doppler shows correlative increase peak systolic velocity (PSV) at the level of the plaque, measuring 504 cm/s. (C) Spectral Doppler of segmental artery demonstrates a tardus-parvus waveform with characteristic delayed systolic upstroke.

venous flow are seen at and distal to the site of occlusion. In patients with limited acoustic window or in challenging cases, further evaluation with MRA or digital subtracted angiography can be performed for more definitive diagnosis of RAT evidenced by diminished or absent flow to the allograft and an abrupt cutoff in the transplant renal artery.[77] It should be noted that absence of blood flow on Doppler in the renal artery may also be a sign of acute rejection. Therefore, CEUS increases confidence in the diagnosis of this severe complication.[78]

Transplant RVT usually seen within the first 2 weeks after surgery and is a major cause of graft loss requiring prompt treatment. It is reported to occur in less than 5% of adult renal transplant recipients but is associated with early graft failure, especially in pediatric patients.[77] When the renal vein is occluded, the kidney enlarges due to congestion, the renal cortex appears hypoechoic and slightly heterogeneous, and there is absence of flow in the main renal vein on color and spectral Doppler. Arterial flow may demonstrate a characteristic reversal of flow in diastole. Isolated reversal of diastolic flow without venous thrombus is somewhat nonspecific findings, which may be seen in the setting of allograft torsion, severe allograft rejection, external compression of the renal hilum by perinephric fluid collection (Page kidney), or ATN.[79] In some situations, visualization of the renal vein may be challenging due to edema, deep positioning of the transplant, and poor Doppler

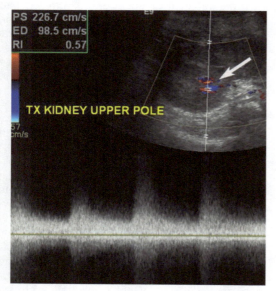

Fig. 33. Transplant arteriovenous fistula (AVF). Color bruit flash artifact (arrow) is identified at the site of an AVF in the transplant. Note high-velocity flow (227 cm/s) at the site of the fistula. (TX = transplant).

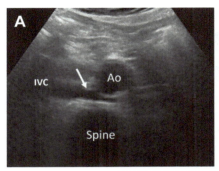
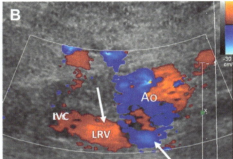
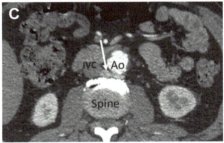

Fig. 34. Retro-aortic left renal vein. (A, B) Grayscale (A) and color Doppler (B) images of the retroperitoneum in transverse plane demonstrate the left renal vein (arrow in A, LRV in B) coursing between abdominal aorta (Ao) and spine (Spine). The venous confluence with the inferior vena cava (IVC in A, B) is also evident. (C) Axial contrast-enhanced ultrasound (CECT) confirms the findings of the retro-aortic renal vein (arrow).

parameter optimization. This can be compensated with the use of CEUS, where absence of venous flow and the presence of pulsatile and high resistance flow in renal parenchyma during the early corticomedullary phase attributable to organ congestion have been reported.[80] Treatment of RVT includes open surgical thrombectomy or endovascular thrombolysis.

SUMMARY

US is essential in the assessment and diagnosis of renal and ureteral pathologies and their management. In many scenarios, it is the first imaging modality and often used as a follow-up examination to evaluate treatment response or stability of previously diagnosed conditions in the native and transplant kidneys. Its advanced techniques, such as microflow imaging, CEUS, and elastography are gaining popularity in the assessment of the vascular patency and complications, renal masses, and chronic renal conditions, respectively. Urinary obstruction, nephrolithiasis, and urinary retention are among most frequent indications for the performance of US. Knowledge of characteristic sonographic appearances and key distinguishing features of various renal and ureteral conditions are paramount in accurate diagnosis and patient management.

CLINICS CARE POINTS

- US is an excelllent tool for grading degree of hydronephrosis.
- US is used for evaluation of immediate post renal transplant complications and serial follow-up imaging.
- Nephrolithiasis is confidently can be detected with ultrasound.
- US is a first line imaging modality for assessment of the renal cysts.
- Contrast-enhanced US is gaining popularity in evaluation of benign and malignant renal masses.

REFERENCES

1. Drudi FM, Cantisani V, Granata A, et al. Multiparametric ultrasound in the evaluation of kidney disease in elderly. J Ultrasound 2020;23(2):115–26.
2. Siracusano S, Bertolotto M, Ciciliato S, et al. The current role of contrast-enhanced ultrasound (CEUS) imaging in the evaluation of renal pathology. World J Urol 2011;29(5):633–8.
3. Peride I, Radulescu D, Niculae A, et al. Value of ultrasound elastography in the diagnosis of native kidney fibrosis. Med Ultrason 2016;18(3):362–9.

4. Roseman DA, Hwang SJ, Oyama-Manabe N, et al. Clinical associations of total kidney volume: the Framingham Heart Study. Nephrol Dial Transplant 2017; 32(8):1344–50.
5. Gulati M, Cheng J, Loo JT, et al. Pictorial review: renal ultrasound. Clin Imaging 2018;51:133–54.
6. Algin O, Ozmen E, Gumus M. Hypertrophic columns of bertin: imaging findings. Eurasian J Med 2014; 46(1):61–3.
7. Yeh HC, Halton KP, Shapiro RS, et al. Junctional parenchyma: revised definition of hypertrophic column of Bertin. Radiology 1992;185(3):725–32.
8. Dias T, Sairam S, Kumarasiri S. Ultrasound diagnosis of fetal renal abnormalities. Best Pract Res Clin Obstet Gynaecol 2014;28(3):403–15.
9. Hansen KL, Nielsen MB, Ewertsen C. Ultrasonography of the kidney: a pictorial review. Diagnostics (Basel) 2015;6(1):2.
10. Zelenko N, Coll D, Rosenfeld AT, et al. Normal ureter size on unenhanced helical CT. AJR Am J Roentgenol 2004;182(4):1039–41.
11. Dalla-Palma L, Bazzocchi M, Pozzi-Mucelli RS, et al. Ultrasonography in the diagnosis of hydronephrosis in patients with normal renal function. Urol Radiol 1983;5(4):221–6.
12. Ather MH, Jafri AH, Sulaiman MN. Diagnostic accuracy of ultrasonography compared to unenhanced CT for stone and obstruction in patients with renal failure. BMC Med Imaging 2004;4(1):2.
13. William D, Middleton ABK, Hertzberg BS, et al, editors. Ultrasound: the requisites. 2nd edition. MO, USA: Mosby; 2004. p. 175–9.
14. Rokni E, Zinck S, Simon JC. Evaluation of stone features that cause the color Doppler ultrasound twinkling artifact. Ultrasound Med Biol 2021;47(5): 1310–8.
15. Ripolles T, Martinez-Perez MJ, Vizuete J, et al. Sonographic diagnosis of symptomatic ureteral calculi: usefulness of the twinkling artifact. Abdom Imaging 2013;38(4):863–9.
16. de Bessa J Jr, Denes FT, Chammas MC, et al. Diagnostic accuracy of color Doppler sonographic study of the ureteric jets in evaluation of hydronephrosis. J Pediatr Urol 2008;4(2):113–7.
17. Chi AC, Flury SC. Urology patients in the nephrology practice. Adv Chronic Kidney Dis 2013;20(5):441–8.
18. Alshoabi SA. Association between grades of Hydronephrosis and detection of urinary stones by ultrasound imaging. Pak J Med Sci 2018;34(4):955–8.
19. Bosniak MA. The current radiological approach to renal cysts. Radiology 1986;158(1):1–10.
20. Cramer MT, Guay-Woodford LM. Cystic kidney disease: a primer. Adv Chronic Kidney Dis 2015; 22(4):297–305.
21. Sekine A, Hidaka S, Moriyama T, et al. Cystic kidney diseases that require a differential diagnosis from autosomal dominant polycystic kidney disease (ADPKD). J Clin Med 2022;11(21):6528.
22. Bausch B, Jilg C, Glasker S, et al. Renal cancer in von Hippel-Lindau disease and related syndromes. Nat Rev Nephrol 2013;9(9):529–38.
23. Cinque A, Minnei R, Floris M, et al. The clinical and molecular features in the VHL renal cancers; close or distant relatives with sporadic clear cell renal cell carcinoma? Cancers (Basel) 2022;14(21):5352.
24. Choyke PL, Glenn GM, Walther MM, et al. Hereditary renal cancers. Radiology 2003;226(1):33–46.
25. Nair N, Chakraborty R, Mahajan Z, et al. Renal manifestations of tuberous sclerosis complex. J Kidney Cancer VHL 2020;7(3):5–19.
26. Urciuoli P, D'Orazi V, Livadoti G, et al. Treatment of renal angiomyolipoma: surgery versus angioembolization. G Chir 2013;34(11–12):326–31.
27. Jinzaki M, Silverman SG, Akita H, et al. Diagnosis of renal angiomyolipomas: classic, fat-poor, and epithelioid types. Semin Ultrasound CT MR 2017;38(1): 37–46.
28. Perez-Ordonez B, Hamed G, Campbell S, et al. Renal oncocytoma: a clinicopathologic study of 70 cases. Am J Surg Pathol 1997;21(8):871–83.
29. Zhao S, Shi J, Yang R, et al. Ultrasonography findings for the diagnosis of renal oncocytoma. J Med Ultrason (2001) 2022;49(2):211–6.
30. Granja MF, O'Brien AT, Trujillo S, et al. Multilocular cystic nephroma: a systematic literature review of the radiologic and clinical findings. AJR Am J Roentgenol 2015;205(6):1188–93.
31. Rumack CM, Willson SR, Charboneau JW. Diagnostic ultrasound. 3rd edition. Amsterdam, Netherlands: Elsevier Health Sciences; 2005.
32. Graumann O, Osther SS, Karstoft J, et al. Bosniak classification system: a prospective comparison of CT, contrast-enhanced US, and MR for categorizing complex renal cystic masses. Acta Radiol 2016; 57(11):1409–17.
33. Herms E, Weirich G, Maurer T, et al. Ultrasound-based "CEUS-Bosniak"classification for cystic renal lesions: an 8-year clinical experience. World J Urol 2023;41(3):679–85.
34. Williams CM, Myint ZW. The role of anticoagulation in tumor thrombus associated with renal cell carcinoma: a literature review. Cancers (Basel) 2023; 15(22):5382.
35. Blitman NM, Berkenblit RG, Rozenblit AM, et al. Renal medullary carcinoma: CT and MRI features. AJR Am J Roentgenol 2005;185(1):268–72.
36. Vikram R, Sandler CM, Ng CS. Imaging and staging of transitional cell carcinoma: part 2, upper urinary tract. AJR Am J Roentgenol 2009;192(6): 1488–93.
37. Zhou C, Urbauer DL, Fellman BM, et al. Metastases to the kidney: a comprehensive analysis of 151

patients from a tertiary referral centre. BJU Int 2016; 117(5):775–82.
38. RW S. Diseases of the kidney and urinary tract. Philadelphia, Pa: Lippincott, Williams & Wilkins; 2001. p. 847–69.
39. Stunell H, Buckley O, Feeney J, et al. Imaging of acute pyelonephritis in the adult. Eur Radiol 2007; 17(7):1820–8.
40. Johnson CM, Wilson DM, O'Fallon WM, et al. Renal stone epidemiology: a 25-year study in Rochester, Minnesota. Kidney Int 1979;16(5):624–31.
41. Cheng PM, Moin P, Dunn MD, et al. What the radiologist needs to know about urolithiasis: part 1–pathogenesis, types, assessment, and variant anatomy. AJR Am J Roentgenol 2012;198(6):W540–7.
42. Stamatelou KK, Francis ME, Jones CA, et al. Time trends in reported prevalence of kidney stones in the United States: 1976-1994. Kidney Int 2003; 63(5):1817–23.
43. Pearle MS, Calhoun EA, Curhan GC, et al. Urologic diseases in America project: urolithiasis. J Urol 2005;173(3):848–57.
44. Evan AP. Physiopathology and etiology of stone formation in the kidney and the urinary tract. Pediatr Nephrol 2010;25(5):831–41.
45. Flannigan R, Choy WH, Chew B, et al. Renal struvite stones–pathogenesis, microbiology, and management strategies. Nat Rev Urol 2014;11(6):333–41.
46. Alic J, Heljic J, Hadziosmanovic O, et al. The efficiency of extracorporeal shock wave lithotripsy (ESWL) in the treatment of distal ureteral stones: an unjustly forgotten option? Cureus 2022;14(9):e28671.
47. Karunarathne S, Udayakumara Y, Govindapala D, et al. Medullary nephrocalcinosis, distal renal tubular acidosis and polycythaemia in a patient with nephrotic syndrome. BMC Nephrol 2012;13:66.
48. System USRD. Annual data report: epidemiology of kidney disease in the United States. 10/31/23. Bethesda, MD: National Institutes of Health, National Institute of Diabetes and Digestive and Kidney Diseases; 2023.
49. Stevens PE, Levin A, Kidney Disease: Improving Global Outcomes Chronic Kidney Disease Guideline Development Work Group Members. Evaluation and management of chronic kidney disease: synopsis of the kidney disease: improving global outcomes 2012 clinical practice guideline. Ann Intern Med 2013;158(11):825–30.
50. Kuttancheri T, Krishnan K, Das SK, et al. Shear wave elastography: usefulness in chronic kidney disease. Pol J Radiol 2023;88:e286–93.
51. Cosgrove D, Piscaglia F, Bamber J, et al. EFSUMB guidelines and recommendations on the clinical use of ultrasound elastography. Part 2: clinical applications. Ultraschall Med 2013;34(3):238–53.
52. Saftoiu A, Gilja OH, Sidhu PS, et al. The EFSUMB guidelines and recommendations for the clinical practice of elastography in non-hepatic applications: update 2018. Ultraschall Med 2019;40(4): 425–53.
53. Cotoi L, Borcan F, Sporea I, et al. Shear wave elastography in diagnosing secondary hyperparathyroidism. Diagnostics (Basel) 2019;9(4):213.
54. Degrassi F, Quaia E, Martingano P, et al. Imaging of haemodialysis: renal and extrarenal findings. Insights Imaging 2015;6(3):309–21.
55. Clingan MJ, Zhang Z, Caserta MP, et al. Imaging patients with kidney failure. Radiographics 2023;43(5): e220116.
56. Tsuzuki T, Iwata H, Murase Y, et al. Renal tumors in end-stage renal disease: a comprehensive review. Int J Urol 2018;25(9):780–6.
57. Berkenblit R, Ricci Z, Kanmaniraja D, et al. CT features of acquired cystic kidney disease-associated renal cell carcinoma. Clin Imaging 2022;83:83–6.
58. Schieda N, Davenport MS, Krishna S, et al. Bosniak classification of cystic renal masses, version 2019: a pictorial guide to clinical use. Radiographics 2022; 42(1):E33.
59. Silverman SG, Pedrosa I, Ellis JH, et al. Bosniak classification of cystic renal masses, version 2019: an update proposal and needs assessment. Radiology 2019;292(2):475–88.
60. Cokkinos D, Antypa E, Stefanidis K, et al. Contrast-enhanced ultrasound for imaging blunt abdominal trauma - indications, description of the technique and imaging review. Ultraschall Med 2012;33(1): 60–7.
61. Afaq A, Harvey C, Aldin Z, et al. Contrast-enhanced ultrasound in abdominal trauma. Eur J Emerg Med 2012;19(3):140–5.
62. Revzin MV, Pellerito JS, Nezami N, et al. The radiologist's guide to duplex ultrasound assessment of chronic mesenteric ischemia. Abdom Radiol (NY) 2020;45(10):2960–79.
63. Revzin MV, PJIJSP MD. Introduction to vascular ultrasonography. 7th Edition ed. Elsevier; 2019. p. 615–53.
64. Fernandez T, Sebastia C, Pano B, et al. Contrast-enhanced US in renal transplant complications: overview and imaging features. Radiographics 2024;44(6):e230182.
65. Sidhu PS, Cantisani V, Dietrich CF, et al. The EFSUMB guidelines and recommendations for the clinical practice of contrast-enhanced ultrasound (CEUS) in non-hepatic applications: update 2017 (long version). Ultraschall Med 2018;39(2):e2–44.
66. Expert Panel on Urologic I, Taffel MT, Nikolaidis P, et al. ACR appropriateness criteria((R)) renal transplant dysfunction. J Am Coll Radiol 2017;14(5S): S272–81.
67. Wang X, Yu Z, Guo R, et al. Assessment of postoperative perfusion with contrast-enhanced ultrasonography in kidney transplantation. Int J Clin Exp Med 2015;8(10):18399–405.

68. Miller A 3rd, Scanlan RA, Lee JS, et al. Volatile compounds produced in sterile fish muscle (Sebastes melanops) by Pseudomonas perolens. Appl Microbiol 1973;25(2):257–61.
69. Como G, Da Re J, Adani GL, et al. Role for contrast-enhanced ultrasound in assessing complications after kidney transplant. World J Radiol 2020;12(8):156–71.
70. David E, Del Gaudio G, Drudi FM, et al. Contrast enhanced ultrasound compared with MRI and CT in the evaluation of post-renal transplant complications. Tomography 2022;8(4):1704–15.
71. Bruno S, Remuzzi G, Ruggenenti P. Transplant renal artery stenosis. J Am Soc Nephrol 2004;15(1):134–41.
72. Fervenza FC, Lafayette RA, Alfrey EJ, et al. Renal artery stenosis in kidney transplants. Am J Kidney Dis 1998;31(1):142–8.
73. de Morais RH, Muglia VF, Mamere AE, et al. Duplex Doppler sonography of transplant renal artery stenosis. J Clin Ultrasound 2003;31(3):135–41.
74. Al-Katib S, Shetty M, Jafri SM, et al. Radiologic assessment of native renal vasculature: a multimodality review. Radiographics 2017;37(1):136–56.
75. Ayvazoglu Soy EH, Akdur A, Kirnap M, et al. Vascular complications after renal transplant: a single-center experience. Exp Clin Transplant 2017;15(Suppl 1):79–83.
76. Srivastava A, Kumar J, Sharma S, et al. Vascular complication in live related renal transplant: an experience of 1945 cases. Indian J Urol 2013;29(1):42–7.
77. Browne RF, Tuite DJ. Imaging of the renal transplant: comparison of MRI with duplex sonography. Abdom Imaging 2006;31(4):461–82.
78. Akbar SA, Jafri SZ, Amendola MA, et al. Complications of renal transplantation. Radiographics 2005;25(5):1335–56.
79. Lockhart ME, Wells CG, Morgan DE, et al. Reversed diastolic flow in the renal transplant: perioperative implications versus transplants older than 1 month. AJR Am J Roentgenol 2008;190(3):650–5.
80. Alvarez Rodriguez S, Hevia Palacios V, Sanz Mayayo E, et al. The usefulness of contrast-enhanced ultrasound in the assessment of early kidney transplant function and complications. Diagnostics (Basel) 2017;7(3):53.

Bowel Ultrasound

Alexandra Medellin, MD[a,*], Stephanie R. Wilson, MD[a,b,1]

KEYWORDS

- Ultrasound • Bowel • Intestinal • Inflammatory bowel disease • Bowel neoplasm

KEY POINTS

- High-resolution ultrasound (US) allows for excellent detection of bowel pathology and its complications.
- Multiple publications have demonstrated that US is comparable in performance to computed tomography and MR imaging for the assessment of inflammatory bowel disease, supporting the choice of US as a first-line investigation.
- US is sensitive in the detection of mural and mesenteric inflammation allowing for a subjective and objective assessment of disease activity and therapeutic response that can be followed overtime.
- New US techniques such as contrast-enhanced ultrasound and elastography are now providing an objective evaluation of the mural perfusion and intestinal stiffness, important in the evaluation of strictures.

 Video content accompanies this article at http://www.radiologic.theclinics.com.

INTRODUCTION

Sonographic evaluation of the intestine is rapicly growing in popularity due to its safety, noninvasive nature, accessibility, and high acceptance by patients. Bowel or intestinal ultrasound is increasingly recognized as a valuable imaging modality for the evaluation of patients with inflammatory bowel disease (IBD)[1] where frequent examinations are needed to monitor disease and therapeutic response. Today, disease management has changed from treating patient's symptoms to recognition that surveillance imaging regarding symptomatology should be the preferred standard of care. This acknowledges that patients' symptoms are often not a reflection of their disease.[2,3] Specially, in IBD, the young age of onset, the chronic nature of the disease, its significant complications, and fluctuating nature of the disease make this radiation-free technique a particularly desirable and important imaging modality. In addition, ultrasound (US) can evaluate all small bowel segments including those proximal loops not assessed by endoscopy and shows the terminal ileum (TI) in those with failed intubation at endoscopy.

Current state-of-the-art US equipment allows for exceptional detailed evaluation of the bowel wall, mesentery, and surrounding peritoneum. The spatial resolution in grayscale US permits detailed identification of the normal bowel wall layers, without requirement for contrast enhancement to detect subtle transmural and mesenteric changes.

Real-time performance gives an advantage to the US operator to directly communicate with the patient regarding ongoing and acute symptomatology often influencing the examination performance. For instance, correlation of an identifiable sonographic abnormality with a focal area of tenderness directs the remaining of the examination. One of the most desirable advantages of US over other imaging techniques is its dynamic

---

[a] Department of Radiology, Cumming School of Medicine, University of Calgary; [b] Department of Radiology and Medicine, Division of Gastroenterology, Cumming School of Medicine, University of Calgary
[1] Present address: 1403 29 Street, Northwest, Calgary, Alberta, T3H5J4, Canada
* Corresponding author. 1403 29 Street. Northwest, Calgary, Alberta, T3H5J4, Canada.
E-mail address: alexandra.medellin@ucalgary.ca

capability. This allows for the assessment of bowel motility, compliance, detection of fixed or transient changes, and recognition of dysfunctional peristalsis, all important observations as diagnostic clues for disease. For instance, the detection of fluid-filled dysfunctional loops of peristaltic bowel in a patient with bloating will direct the search for the cause of obstruction.

Detection of mural inflammation is vital for the assessment of disease activity in IBD. Color Doppler imaging (CDI) displays mural and mesenteric vascularity. However, CDI only detects large vessels with fast flow and may be compromised by obesity and deep position of abnormal segments causing poor flow detection. Therefore, it is advocated that contrast-enhanced ultrasound (CEUS) is a necessary addition to brightness mode (B-mode) imaging in these scenarios. CEUS allows for mural blood flow detection at the microcirculatory level and provides objective measurements of mural flow that can be followed overtime for disease activity assessment and therapeutic response.[4,5]

In addition, the increasing popularity of shear wave elastography (SWE) for the evaluation of tissue stiffness has sparked interest to use this technique in the assessment of strictures in IBD.[6,7] Strictures are characterized by the presence of inflammation, muscular hypertrophy, and fibrotic components in various degrees.[8] In combination, these US techniques provide all the necessary tools for stricture characterization.

Although sonographic evaluation predominantly focused on changes of the small and large bowel, it may be also expand to evaluate for perianal disease[9] for detection of fistulas and inflammatory masses with great resolution.

The importance of bowel US goes beyond IBD. The US has long been used as the first-line imaging modality for the evaluation of abdominal pain in the acute setting to detect common conditions such as appendicitis, diverticulitis, or enteritis. However, most routine abdominal-pelvic US examinations have focused on the solid organs and in most cases excluded the bowel due to the traditional view that gas does not allow for intestinal visualization. The authors prefer that this practice should be improved with the addition of a quadrant survey to detect any potential abnormal bowel segment that may direct the need for a more detailed bowel assessment.

NORMAL ANATOMY AND IMAGING TECHNIQUES

Conventional grayscale US, with high-resolution imaging, shows normal bowel wall as a multilayered cylindrical structure, which shows a diagnostic gut signature with 5 layers that alternate in echogenicity with the recognition that the hypoechoic (black) layers represent muscular components. From the lumen to the outer layer, they are as follows: (1) mucosa—echogenic, (2) muscularis mucosa—hypoechoic (not always visible or very thin), (3) submucosa—echogenic (most obviously recognized), (4) muscularis propria—hypoechoic (well seen), (5) serosa or adventitia—hyperechoic (normally difficult to visualize; **Fig. 1**A–D).

The exceptional depiction of the wall layers by US gives this modality an advantage over other cross-sectional imaging techniques that require contrast enhancement for bowel layer differentiation. Visualization of the gut signature may vary depending on the transducer resolution and body habitus. Normal bowel is compliant and easy to compress during the sonographic evaluation, with wall measuring less than 3 mm.[10] The normal colonic wall may vary in thickness depending on the degree of colonic distension with normal average thickness of less than 3 mm if well-distended and less than 5 mm if not.

Specific features to aid in identifying a bowel segment include recognition of rugae in the stomach, valvulae conniventes in the small bowel, and haustra in the colon.

Normal mural vascularity of the bowel is evaluated with CDI using subjective observations of the extent and number of vessels present within the bowel wall.[11] A normal bowel loop should only show a few color signals within the wall, whereas excess signal is associated with either neoplastic or inflammatory pathology.

Sonographic Technique

Grayscale and Doppler assessment

It is our preference to perform routine bowel examinations after 6 hours of fasting. This shows the bowel in a normal resting physiologic state, avoiding overestimation of vascularity due to a postprandial or functional hyperemia, and avoids fluid-filled loops of peristaltic bowel that may follow a large meal.

Initially, a survey of the bowel is performed using a standard low-frequency convex probe (3–8 MHz). With the patient in a supine position, the probe is placed on the abdomen, and with constant pression, the probe is moved to cover all segments of the bowel using a systematic approach. This technique allows for adequate detection of normal or abnormal bowel segments, assists anatomic localization of an affected loop, and excludes any abnormal deep segments or complications.

There are 2 approaches for bowel scanning that are largely motivated by personal preference of

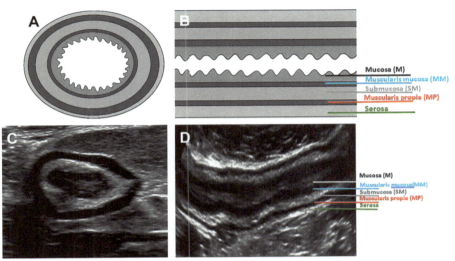

Fig. 1. Normal bowel wall layers. (*A*) Axial and (*B*) long-axis drawing of the bowel showing 5 recognizable layers. (1) Mucosa (M); (2) muscularis mucosa (MM); (3) submucosal (SM); (4) muscularis propria (MP); and (5) serosa (S). Bottom-axial US image of the small bowel (left); and corresponding US long-axis view (right); (*C*) axial and (*D*) long-axis US images showing the normal bowel layers.

the operator. (1) The most frequently used in the acute setting starts at the right upper quadrant (RUQ) (hepatic flexure of the colon). A downward motion of the probe allows assessment of the ascending colon, cecum, TI, and appendix. This is followed by sequential scanning of the entire colon from the RUQ forward to the level of the rectum. Then, a sweeping motion of the abdomen is used for survey of the small bowel. (2) Starts at the rectum (using the bladder as a sonographic window) and then following the entire colon in a retrograde fashion from the suprapubic region to the right lower quadrant to also included the appendix and TI (Video 1). Then a survey of the entire small bowel is performed. This scanning technique is particularly helpful in patients with prior surgeries to assist in the localization of the anastomosis.

After the bowel is surveyed, a higher frequency probe, either curvilinear and/or linear probe (7–18 MHz), is used for a more detailed evaluation of the bowel wall, mesentery, and vascularity. High-frequency probes best delineate the wall layers, detailing transmural disease, serosal abnormalities, sinus tracts, and fistulas. In children and slim individuals, a high-frequency linear probe can be used to perform the entire examination.

If there are localized symptoms in the upper abdomen, a search for the stomach and duodenum is performed. The stomach is generally collapsed in a fasting state and should not show any mural thickening. Some authors suggest oral water ingestion to distend the stomach and upper gastrointestinal (GI) tract to confirm a persistent abnormality. However, ingested air may make this an inconsistent procedure.

All segments of the bowel are imaged using grayscale and Doppler imaging in the axial and longitudinal planes. It is important to optimize Doppler imaging for the detection of low-velocity flow or to use new microcirculation techniques to properly detect mural flow.

Representative images and cine-clips of the affected segment and TI are recorded and stored. Cine-clips are essential for documentation of disease extent, and detection of transition points, subtle mural changes, sinus tracts and fistulas that may have been missed by the operator at the time of the examination. One of the most important contributions of cine-clips is the assessment of bowel motility with identification of normal, excess, or dysfunctional peristalsis. This is essential for the detection of strictures and mechanical bowel obstruction.

Endovaginal scanning

Another important technique in female patients is the addition of endovaginal (EV) scanning, because the cecum, TI, and appendix in some patients are located within the pelvis and can only be seen using an EV approach.

The use of an EV probe allows exceptional visualization of the pelvic loops, and it is sensitive for the detection of abnormal pelvic segments that are not visible by the transabdominal approach (**Fig. 2**A–D and Videos 2 and 3).

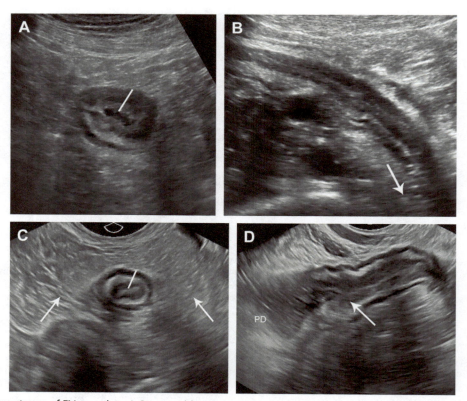

Fig. 2. Importance of EV scanning. A 61 year old woman with crohn's disease (CD) presents for evaluation of disease extent and activity. (A) Axial transabdominal US of the RLQ shows abnormal TI with mural thickening of 8 mm (bar). (B) The abnormal TI segment dives down into the pelvis where it is no longer visible with a transabdominal approach. (C) Axial EV scan shows the nonvisible segment of distal ileum within the pelvis demonstrating wall thickening (bar), and abundant echogenic inflammatory fat (arrows). (D) Long-axis EV image shows a stricture with a transition point (arrow) and a prestenotic fluid-filled dilated segment (PD). Cine-clip shows dysfunctional peristalsis with to-and-fro peristalsis, only visible with the EV scan (Video 2).

Transperineal scanning

Performed in patients with perianal symptoms, a transperineal scan provides excellent visualization of the anal canal and perianal soft tissues to approximately the level of the anorectal junction. A conventional probe with a plastic cover and abundant gel inside and outside the cover is used. The procedure is initiated in a lithotomy position. A high-frequency linear or curvilinear probe is placed on the perineum between the anal canal and vagina in women and between the scrotum and anus in men. Imaging is performed in the axial and sagittal planes, while maintaining the probe position on the perineum and sweeping from left to right for sagittal and top to bottom for axial imaging. Cine-clips in both planes are recorded.

Ostomy scanning

Ostomy evaluation is also an important component of the bowel assessment. A small footprint probe is placed within the ostomy ring over the bag to visualize the ostomy loop. If this is not possible, the probe then needs to be placed next to the ostomy ring and angle toward the opening until the ostomy loop is well visualized in the field-of-view.

Contrast-enhanced ultrasound

CEUS should be performed on the most abnormal bowel segment, commonly in a long-axis view to facilitate CEUS quantification. Microbubble contrast agents are injected intravenously and a 2 minute videoclip is recorded (Video 4). For mural quantification, proprietary software is used to measure the degree of wall enhancement by placing a region of interest (ROI) within the bowel wall. This creates an enhancement curve or time-intensity curve that allows for the determination of peak enhancement (PE) and area under the curve (AUC) as expression of mural vascularity[4,12] and disease activity. CEUS is also used for assessment and characterization of inflammatory masses and neoplasms.

Shear wave elastography

Bowel wall stiffness plays an important role in the evaluation of strictures, specially to assist in the management and assessment of treatment response.[7] SWE of the bowel is challenging due to the small size of the target, sonographic compression, bowel motility, adjacent bowel gas, and patient breathing. Nonetheless, investigators have reported optimism for the value of SWE in the assessment of bowel strictures.[8]

SWE is performed using the axial plane of the stricture segment to include as much bowel wall as possible while avoiding lumen and perienteric tissues. An ROI is placed within the abnormal bowel wall, and at least 4 SWE samples are recorded in m/s. Although specific thresholds have not been published, we propose that values greater than 2 m/s will denote significant mural stiffness.

CLINICAL APPLICATIONS
Acute Abdominal Pain

In the acute setting, US has been commonly used for the evaluation of acute right lower quadrant (RLQ) or left lower quadrant (LLQ) pain. The most common indications include suspected acute appendicitis, diverticulitis, pyloric stenosis, and intussusception, especially in children and young adults. However, other acute intestinal conditions can also be recognized during any sonographic assessment including omental infarcts, mesenteric adenitis with terminal ileitis, acute typhlitis, irritable bowel syndrom (IBD), peptic ulcer disease, and enteritis. Therefore, US evaluation in the acute setting should not be limited to the assessment of the appendix or the area of concern alone. If the etiology is not found with the initial inspection, the sonographic evaluation should be expanded to include the cecum, TI, and a short survey of the small bowel. In patients with diffuse abdominal pain and bloating, a close survey of the bowel is also necessary to detect signs of mechanical bowel obstruction such as dilated segments, dysfunctional peristalsis, or narrowing.

It is known that US has the advantage of having direct input from the patient to localize the area of pain to guide the sonographic assessment. For instance, if pain is localized in the LLQ, the most common explanation is acute diverticulitis (**Fig. 3**A, B). A diverticulum in US is seen as an outpouching beyond the bowel serosa that can be filled with intestinal content or air appearing as a bright echo with distal shadowing (**Fig. 4**A). Bacterial overgrowth within the diverticula causes inflammatory changes/acute diverticulitis. This is characterized by hyperemia of the diverticulum and surrounding mesenteric inflammatory changes in the early stage.

This can progress to involve a segment of the colon with mural thickening and hyperemia. Localized perforations can occur where echogenic foci representing air are seen adjacent to the inflamed diverticula or colon. An important complication that needs to be recognized is the presence of an abscess (**Fig. 4**B, C). This can appear as a complex fluid collection with peripheral vascularity on CDI or CEUS or as a hypoechoic area within the inflammatory fat. Acute diverticulitis can occur in any part of the intestine; therefore, a careful search of the bowel at the area of pain may help to identify this condition.

Acute appendicitis remains today as the most common cause of the so-called acute abdomen. Images are characterized by demonstration of a dilated appendix, more that 7 to 8 mm in diameter, a fluid-filled lumen with or without appendicolith, periappendiceal inflammatory fat, and hyperemia.[13] Detailed evaluation of the entire appendix, with a focus on the detection of the tip and its wall, is important to identify complications, such as perforation and abscess.

Granulomatous appendicitis is a self-limited process that is treated conservatively. US will nicely demonstrate an increased diameter of the appendix, predominantly related to mural thickening and inflammatory change.[14] The lumen is collapsed a differentiating feature from suppurative appendicitis where the lumen is dilated by fluid/pus most commonly due to an obstructing appendicolith.

Epiploic appendagitis and mesenteric infarcts can also be the cause of localized pain. On US, both are fat-containing echogenic masses and are differentiated only by the location of the mass. Epiploic appendagitis is intimately adjacent to the antimesenteric border of the colon, while mesenteric infarcts are typically located further from the colon.[15]

In children and young adult, intussusception is a common cause of patient's abdominal pain. This is easily recognized on US by the "target sign" in axial view that represents the invagination of one bowel segment within another. In long axis, it has a "pitch-fork" appearance. In children, intussusception is mostly idiopathic; however, in adults, a close search for a lead point is necessary.

Although much less common today, peptic ulcer disease may be a cause of upper abdominal pain. Ulcers can be recognized as bright echoes with ring-down artifact either within or beyond the wall at the area of pain. Peri-enteric fluid and inflammatory fat can also be seen (**Fig. 5**A, B, Video 5).

Inflammatory Bowel Disease

Currently, bowel US plays an invaluable role in the assessment of IBD and its complications.[16,17] It

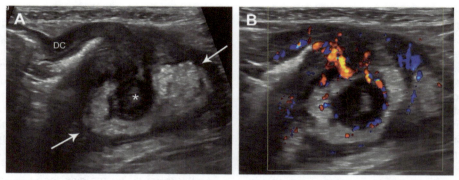

Fig. 3. Acute diverticulitis in a 73 year old woman who presented to ER with acute LLQ pain. (*A*) Grayscale long-axis view of the descending colon (DC) shows an inflamed diverticulum (*) with marked surrounding inflammatory fat. The diverticulum and adjacent colonic wall show mural thickening. (*B*) CDI confirms severe vascularity/inflammation.

can be used as the first-time examination at the time of diagnosis, for routine monitoring of disease activity, during acute flares, or for evaluation of therapeutic response.

In addition, US may be utilized to evaluate a broad range of gastrointestinal symptoms in patients with IBD or irritable bowel syndrome (IBS) such as abdominal pain, abdominal distension, diarrhea, or stool habit changes. In patients with IBD, the focus of the US examination is to detect any signs of active inflammation, while in IBS, it is to exclude the presence of IBD as the cause of patient's symptoms.

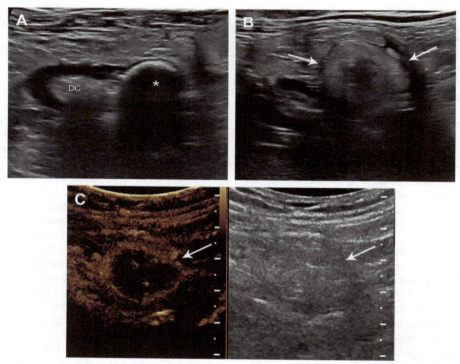

Fig. 4. Acute diverticulitis with abscess. A 72 year old man with known diverticular disease presents with LLQ pain and fever. (*A*) Axial grayscale image of the descending colon (DC) shows a bright curvilinear echo representing air within a large diverticulum (*). (*B*) Adjacent to the diverticulum, there is mixed echogenic inflammatory mass with central hypoechoic components (*arrows*). (*C*) CEUS dual screen shows on the left the inflammatory mass (*arrows*) with central avascular component and peripheral rim of hyperenhancement consistent with an abscess. On the right, low mechanical index (MI) poor grayscale correlate.

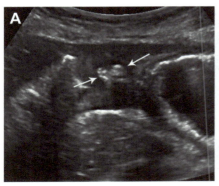 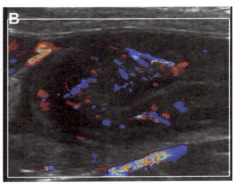

Fig. 5. Peptic ulcer disease. A 50 year old woman presented to ER with epigastric/RUQ pain for 4 days. (*A*) Grayscale long-axis view of the antrum of the stomach shows persistent mural thickening with black walls with a central area of echogenic gas representing the ulcer (*arrows*). (*B*) CDI confirms significant hyperemia within this segment (Video 3).

Bowel wall thickening is known to be the most reliable sign indicating active disease.[16] Normal bowel wall should not measure more than 3 to 4 mm in thickness. Any abnormal segments and their adjacent mesentery should be evaluated closely for signs of active inflammation, transmural disease, or complications.[18]

Active inflammation in inflammatory bowel disease

There are a number of sonographic parameters used to determinate disease activity, including wall thickening, mural vascularity on CDI, and the presence of mesenteric fatty proliferation (**Fig. 6**A–C). Mural thickening, as an objective observation, is considered an accurate measurement reflecting active inflammation that can be followed overtime. However, mural vascularity on CDI and fatty proliferation are more subjective observations and may be operator dependent. In our institution, a US global assessment (USGA) of disease activity is used to assist in the determination and grading of inflammatory activity in a more standardized way. USGA parameters and PE values on CEUS have been correlated with the degree of mural inflammation at endoscopy, and they assist in the evaluation of therapeutic response or disease progression (**Table 1**).[19]

In our experience, bowel wall thickening may completely resolve in some patients with IBD after adequate treatment. However, in others, mural wall thickening may persist without the presence of active inflammatory change. This may be due to the presence of submucosal fatty deposition or muscular hypertrophy.[20,21] In these instances, CDI and CEUS play a key role in the confirmation or exclusion of mural vascularity reflecting active disease.[22] However, CDI can only identify large-size and medium-size vessels with fast flow, and its detection can be affected by high body mass index (BMI) and/or deep loop location. This is important to acknowledge when an abnormally thickened segment is visualized, but no color Doppler signal is captured. The lack of CDI may be due to a true lack of vascularity (remission) or be secondary to technical factors limiting its detection. Therefore, activity is deemed indeterminate with grayscale and CDI findings alone. In this instance, CEUS is an indispensable addition allowing for more sensitive detection of mural microvascularity. CEUS also provides objective quantification values that can be graded and followed overtime[19,23] (**Fig. 6**D, E).

An essential part of the mural assessment is the detailed observation of the bowel wall layers. Presence of wall layer destruction in patients with IBD (**Fig. 7**A) will suggest a severe transmural process, either secondary to high degree of inflammation[24] or a stricture. The identification of wall layer destruction should instigate the US operator to perform a closer look of the serosa for evidence of disruption that will suggest perforation or fistula. However, it should be remembered that wall layer disruption can also be seen with other infiltrative processes including neoplasm.

While assessing the bowel wall, it is also important to recognize other changes such as echogenic thicken submucosa reflecting fatty deposition (**Fig. 7**B), which can be observed in chronic changes and individuals with obesity. Thickening of the muscular layer will suggest muscular hypertrophy, an important observation in stricturing Crohn's disease (CD) and diverticulosis.

Other wall observations visible with US are mucosal ulcerations, intramural abscess, sinus tracts, and serosal disruptions or spiculations. Ulcerations show a variety of appearances but are most often recognized by the presence of air in

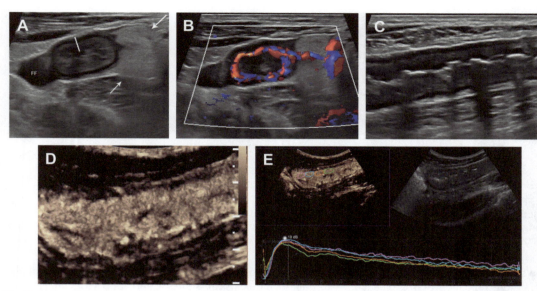

Fig. 6. Active IBD. A 38 year old man with crohn's disease (CD) for 4 years and prior bowel resection presents for bowel assessment. (*A*) Axial grayscale of the NeoTI in the RUQ shows moderate mural thickening of 7 mm (bar) and moderate adjacent echogenic inflammatory fat (*arrows*). Trace of free fluid (FF) is also present. (*B*) CDI shows severe mural and mesenteric vascularity. (*C*) Long-axis view of the same segment shows mural thickening with some layer destruction. (*D*) There is transmural hyperenhancement on CEUS. (*E*) CEUS dual screen with quantification at the bottom from 4 ROIs (color circles) confirms moderate active disease with PE of 19 dB. Reproducibility of the ROI TICs is excellent.

abnormal locations (within the wall, close to the serosal surface, or within the peri-enteric soft tissue; **Fig. 7**C, D). Occasionally, air can travel or dissect the bowel wall seen as a linear echo along the wall. If gas is seen near the serosa, an impending or localized perforation would be the concern (**Fig. 8**A, B).

In patients with IBD, the extent of disease needs to be documented using cine-clips. A continuous video of the affected segment is recorded showing

Table 1
Ultrasound global assessment of disease activity

Ultrasound Features of Activity	Classification			
	Inactive	Mild	Moderate	Severe
Wall Thickness mm	< 4	4.0–6.0	6.1–8.0	> 8
Color Doppler imaging	• Absent	• Small regions of color • No vessel structure	• Medium vessel length	• Circumferential vessels • ± mesenteric vessels
Inflammatory fat	• Perienteric region resembles normal mesenteric fat	• Masslike • Slightly echogenic • LESS AREA than the bowel on axial view	• Masslike • More echogenic • EQUAL AREA to the bowel on axial view	• Masslike • Significantly echogenic • GREATER AREA than bowel on axial view
With integration of contrast-enhanced ultrasound (CEUS)—Peak enhancement				
CEUS Peak dB	Absent—15 dB	15—18 dB	18—23 dB	> 23 dB

From Medellin A, Merrill C, Wilson SR. Role of Contrast-enhanced ultrasound in evaluation of the bowel. Abdom Radiol (NY). 2018 Apr;43(4):918–933; with permission.

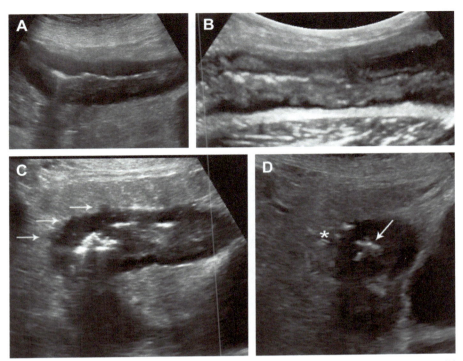

Fig. 7. Mural changes in different patients. (*A*) Wall layer destruction. (*B*) Echogenic submucosal proliferation. (*C*) Axial views show complete wall layer destruction, serosa spiculation (*arrows*), (*D*) mural ulcerations (*arrow*) and localized perforation (*) in the same patient as C.

the areas of transition from normal to abnormal and the length of the affected segment is estimated. Any skip segments or sacculations are also recorded.

Inflammatory Bowel Disease Complications

Sinus tracts and fistulas

During any bowel assessment, a careful search of the mesentery of the adjacent abnormal segment must be performed to detect any penetrating disease. Sinus tracts and fistulas are important findings to be recognized, but they can be very subtle and easy to miss. The presence of any serosal spiculation or disruption should prompt the operator to meticulously look for any hypoechoic tracts, free fluid, or free air.

Sinus tracts are blind-ended hypoechoic tracts, while fistulas communicate between 2 epithelial surfaces/organs: entero-enteric (**Fig. 8**C, D, Video 6), enterocutaneous, enterovaginal, or enterovesical.[25] Fistulas can be open with gas and fluid transversing them or closed with no material seen within. The entire length of the fistula needs to be evaluated, including the connecting organs for abnormal mural thickening, inflammatory change, and other complications such as abscesses. Fistulas can also be complex, connecting various adjacent loops or present with a central converging hypoechoic inflammatory mass most commonly described as a "star" shape appearance. If cicatrization is present, bowel retraction and fixed angulations are frequently seen.

Perianal disease in IBD is generally complex with multiple fistulas tracts and inflammatory changes. If present at initial diagnosis, perianal disease confers a poor prognosis. Complex transsphincteric fistulas can extend to the deep tissues including buttocks, perineum, scrotum labia, and vagina. It is important to denote the origin of the fistula, using a clock-face position, the tract of the fistula, and any external openings. Any inflammatory masses need to be characterized with CEUS as abscess or phlegmonous.

Inflammatory masses

Inflammatory complications are common in IBD (**Fig. 8**E), but their nomenclature remains controversial. Although there is a preference by some to classify these as inflammatory masses and abscesses,[26,27] we prefer, from our US experience, an overall category of inflammatory masses that includes both abscesses and phlegmons. This preference is based on our extensive experience showing that the original US grayscale imaging is often indeterminate as to whether or not there is

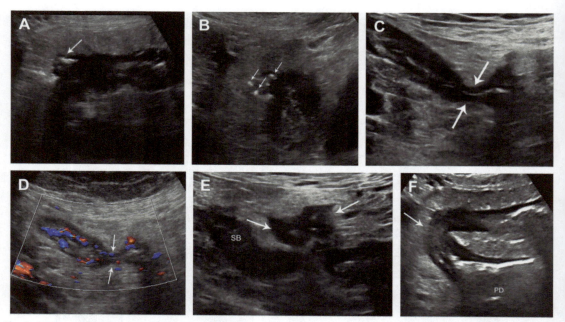

Fig. 8. IBD complications in a patient with CD. (*A*) Localized perforation. (*B*) Same patient as in A, grayscale shows free air (*arrows*) within the inflamed mesentery. (*C*) Long-axis view shows an open enteroenteric fistula (*arrows*) with gas along the tract. (*D*) CDI of the same segments and fistula (*arrows*) as in C shows mural vascularity with inflammatory changes along the fistula. (*E*) Inflammatory mass. Long-axis view shows hypoechoic irregular mass adjacent to a small bowel loop (SB) with active inflammation. Centrally it contains a bubble of gas, and it is surrounded by inflammatory fat. (*F*) Fixed angulation (*arrow*) causing incomplete mechanical bowel obstruction (IMBO), note the prestenotic dilatation (PS).

drainable pus. Further, it is only with the addition of CEUS that we can distinguish the vascular phlegmon from the avascular abscess.[28]

Imaging distinction between a phlegmon and an abscess is important, as patients with IBD on aggressive treatment regimens often do not present with typical infective symptoms. Therefore, the evolution of an inflammatory mass, from a mass-like reactive inflammation (phlegmon) to a well-organized abscess, has management implications (either medical or with a placement of a drain).

On B-mode, phlegmons and abscesses present as similar hypoechoic or mixed echogenic masses, which are difficult to differentiate. CEUS is the preferred modality to differentiate an inflammatory phlegmon and an abscess, as it is more sensitive than CDI. Phlegmons are hypervascular representing inflammatory changes (**Fig. 9**A, B) and show homogeneous hyperenhancement with no discrete wall. On the contrary, abscesses will have avascular components reflecting pus and show a peripheral rim of reactive inflammation.

Strictures

Strictures in US are seen as persistent areas of luminal narrowing with associated wall thickening with or without proximal bowel dilatation.[21] Real-time US is invaluable to differentiate a transient observation from a true narrowing that shows abnormal mural thickening and luminal narrowing of various degrees. US can dynamically assess for the motion of intestinal contents. Evidence of any dysfunctional peristalsis or hyperperistaltic loops should trigger a close examination of the bowel for any evidence of disease or a stricture segment. Most strictures are predominantly composed of inflammation, muscular hypertrophy, or a combination of both.[20,21] In recent years, we have integrated CEUS and SWE in the evaluation of strictures.[8] This allows for detection of mural inflammation and stiffness. Most strictures have mixed components,[21] but any high values on SWE would suggest a very stiff bowel wall that may not respond to medical therapy[29] (**Fig. 10**A–D).

Bowel obstruction

Bowel obstruction may be due to a stricture segment, fixed angulation (**Fig. 8**F), and bowel retraction in patients with IBD, but it is most commonly secondary to adhesions. Currently, a prestenotic loop greater that 3 cm in diameter is generally considered abnormal in computed tomography (CT) and MR imaging publications.[27] However, we believe that the absolute criteria for

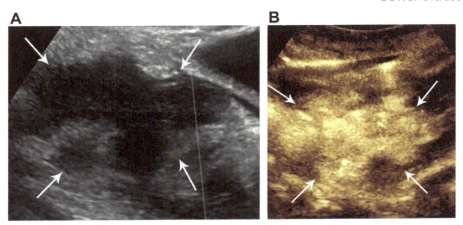

Fig. 9. Inflammatory mass. A 20 year old man was newly diagnosed with CD. (*A*) During US assessment, a hypoechoic irregular mass-like area (*arrows*) was discovered adjacent to an abnormal long segment of bowel with active inflammation (not shown). (*B*) CEUS nicely shows that this represents a phlegmon with homogenous enhancement. No avascular components are present to suggest an abscess.

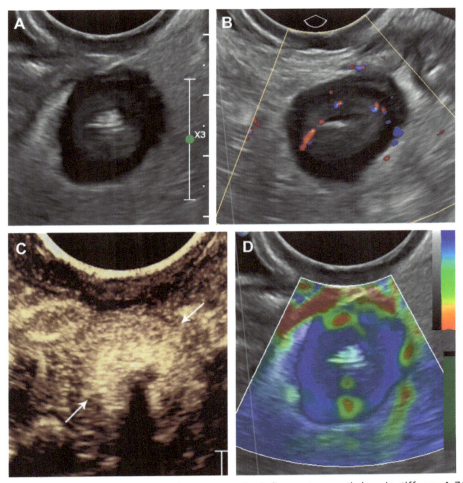

Fig. 10. Sigmoid colon stricture with a mixed pattern, active inflammatory, and chronic stiffness. A 74 year old woman presents for assessment for possible IBD. (*A*) Axial EV grayscale shows a short stricture segment with severe wall thickening of 8 mm and surrounding inflammatory fat. (*B*) Axial CDI shows some vascularity in the wall, but it is less than expected when compared to the wall thickness. (*C*) CEUS shows significant transmural enhancement with PE of 25 dB (time intensity curve no shown) confirming severe active inflammation. (*D*) SWE shows mixed changes with soft components (blue) and stiff mural areas (red) measuring up to 2.8 m/s suggesting very stiff bowel.

the stricture and prestenotic segment may be lower/different for US, as the real-time demonstration of abnormal luminal apposition, with a preceding segment showing fluid content, dysfunctional peristalsis with to-and-fro activity and often squirting luminal content is more convincing for bowel obstruction than absolute measurement obtained at a single point of time.

Occasionally, particulate material,echogenic content or bezoars can also be visualized suggesting a long-standing stagnation of the intestinal contents.

Inflammatory Bowel Disease Assessment of Therapeutic Response

Assessment of therapeutic response in US relies upon the USGA parameters of disease activity. Grayscale findings and degree of CDI are compared to prior studies to characterize any interval improvement or worsening.[30] A challenge arises when there is persistent mural thickening with no CDI, and therefore, disease activity is indeterminate with B-mode US alone. This may be due to poor technical sensitivity of CDI or real remission. In this instance, CEUS should be performed to better evaluate for mural perfusion at the capillary level. CEUS is more sensitive for the detection of mural flow at the microcirculatory level and allows for a subjective and objective evaluation. The most commonly used quantification parameters are PE and AUC.

BOWEL INFECTIONS

Acute infections such as typhlitis and pseudomembranous colitis also show mural wall thickening and inflammatory changes. Location and distribution of the findings give a diagnostic clue. In the case of pseudomembranous colitis, the presence of an exaggerated haustral thickening or a nonhomogeneous thickening of the submucosal layer with luminal apposition may be a diagnostic indicator.

Intestinal tuberculosis, although uncommon in North America, may occur and is occasionally missed since it is not routinely considered and can mimic other bowel conditions, including IBD.[31] Any circumferential wall thickening with hypoechoic (black) walls at the cecum or TI, in association with prominent lymphadenopathy with signs of necrosis, should lead to consideration of tuberculosis anywhere in the world.[32]

BOWEL NEOPLASMS

US is not used as the first modality for the evaluation of bowel malignancies; although neoplasms may be incidentally discovered during a routine US. Bowel masses are frequently black on US and have increased conspicuity, as compared to their appearance on CT and MR scans. The best diagnostic clue is a focal asymmetric thickening of the bowel wall or a luminal or mural mass. Suspected mural masses or mural thickening are evaluated with CEUS to determinate their vascularity and washout characteristics.[32]

The excellent spatial resolution of US allows for localization of the mass in relation to the bowel wall and detection of other important features such as mass ulceration, wall destruction/invasion, or luminal dilatation, assisting in the differential diagnosis. In the setting of neoplasm, bowel wall layer destruction is most commonly seen with lymphoma and adenocarcinoma. Detailed descriptions of multiple bowel neoplasms on US can be found in multiple publications.[32]

A pitfall in the interpretation of thickening of the bowel wall is an endometrial plaque or seeding that mimics serosal metastasis and primary wall neoplasms. On grayscale, endometriosis deposits are hypoechoic masses with a variable vascularity, which depends on the women's day of cycle and the amount of stromal and glandular components.

Mucocele of the appendix is relatively uncommon but can be encountered when evaluating the appendix for other reasons. A benign mucocele shows a dilated segment of the appendix, related to buildup of mucus distal to an area of inflammatory scarring that blocks the lumen. Patients are generally asymptomatic. The neoplastic varieties include primary mucous cystadenoma and cystadenocarcinoma and typically appear as a large, hypoechoic, well-defined cystic mass often with calcifications. CEUS allows for differentiation of a benign and a malignant lesion by demonstrating the vascular components in the neoplasm.

SUMMARY

High-resolution US allows for excellent detection of bowel pathology and its complications. US is safe, accurate, and highly accepted by patients and can be performed as a frequent examination without risks associated with ionizing radiation. This makes US a recommended first-line imaging modality for the assessment of acute abdominal pain and IBD. Detection of mural and mesenteric changes is the most important observations leading to the recognition of inflammatory or neoplastic processes and their complications. EV and perianal scanning increase the detection of abnormal segments deep within the pelvis and exceptionally evaluate perianal disease. Their addition to any bowel examination is essential depending upon patient symptoms.

In recent years, newer US techniques have been used for the evaluation of IBD. CEUS is now an essential addition for the evaluation of disease activity and inflammatory masses. In combination, CEUS and elastography show mural perfusion and intestinal stiffness, as important components in the assessment of structuring Crohn's disease. CEUS also provides objective measurements of mural vascularity that can be followed overtime, desirable for the determination of therapeutic response. Although there is still controversy on the capabilities of these 2 techniques, CEUS and SWE demonstrate great potential for the evaluation of disease activity, characterization of strictures, and evaluation of treatment response in patients with IBD.

CLINICS CARE POINTS

- US is a safe and accurate modality, highly accepted by patients, and performed as a frequent examination without risk of ionizing radiation.
- US is sensitive in the detection of mural and mesenteric inflammation.
- Bowel wall thickening and/or loss of wall layer definition are the most important observations suggesting bowel pathology.
- US allows direct evaluation of the symptomatic area.
- Real-time dynamic US is incomparable for showing functional and morphologic changes of bowel disease.
- The addition of EV examinations in many women increases the detection of disease in the deep pelvis.
- Transperineal scans allow for excellent visualization of the anal canal.
- New techniques such as CEUS and SWE now provide a more objective evaluation of mural perfusion and intestinal stiffness, which represent important factors in the characterization of strictures.

DISCLOSURE

A. Medellin has nothing to disclose. S.R. Wilson: Advisory board, Definity. Lantheus Medical Imaging; Speaker's bureau, Philips; Equipment support Siemens, Samsung and Philips.

SUPPLEMENTARY DATA

Supplementary data to this article can be found online at https://doi.org/10.1016/j.rcl.2024.08.002.

REFERENCES

1. Maconi G, Nylund K, Ripolles T, et al. EFSUMB recommendations and clinical guidelines for intestinal ultrasound (GIUS) in inflammatory bowel diseases. Ultraschall der Med 2018;39(3):304–17.
2. Nardone OM, Calabrese G, Testa A, et al. The impact of intestinal ultrasound on the management of inflammatory bowel disease: from established facts toward new horizons. Front Med 2022; 9(May):1–9.
3. Dolinger MT, Kayal M. Intestinal ultrasound as a non-invasive tool to monitor inflammatory bowel disease activity and guide clinical decision making. World J Gastroenterol 2023;29(15):2272–82.
4. Medellin-Kowalewski A, Wilkens R, Wilson A, et al. Quantitative contrast-enhanced ultrasound parameters in Crohn disease: Their role in disease activity determination with ultrasound. Am J Roentgenol 2016;206(1):64–73.
5. Medellin A, Merrill C, Wilson SR. Role of contrast-enhanced ultrasound in evaluation of the bowel. Abdom Radiol 2017. https://doi.org/10.1007/s00261-017-1399-6.
6. Dillman JR, Smith E, Sanchez RJ, et al. Pediatric small bowel crohn disease: correlation of US and MR enterography 1. Radiographics 2015. https://doi.org/10.1148/rg.2015140002.
7. Dillman JR, Stidham RW, Higgins PDR, et al. US elastography-derived shear wave velocity helps distinguish acutely inflamed from fibrotic bowel in a Crohn disease animal model. Radiology 2013; 267(3):757–66.
8. Lu C, Gui X, Chen W, et al. Ultrasound shear wave elastography and contrast enhancement: effective biomarkers in Crohn's disease strictures. Inflamm Bowel Dis 2017;0(0):1–10.
9. Stewart1 LK, Wilson1 SA. Transvaginal sonography of the anal sphincter: reliable, or not?. Available at: www.ajronline.org.
10. Fernandes T, Oliveira MI, Castro R, et al. Bowel wall thickening at CT: Simplifying the diagnosis. Insights Imaging 2014;5(2):195–208.
11. Sasaki T, Kunisaki R, Kinoshita H, et al. Doppler ultrasound findings correlate with tissue vascularity and inflammation in surgical pathology specimens from patients with small intestinal Crohn's disease. BMC Res Notes 2014;7(1):363.
12. Romanini L, Passamonti M, Navarria M, et al. Quantitative analysis of contrast-enhanced ultrasonography of the bowel wall can predict disease activity in inflammatory bowel disease. Eur J Radiol 2014.

13. Jeffrey RB. Acute appendicitis:high-resolution real-time US findings. Radiology 1987;163(1):11–4.
14. Higgins MJ, Walsh M, Kennedy SM, et al. Granulomatous appendicitis revisited:report of a case. Dig Surg 2001;18(3).
15. Menozzi G, Maccabruni V, Zanichelli M, et al. Contrast-enhanced ultrasound appearance of primary epiploic appendagitis. J Ultrasound 2014; 17(1):75–6.
16. Frias-Gomes C, Torres J, Palmela C. Intestinal ultrasound in inflammatory bowel disease: a valuable and increasingly important tool. GE Port J Gastroenterol 2022;29(4):223–39.
17. Fraquelli M, Colli A, Casazza G, et al. Role of US in detection of Crohn disease: meta-analysis. Radiology 2005;236(1):95–101.
18. Lin WC, Chang CW, Chen MJ, et al. Intestinal ultrasound in inflammatory bowel disease: A novel and increasingly important tool. J Med Ultrasound 2023;31(2):86–91.
19. Medellin A, Merrill C, Wilson SR. Role of contrast-enhanced ultrasound in evaluation of the bowel. Abdom Radiol 2018;43(4):918–33.
20. Lu C, Gui X, Chen W, et al. Ultrasound shear wave elastography and contrast enhancement: effective biomarkers in Crohn's disease strictures. Inflamm Bowel Dis 2017;23(3):421–30.
21. Sleiman J, Chirra P, Gandhi NS, et al. Crohn's disease related strictures in cross-sectional imaging: More than meets the eye? United Eur Gastroenterol J 2022;10(10):1167–78.
22. Spalinger J, Patriquin H, Marie-Claude M, et al. Doppler US in patients with crohn disease:vessel density in the diseased bowel refects diasese activity. Radiology 2000;217(3):787–91.
23. Ripollés T, Rausell N, Paredes JM, et al. Effectiveness of contrast-enhanced ultrasound for characterisation of intestinal inflammation in Crohn's disease: A comparison with surgical histopathology analysis. J Crohn's Colitis 2013;7(2):120–8.
24. Jauregui-Amezaga A, Rimola J. Role of intestinal ultrasound in the management of patients with inflammatory bowel disease. Life 2021;11(7):1–14.
25. Rieder F, Bettenworth D, Ma C, et al. An expert consensus to standardise definitions, diagnosis and treatment targets for anti-fibrotic stricture therapies in Crohn's disease. Aliment Pharmacol Ther 2018;48(3):347–57.
26. Bruining DH, Zimmermann EM, Loftus EV, et al. Consensus recommendations for evaluation, interpretation, and utilization of computed tomography and magnetic resonance enterography in patients with small bowel crohn's disease. Gastroenterology 2018;154(4):1172–94.
27. Guglielmo FF, Anupindi SA, Fletcher JG, et al. Small bowel crohn disease at CT and MR enterography: Imaging atlas and glossary of terms. Radiographics 2020;40(2):354–75.
28. Ripollés T, Martínez-Pérez MJ, Paredes JM, et al. Contrast-enhanced ultrasound in the differentiation between phlegmon and abscess in Crohn's disease and other abdominal conditions. Eur J Radiol 2013; 82(10):e525–31.
29. Ding SS, Fang Y, Wan J, et al. Usefulness of strain elastography, ARFI imaging, and point shear wave elastography for the assessment of crohn disease strictures. J Ultrasound Med 2019 Nov;38(11): 2861–70.
30. Ilvemark JFKF, Hansen T, Goodsall TM, et al. Defining transabdominal intestinal ultrasound treatment response and remission in inflammatory bowel disease: systematic review and expert consensus statement. J Crohn's Colitis 2022;16(4):554–80.
31. Kilcoyne A, Kaplan JL, Gee MS. Inflammatory bowel disease imaging: Current practice and future directions. World J Gastroenterol 2016. https://doi.org/10.3748/wjg.v22.i3.917.
32. Rumack CLD. Diagnostic ultrasound. 2. 6th Edition 2023.

Emerging Techniques in Pediatric Ultrasound, with Emphasis on Infants

Jeffrey J. Tutman, MD[a], Catalina Le Cacheux, MD[b,c], Judy H. Squires, MD, FSRU[b,c,*]

KEYWORDS

- Infant • Ultrasound • Necrotizing enterocolitis • Malrotation • Midgut volvulus • CEUS
- Congenital hepatic hemangioma • Infantile hepatic hemangioma

KEY POINTS

- Necrotizing enterocolitis (NEC) is a potentially devastating disease of infants. In conjunction with radiographs, ultrasound of the bowel, mesentery and peritoneal cavity, and abdominal wall may help in diagnosis and management.
- Ultrasound is increasingly important in the diagnosis of malrotation with midgut volvulus, with findings including proximal duodenal dilation and clockwise swirling of bowel and mesentery around the superior mesenteric artery.
- Liver lesions in infants are different from those found in older patients. Contrast-enhanced ultrasound (CEUS) is increasingly used for definitive characterization due to the specific appearance of different lesions.

 Video content accompanies this article at http://www.radiologic.theclinics.com.

INTRODUCTION

Ultrasound is an important modality for the assessment of pediatric patients and the number of clinical uses continues to increase. In this review, several emerging applications of ultrasound in pediatric patients are detailed, focusing on diseases impacting infants, including necrotizing enterocolitis, malrotation with midgut volvulus, and liver lesion characterization.

NECROTIZING ENTEROCOLITIS
Background

Necrotizing enterocolitis (NEC) is a gastrointestinal emergency in newborns and is potentially a devastating disease. Most cases occur in very low birth weight (<1500 g) infants born at less than 32 weeks' gestation, but it is important to note that NEC can occur in term infants, particularly those who have experienced an ischemic event, such as patients with congenital heart disease.[1-3] The true incidence of NEC is unknown; however, estimates range from 1 to 3 cases per 1000 live births or up to 7% of infants with birth weight between 500 and 1500 g, and death rates are reported to be as high as 50%.[2,3] There is substantial long-term morbidity in survivors of NEC, who often require prolonged hospitalization and suffer from continued intestinal, neurodevelopmental, and growth complications of the disease.[2]

---

[a] Department of Radiology, University of Colorado School of Medicine and Children's Hospital of Colorado, Box 125, Aurora, CO 80045, 80920, USA; [b] Department of Radiology, UPMC Children's Hospital of Pittsburgh, 4401 Penn Avenue, 2nd Floor Radiology, Pittsburgh, PA 15224, USA; [c] Department of Radiology, University of Pittsburgh School of Medicine, 200 Lothrop Street, First Floor PUH, Suite E-174, Pittsburgh, PA 15213, USA
* Corresponding author.
E-mail address: Judy.Squires@chp.edu

NEC is an evolving process of unknown but likely multifactorial etiology, characterized by ischemic necrosis of the intestinal mucosa and severe inflammation, which leads to an extension of enteric gas-forming bacteria into the bowel wall and into the portal venous system or may cause intestinal perforation. NEC most commonly affects the terminal ileum and proximal colon.[4]

Treatment of NEC involves bowel rest with parenteral feeds, gastric decompression, antibiotic therapy, fluid replacement, and close monitoring to ensure surgical intervention is not required. Evidence of bowel perforation is currently the only widely accepted indication for surgical intervention.[2] Acute complications of NEC include sepsis, cardiorespiratory failure, prolonged hospitalization, and death.[2] Long-term complications include postischemic stricture formation, altered bowel motility, adhesions that may lead to bowel obstructions, and short bowel syndrome and/or intestinal failure as a result of resection of involved bowel segments.[2]

The clinical presentation includes feeding intolerance, abdominal distention, abdominal discoloration, bloody stools, and vital sign instability; however, these signs may be very subtle and are not specific for NEC.[2,5] Therefore, imaging often plays a crucial role in the assessment of infants with concern for possible NEC.

Diagnostic Performance of Ultrasound

Radiographs have traditionally been the mainstay to assess infants with clinical concern for NEC. Sequential evaluation of the bowel gas pattern and appearance overtime may be helpful. Dilated and elongated bowel loops raise concern on radiographs for NEC, with a fixed loop of bowel (a bowel loop that does not change in appearance overtime on radiographs) additionally concerning.[6] Intramural gas (pneumatosis intestinalis or coli), portal venous gas, and pneumoperitoneum may also be seen in association with NEC but are not specific for NEC.[2,6,7] Importantly, the most common clinical staging system, the modified Bell staging, uses radiographs as part of the staging criteria.[2]

Ultrasound is gaining acceptance by neonatologists and pediatric surgeons and is currently predominantly used in conjunction with radiographs to assist in the clinical diagnosis, management, and follow-up of infants at risk for NEC. Faingold and colleagues[4] demonstrated that the absence of bowel wall perfusion at color Doppler ultrasound (US) is more sensitive and specific than the presence of free air at abdominal radiography in the detection of necrotic bowel in NEC. Color Doppler US findings were also shown to be more accurate than the Bell staging and abdominal radiography in the prediction of necrosis in neonates with NEC and therefore may alter clinical staging and management.[4]

Cuna and colleagues[1] evaluated ultrasound findings compared to patient outcomes in a meta-analysis and demonstrated an association of focal fluid collections, complex ascites, absent bowel peristalsis, pneumoperitoneum, bowel dilation, bowel wall absent perfusion, or bowel wall thinning, thickening, or abnormal echogenicity were all associated with poorer outcomes, specifically death and surgery requirement. Infants with NEC requiring surgical management have also been shown to have worse outcomes. Conversely, when portal venous gas, pneumatosis intestinalis, increased bowel wall perfusion, and simple ascites were independently compared with the need for surgery or death, there was no significant association.[1]

Finally, Le Cacheux and colleagues[8] reported an association of mesenteric thickening, hyperechogenicity of intraluminal bowel content, edema and hyperemia of the abdominal wall, and poor intestinal wall definition that are also associated with poorer patient outcomes, including patient death and short-term or long-term surgery requirement.

Patient Preparation

Patients with clinical concern for NEC will typically be cared for in the neonatal intensive care unit, and examinations are performed portably. No specific patient preparation is needed; however, patients are often fasting for treatment of suspected NEC.

Ultrasound Scanning Protocol

Comparison with preceding radiographs may be helpful to focus on specific areas of concern. A small footprint curved array (microconvex) mid-frequency (4–10 MHz) transducer is useful to assess the abdomen with a larger field of view for an overall assessment, to scan beneath ribs and the xyphoid, and to compress gas away from areas of interest. This should be followed by a linear high-frequency (6–20 MHz) transducer to assess structures in greater detail and for Doppler evaluation. Some authors advocate for an "outside-to-in" imaging approach moving from the colon to the small bowel, while others prefer to trace the course of bowel, followed by quadrant assessment. The structures to be evaluated are detailed in **Table 1**. Both still and cinematic "cine" images should be saved if possible, including cinematic images with the transducer stationary to evaluate for bowel peristalsis. A shortened protocol can be considered for specific problem-solving, in limited resource settings, or for follow-up examinations.[9]

Table 1
Suggested protocol for the evaluation of infants with known or suspected necrotizing enterocolitis

	Structure	Findings Assessed
Grayscale Assessment	Abdominal wall	Edema
	Peritoneal cavity	Free fluid
		Septated fluid
		Debris-containing fluid
		Focal fluid collection(s)
		Pneumoperitoneum
	Bowel wall	Thickening (>3 mm)
		Thinning (<1 mm)
		Peristalsis
	Bowel lumen	Dilation
		Hyperechoic contents
	Mesentery	Thickening
	Portal vein branches	Gas
Color or Power Doppler Assessment	Abdominal wall	Hyperemia
	Bowel wall	Hyperemia
		Hypoperfusion
		No perfusion
	Mesentery	Hyperemia
	Portal vein branches	Gas
		Spectral Doppler may be helpful to distinguish gas from rouleaux formation

Ultrasound Findings

Abdominal wall
NEC causes abdominal wall edema and hyperemia, usually following the distribution of the diseased bowel. Abdominal wall edema is seen sonographically as thickening and increased echogenicity, progressing to reticular strands of fluid separating the subcutaneous tissues resembling a mosaic pattern of fluid and fat.[8] Hyperemia is also a common finding and is best assessed with the linear probe.

Peritoneal cavity
The entire peritoneal cavity should be assessed, most often by dividing the abdomen into 4 quadrants and carefully evaluating each quadrant. Septated fluid, debris-containing fluid, and focal fluid collections are associated with poorer outcomes in NEC.[1] Evaluation of fluid should include an attempt to visualize linear echogenic foci, turbid, or punctate echoes (debris) within abdominal cavity fluid. Focal fluid collections may closely approximate and mold to the shape of a loop of the bowel or may be located within thickened mesentery, making distinction among bowel wall, mesentery, and fluid collection challenging, particularly for echogenic fluid. Lack of color Doppler signal can be helpful for diagnosing fluid. A complex collection adjacent to an avascular or otherwise abnormal-appearing bowel loop (see Bowel section) should raise concern for bowel perforation. Pneumoperitoneum, even in small quantities, can be readily visualized at ultrasound, and its presence suggests bowel perforation.[5]

Mesentery Normally, the mesentery in infants is a thin structure and is inconspicuous at ultrasound. When visible, the normal appearance is a fine hypoechoic structure softly laced between small bowels. Abnormal mesentery in the setting of NEC is thickened, hyperechoic or heterogeneous, and hypervascular, with at times a mass-like appearance, causing splaying of bowel loops (**Fig. 1**). In later stages of NEC, the mesentery becomes fingerlike or bandlike, with spongiform projections causing tethering of bowel loops.[8]

Bowel
Bowel peristalsis Normal small bowel will demonstrate normal peristalsis, defined as at least 10 contractions per minute.[4] Peristalsis may be decreased or absent in the setting of NEC. However, caution should be used in patients treated by paralytic agents that may impact bowel peristalsis.

Bowel wall echogenicity, distinction, thickness, and perfusion Normal bowel wall will have a stratified appearance of bowel wall layers (also called gut signature) and measures about 1.7 mm in thickness. Bowel wall of loops affected by NEC may have a loss of the normal distinction between bowel wall layers, have a general poorly defined appearance,

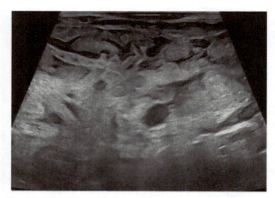

Fig. 1. A 14 day old former 29 week gestational age girl with clinical diagnosis of NEC. Transverse grayscale ultrasound of the midline upper abdomen demonstrates edematous, thickened, hyperechoic mesentery splaying bowel loops.

and/or demonstrate increased echogenicity.[8] Bowel wall thickening (thickness >3 mm) or thinning (thickness <1 mm) may be seen. With increased disease severity, thick hyperemic bowel progresses to thin avascular bowel prior to possible perforation (Fig. 2).[5] Hyperemia is defined as striated ("zebra" appearance), complete ring of bowel wall flow, and/or Y-shaped flow related to distal mesenteric and subserosal vessel flow.[4]

Bowel content Intraluminal content of the bowel normally is fluid and air. Intraluminal content is considered abnormal when the echogenicity is greater than the adjacent intestinal wall, liver, and spleen.[8] The proposed etiology is that bowel impacted by NEC contains sloughed mucosa, muscle, and submucosa layers, as well as mucin, hemorrhage, and inflammatory debris (Fig. 3). Care should be taken not to confuse intraluminal milk or formula content with the abnormal content of NEC.

Bowel wall pneumatosis Pneumatosis is nonspecific and is not always seen in the setting of NEC, and the severity does not correlate with disease severity.[5] Therefore, although ultrasound performed for NEC should include assessment for pneumatosis, interpretation should be made in conjunction with clinical context and with incorporation of all sonographic findings. Air within bowel wall will be visible as echogenic foci or a complete bright rim in both the nondependent and dependent portions of the bowel wall (Fig. 4). Evaluating the deep wall of bowel is helpful to ensure air is truly air located within bowel wall, rather than small foci of air located within the projections of the valvulae conniventes, which is a normal finding. Assessing the appearance of the bowel wall with transducer held stationary while the underlying bowel peristalses can also be helpful to distinguish intraluminal air from intramural air, because pneumatosis will remain in a fixed position within the bowel wall, while intraluminal content will move.

Portal venous gas Portal venous gas is not specific for NEC but rather is more commonly secondary to an umbilical catheter. Like pneumatosis intestinalis, the quantity of portal venous gas and its resolution do not correlate with clinical status in infants with NEC.[5] At ultrasound, portal venous gas may

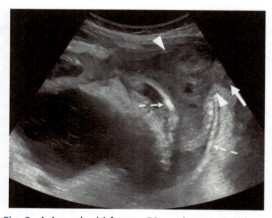

Fig. 2. A 1 week old former 29 week gestational age boy with rapid clinical deterioration, distended abdomen, and bloody stools. Sagittal grayscale ultrasound demonstrates frank bowel perforation (*arrowheads*), complex fluid (*solid arrow*), and pneumatosis intestinalis (*dashed arrows*).

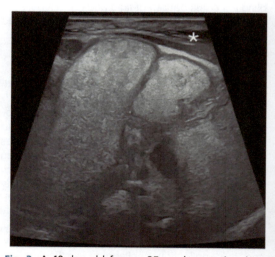

Fig. 3. A 40 day old former 25 week gestational age infant boy with abdominal distention, bloody stools, and clinical diagnosis of NEC. Transverse grayscale ultrasound demonstrates hyperechogenic intraluminal content and abdominal wall edema (*asterisk*).

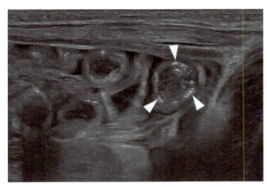

Fig. 4. A 2 week old former 26 week gestational age infant boy with abdominal distention, clinical concern for NEC and pneumatosis intestinalis questioned on radiographs. Transverse grayscale ultrasound demonstrates pneumatosis intestinalis (*arrowheads*).

be seen as mobile foci of air, with characteristic spectral Doppler spikes.[5] Gas may be seen peripherally in portal venules as linear branching echogenic foci or may reach the liver parenchyma level, described as a "fruit-pulp" pattern.[10]

ULTRASOUND OF MALROTATION AND MIDGUT VOLVULUS
Background

Midgut malrotation is an anomaly of fetal development, resulting in abnormalities in bowel rotation and fixation. Midgut volvulus is a rare, life-threatening complication of midgut malrotation, characterized by the abnormal twisting of the midgut around its mesenteric axis resulting in closed-loop obstruction. Malfixation of the midgut leads to a narrow mesenteric root, which is then prone to volvulus. The incidence of midgut volvulus is not clearly established but has been estimated at approximately 1 in 6000 live births.[11]

Infants with midgut volvulus most commonly present within the first month of life, with the majority presenting within the first year.[12–14] Bilious emesis is the classic symptom associated with midgut volvulus, and hemodynamic instability, abdominal distension, and/or peritonitis may also be present.

Prompt surgical intervention is essential in the management of midgut volvulus to prevent bowel ischemia and necrosis. Surgical treatment typically involves derotation of the twisted bowel followed by assessment for bowel viability, with resection of nonviable bowel, followed by a Ladd procedure to prevent future volvulus. Delayed diagnosis or surgery may result in extensive bowel infarction and development of short bowel syndrome; therefore, rapid diagnosis and intervention are critical.

Diagnostic Performance of Ultrasound

Radiographic and/or fluoroscopic evaluation of the upper gastrointestinal tract has long been the mainstay in the evaluation of midgut volvulus.[15,16] The sonographic diagnosis of midgut volvulus was initially described in the 1980s, but the diagnostic performance of the examination has historically been unclear.[17–19] Only in recent years has increasingly robust evidence supported the use of ultrasound as a potential first-line imaging modality in the evaluation of midgut volvulus.

Ultrasound offers several advantages to fluoroscopy, including being readily available, portable, and lacking ionizing radiation. Many pediatric facilities have more robust sonographer coverage as compared to fluoroscopy coverage, which generally requires an in-house or on-call radiologist, and depending on local institutional models; ultrasound may offer a more expeditious diagnosis compared to fluoroscopy.[20] A recent meta-analysis has demonstrated similar diagnostic performance of ultrasound and fluoroscopy for the evaluation of malrotation with or without midgut volvulus. Ultrasound demonstrated a sensitivity of 94% and specificity of 100%, compared to sensitivity and specificity of 91% and 94% for fluoroscopic upper gastrointestinal (GI) series.[21]

Comparatively, other modalities such as radiography or computed tomography (CT) may sometimes be employed but are less sensitive and expose the patient to ionizing radiation. Radiography is commonly utilized in the workup of the vomiting infant and may demonstrate features of upper gastrointestinal obstruction. However, it is not specific for the diagnosis of midgut volvulus, and radiographs may be normal. CT is rarely obtained but may be used in cases of diagnostic uncertainty or at centers without dedicated pediatric imagers. Diagnostic laparoscopy remains the reference standard for definitive diagnosis and management.

Patient Preparation

No specific patient preparation is needed. Some advocate for enteric fluid administration to improve visualization of the duodenum, which can improve diagnostic accuracy, but at the cost of potentially increasing time to complete the examination if an enteric tube is not already in place.[22]

Ultrasound Scanning Protocol

Ultrasound protocol should utilize a high-frequency linear transducer to assess the superior mesenteric vasculature and the duodenum. The use of a small-footprint microconvex mid-frequency (4–10 MHz) transducer may also be beneficial, especially to apply graded compression as needed to displace bowel gas. The course of the duodenum should be assessed, and the left renal vein can be used as an anatomic landmark when the entirety is not well seen.[23] Cinematic imaging with and without color Doppler imaging should be performed from the origin of the superior mesenteric artery (SMA) to the urinary bladder to assess for abnormal clockwise mesenteric swirling and to assess the orientation of the SMA and superior mesenteric vein (SMV). The expected normal location of the cecum in the right lower quadrant should be assessed[24] (**Table 2**).

Ultrasound Findings

Familiarity with the normal anatomy is crucial. With normal bowel rotation, the third portion of the duodenum has a retroperitoneal course between the aorta and the SMA near the left renal vein level. The SMA should normally be located to the left of the SMV (**Fig. 5** and Videos 1 and 2). Normal counterclockwise swirling of the jejunal branches of the SMV can be seen as a normal variant and should not be confused with midgut volvulus.

Malrotation may be seen with or without midgut volvulus. When malrotation is present, the duodenum is intraperitoneal in location, coursing anterior to the SMA. The SMV can be located anterior or to the left of the SMA. The cecum may be abnormally positioned, or small bowel loops may be seen filling the right lower quadrant.

Ultrasound findings suggestive of concomitant midgut volvulus include the "whirlpool sign," characterized by clockwise swirling of the mesentery around the SMA, correlating with the "corkscrew sign" demonstrated on fluoroscopy (**Fig. 6** and Video 3 and **Fig. 7** and Videos 4 and 5). Features such as bowel wall thickening, dilated duodenum proximal to the volvulus, and absent peristalsis may also be present at ultrasound.[22]

ULTRASOUND FOR CHARACTERIZATION OF NEONATAL LIVER LESIONS

In an infant, the most commonly encountered liver lesions have a nonspecific ultrasound appearance and are congenital hemangioma, infantile hemangiomas, hepatoblastoma, and metastasis.[25] The use of contrast-enhanced ultrasound (CEUS) to definitively characterize liver lesions is increasing because, like for other uses of ultrasound, there is no utilization of ionizing radiation, no need for sedation, and critically ill infants (such as those with large congenital hemangiomas) can be imaged portably.[26] Importantly, most liver lesions encountered in infants do not occur in adult patients; therefore, familiarization with the appearance of each is paramount. In particular, although the term "hemangioma" is used throughout the literature to describe vascular malformations encountered in teenagers and adults, this is a misnomer because these are best characterized as vascular malformations (usually slow flow or venous malformations) based on the current International Society for the Study for Vascular

Table 2
Suggested protocol for the evaluation of infants with suspected malrotation and midgut volvulus

	Structure	Findings Assessed
Grayscale Assessment	Superior mesenteric artery (SMA) and superior mesenteric vein (SMV)	Ensure SMV is located to right of SMA
	1st to 2nd duodenum portions	Evaluate for dilation, raising concern for obstruction if present
	3rd duodenum portion	Ensure retroperitoneal course, completely crossing midline between the SMA and aorta
	Mesenteric pedicle cine	Assessing for clockwise "whirlpool" of volvulus
	Cecum, terminal ileum, and/or appendix	Ensure normal location in right lower abdominal quadrant
Color or Power Doppler assessment	SMA and SMV	Ensure patency. Also, helpful to ensure "whirlpool" is mesentery and vessel rather than intussusception

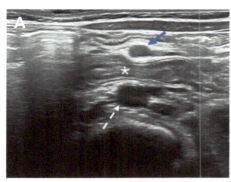
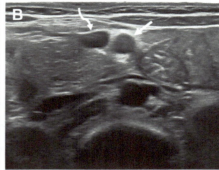

Fig. 5. Normal healthy infant midgut anatomy. (A) Transverse grayscale image demonstrates the normal retroperitoneal course of the third portion of the duodenum (asterisk) between the aorta (dashed arrow) and SMA (solid arrow). (B) Transverse grayscale image more superior, near the origin of the SMA, demonstrating normal orientation with the SMV (curved arrow) located to the right of the SMA (straight arrow). The SMA is identifiable by its typical echogenic halo of fat.

Anomalies classification.[26,27] Congenital and infantile hemangiomas are true hemangiomas and are benign vascular neoplasms. Therefore, the appearance at CEUS in the delayed phase may differ from lesions encountered in older patients.

Background

Liver lesions are uncommon in the general population but are relatively frequently seen incidentally when imaging infants. Liver lesion assessment is the most frequent indication for CEUS because sulfur hexafluoride lipid type-A microspheres (Bracco Diagnostics, Monroe Township, NJ, USA) are Food and Drug Administration approved in the United States for intravenous use to characterize liver lesions in patients of all ages.[28]

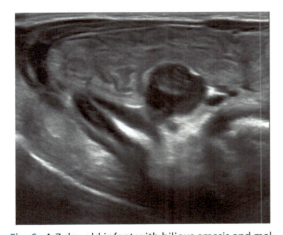

Fig. 6. A 7 day old infant with bilious emesis and malrotation with midgut volvulus. Transverse grayscale image demonstrates absence of cecum/colon in the right lower quadrant, with only small bowel present, supporting a diagnosis of malrotation.

Diagnostic Performance of Ultrasound

Studies have shown the utility of CEUS to distinguish benign from malignant liver lesions in children, with a sensitivity of 84.6% to 100% and specificity of 90.9% to 100%.[29,30]

Patient Preparation and Ultrasound Scanning Protocol

No specific patient preparation is needed. It may be helpful to withhold feeds and then feed the baby during CEUS to help maintain patient immobility and ensure diagnostic arterial phase imaging. The scanning protocol is identical to that recommended by American College of Radiology (ACR) Liver Imaging Reporting and Data System (LI-RADS), with continuous cinematic lesion assessment during the arterial phase and intermittent assessment during delayed phases.[31]

Clinical Features and Ultrasound Findings

Congenital hemangioma

Congenital hemangioma is usually a solitary lesion, is largest in size at birth, and is not associated with cutaneous lesions, unlike infantile hemangiomas. Clinically, patients may present with high-output heart failure due to intralesional shunting and may be critically ill, particularly with large masses. The primary differential diagnosis is hepatoblastoma. At ultrasound, congenital hemangioma typically is heterogeneous in echogenicity, with calcifications possible, and large vessels may be seen. At CEUS, there is globular peripheral hyperenhancement with complete (small lesions) or incomplete (large lesions) fill-in (Fig. 8). There may be washout of internal enhancing areas; however, the peripheral large enhancing vessels should show sustained enhancement in delayed phases, unlike the late

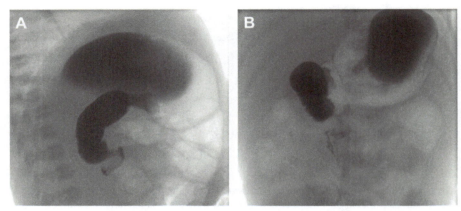

Fig. 7. A 10 day old infant with bilious emesis and malrotation with midgut volvulus. (*A*) Lateral and (*B*) frontal fluoroscopic views show that stomach and proximal duodenum are distended with gas and contrast, with focal transition to collapsed and volvulized mid-duodenum.

portal venous phase washout seen with hepatoblastoma.[28,32] There is currently no treatment of congenital hemangiomas, although embolization of shunts may be attempted if needed.

Infantile hemangiomas

Infantile hemangiomas are not present at birth but rather are seen within the first few weeks to months of life and grow commensurate with the patient over the first years of life. Unlike congenital hemangiomas, infantile hemangiomas are associated with cutaneous infantile hemangiomas, and in fact, when 5 or more cutaneous lesions are present, screening for visceral infantile hemangiomas is recommended. Infantile hemangiomas are typically more homogeneous in appearance than

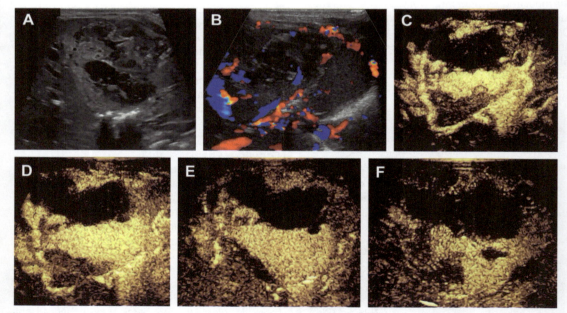

Fig. 8. A 2 day old boy baby delivered preterm at 32 weeks gestational age for nonimmune hydrops fetalis and hepatic congenital hemangioma. (*A*) Transverse grayscale ultrasound demonstrates a heterogeneous mass in the left hepatic lobe, with some vessels seen at color Doppler (*B*). CEUS images at 8 seconds (*C*), 15 seconds (*D*), 1 minute 17 seconds (*E*), and 3 minutes 15 seconds (*F*) following sulfur hexafluoride lipid type-A microsphere contrast injection demonstrate central non-enhancement and large vessels with globular enhancement that remain hyperenhancing compared to adjacent liver.

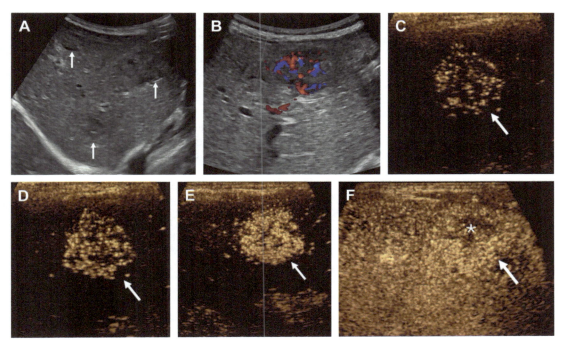

Fig. 9. A 11 month old girl baby with incidental infantile hepatic hemangiomas seen at ultrasound performed due to clinical concern for intussusception. (A) Sagittal grayscale ultrasound demonstrates multiple subtle heterogeneously isoechoic liver lesions (arrows). (B) Transverse color Doppler ultrasound demonstrates hypervascularity. CEUS images at 10 seconds (C), at 10 seconds slightly later (D), 12 seconds (E), and 3 minutes (F) following contrast injection demonstrate very rapid out-to-in enhancement of a representative lesion (arrow), with incomplete central fill-in and some subtle internal washout (asterisk) in delayed phase. Fill-in is so rapid that there is change in enhancement over less than 1 second of imaging.

congenital hemangiomas and are either multifocal or innumerable. At CEUS, there is very rapid peripheral centripetal hyperenhancement, which is often so rapid it may be missed at multiphase CT or MR imaging (**Fig. 9**). There may be hyperenhancement, isoenhancement, or subtle late washout (similar to the appearance of hepatocellular carcinoma).[28] However, the primary differential diagnosis is metastasis. Lack of early, marked washout distinguishes infantile hemangiomas from metastases. When indicated, propranolol is the treatment of choice.

Hepatoblastoma

Hepatoblastoma is the most common primary malignant liver lesion in a young child and should be staged using pretreatment extent of tumor.[33] At CEUS, there is a variable arterial phase appearance;

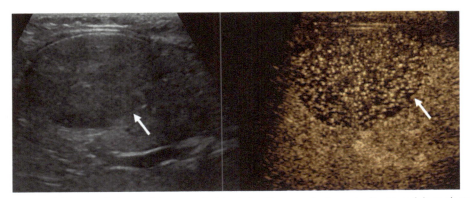

Fig. 10. A 1 year old boy with hepatoblastoma incidentally discovered at renal ultrasound (not shown). Split-screen CEUS image at 2 minutes 14 seconds following contrast injection shows washout of the mass (arrows).

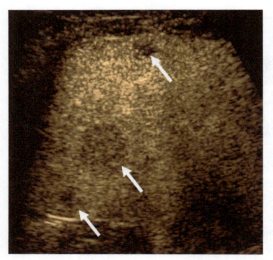

Fig. 11. A 6 month old girl baby with neuroblastoma and hepatic metastases, which demonstrate washout (*arrows*) at 1 minute 17 seconds following contrast injection.

however, there is late portal venous phase washout (Fig. 10) that becomes more pronounced overtime, which is helpful to distinguish from congenital hemangioma.[32] Treatment is based on the Children's Oncology Group recommendations.

Metastases

The most common liver metastases in an infant are from neuroblastoma and Wilms tumor.[26] Like metastases encountered in adult patients, there is a variable appearance of liver metastases at ultrasound and in the arterial phase at CEUS. However, early marked washout at CEUS is characteristic of metastases (Fig. 11) regardless the etiology, which is helpful to distinguish from infantile hemangiomas. Treatment varies depending on the type of primary tumor.

SUMMARY

Ultrasound is an excellent modality to evaluate pediatric patients, and infants in particular, and there are increasing applications in this population. Several of these uses of ultrasound were reviewed, with specific details to help improve the care of infants.

CLINICS CARE POINTS

- In patients with necrotizing enterocolitis (NEC), focal fluid collections, complex ascites, abdominal wall edema, mesenteric edema, pneumoperitoneum, absent bowel peristalsis, bowel dilation, echogenic intraluminal bowel content, absent bowel wall perfusion, and bowel wall abnormalities such as thinning, thickening, abnormal echogenicity, or ill-definition at ultrasound are associated with poor patient outcomes.
- Ultrasound findings of malrotation with midgut volvulus include proximal duodenal dilation and clockwise swirling of bowel and mesentery around the superior mesenteric artery.
- At contrast-enhanced ultrasound (CEUS), congenital hemangiomas can be distinguished from hepatoblastoma by sustained peripheral globular enhancement at delayed imaging. Infantile hemangiomas can be distinguished from metastases by lack of early washout.

DISCLOSURE

The authors have nothing to disclose.

SUPPLEMENTARY DATA

Supplementary data to this article can be found online at https://doi.org/10.1016/j.rcl.2024.07.006.

REFERENCES

1. Cuna AC, Reddy N, Robinson AL, et al. Bowel ultrasound for predicting surgical management of necrotizing enterocolitis: a systematic review and meta-analysis. Pediatr Radiol 2018;48(5):658–66.
2. Neu J, Walker WA. Necrotizing enterocolitis. N Engl J Med 2011;364(3):255–64.
3. Ginglen JG, Butki N. Necrotizing Enterocolitis, . StatPearls. Treasure Island (FL): StatPearls Publishing; 2024.
4. Faingold R, Daneman A, Tomlinson G, et al. Necrotizing enterocolitis: assessment of bowel viability with color Doppler US. Radiology 2005;235(2):587–94.
5. Epelman M, Daneman A, Navarro OM, et al. Necrotizing enterocolitis: review of state-of-the-art imaging findings with pathologic correlation. Radiographics 2007;27(2):285–305.
6. Silva CT, Daneman A, Navarro OM, et al. A prospective comparison of intestinal sonography and abdominal radiographs in a neonatal intensive care unit. Pediatr Radiol 2013;43(11):1453–63.
7. Coursey CA, Hollingsworth CL, Wriston C, et al. Radiographic predictors of disease severity in neonates and infants with necrotizing enterocolitis. AJR Am J Roentgenol 2009;193(5):1408–13.

8. Le Cacheux C, Daneman A, Pierro A, et al. Association of new sonographic features with outcome in neonates with necrotizing enterocolitis. Pediatr Radiol 2023;53(9):1894–902.
9. May LA, Costa J, Hossain J, et al. The role of an abbreviated ultrasound in the evaluation of necrotizing enterocolitis. Pediatr Radiol 2024. https://doi.org/10.1007/s00247-024-05912-w.
10. Pan HB, Huang JS, Yang TL, et al. Hepatic portal venous gas in ultrasonogram–benign or noxious. Ultrasound Med Biol 2007;33(8):1179–83.
11. Alani M, Rentea RM. Midgut Malrotation, . StatPearls. Treasure Island (FL): StatPearls Publishing; 2024.
12. Aboagye J, Goldstein SD, Salazar JH, et al. Age at presentation of common pediatric surgical conditions: Reexamining dogma. J Pediatr Surg 2014; 49(6):995–9.
13. Pickhardt PJ, Bhalla S. Intestinal malrotation in adolescents and adults: spectrum of clinical and imaging features. AJR Am J Roentgenol 2002;179(6): 1429–35.
14. Torres AM, Ziegler MM. Malrotation of the intestine. World J Surg May-Jun 1993;17(3):326–31.
15. Ladd WE. Congenital Obstruction of the Bile Ducts. Ann Surg 1935;102(4):742–51.
16. Simpson AJ, Leonidas JC, Krasna IH, et al. Roentgen diagnosis of midgut malrotation: value of upper gastrointestinal radiographic study. J Pediatr Surg 1972;7(2):243–52.
17. Cohen HL, Haller JO, Mestel AL, et al. Neonatal duodenum: fluid-aided US examination. Radiology 1987;164(3):805–9.
18. Gaines PA, Saunders AJ, Drake D. Midgut malrotation diagnosed by ultrasound. Clin Radiol 1987; 38(1):51–3.
19. Hayden CK Jr, Boulden TF, Swischuk LE, et al. Sonographic demonstration of duodenal obstruction with midgut volvulus. AJR Am J Roentgenol 1984;143(1): 9–10.
20. Nguyen HN, Sammer MB, Bales B, et al. Time-Driven Activity-Based Cost Comparison of Three Imaging Pathways for Suspected Midgut Volvulus in Children. J Am Coll Radiol 2020;17(12):1563–70.
21. Nguyen HN, Kulkarni M, Jose J, et al. Ultrasound for the diagnosis of malrotation and volvulus in children and adolescents: a systematic review and meta-analysis. Arch Dis Child 2021;106(12):1171–8.
22. Nguyen HN, Navarro OM, Bloom DA, et al. Ultrasound for Midgut Malrotation and Midgut Volvulus: AJR Expert Panel Narrative Review. AJR Am J Roentgenol 2022;218(6):931–9.
23. Le Cacheux C, Daneman A. Left renal vein as an anatomical landmark for the evaluation of the midgut anatomy. Pediatr Radiol 2024. https://doi.org/10.1007/s00247-024-05923-7.
24. Nguyen HN, Sammer MBK, Ditzler MG, et al. Transition to ultrasound as the first-line imaging modality for midgut volvulus: keys to a successful roll-out. Pediatr Radiol 2021;51(4):506–15.
25. Vasireddi AK, Leo ME, Squires JH. Magnetic resonance imaging of pediatric liver tumors. Pediatr Radiol 2021. https://doi.org/10.1007/s00247-021-05058-z.
26. Squires JH, McCarville MB. Contrast-Enhanced Ultrasound in Children: Implementation and Key Diagnostic Applications. AJR Am J Roentgenol 2021. https://doi.org/10.2214/AJR.21.25713.
27. Squires JH, Fetzer DT, Dillman JR. Practical Contrast Enhanced Liver Ultrasound. Radiol Clin North Am 2022;60(5):717–30.
28. El-Ali AM, McCormick A, Thakrar D, et al. Contrast-Enhanced Ultrasound of Congenital and Infantile Hemangiomas: Preliminary Results From a Case Series. AJR Am J Roentgenol 2020;214(3):658–64.
29. Wang G, Xie X, Chen H, et al. Development of a pediatric liver CEUS criterion to classify benign and malignant liver lesions in pediatric patients: a pilot study. Eur Radiol 2021;31(9):6747–57.
30. Chen M, Qiu M, Liu Y, et al. Utility of the pediatric liver contrast-enhanced ultrasound criteria in differentiating malignant and benign multifocal lesions. Pediatr Radiol 2023;53(10):2004–12.
31. v2017 ACR CEUS LI-RADS, Available at: https://www.acr.org/-/media/ACR/Files/RADS/LI-RADS/CEUS-LI-RADS-2017-Core.pdf. (Accessed August 13 2024).
32. Anupindi SA, Biko DM, Ntoulia A, et al. Contrast-enhanced US Assessment of Focal Liver Lesions in Children. Radiographics 2017;37(6):1632–47.
33. Schooler GR, Squires JH, Alazraki A, et al. Pediatric Hepatoblastoma, Hepatocellular Carcinoma, and Other Hepatic Neoplasms: Consensus Imaging Recommendations from American College of Radiology Pediatric Liver Reporting and Data System (LI-RADS) Working Group. Radiology 2020;296(3):493–7.

Approach to Evaluating Superficial Soft Tissue Masses by Ultrasound

Pamela Garza-Báez, MD[a], Sandra J. Allison, MD[b,c], Levon N. Nazarian, MD[a,*]

KEYWORDS

- Ultrasound • Soft-tissue lesion • Soft-tissue tumor

KEY POINTS

- This article presents a systematic approach to the ultrasound (US) evaluation of superficial soft tissue masses.
- The clinical history, the location of the lesion and its detailed characterization by US usually leads to a confident diagnosis.
- If there are inconclusive or suspicious findings by US, correlative imaging or a percutaneous biopsy should be performed.

 Video content accompanies this article at http://www.radiologic.theclinics.com.

INTRODUCTION

Sonographic evaluation of superficial soft tissue masses is a common diagnostic challenge in clinical practice. A systematic approach to these masses enables effective diagnosis and minimizes errors. This article presents the authors' preferred approach based on lesion location, grayscale appearance and Doppler features. In many cases a specific diagnosis is possible, but when US findings are inconclusive, US-guided biopsy provides a safe and accurate way to establish the etiology of the mass.

GENERAL APPROACH TO A SUSPECTED SOFT TISSUE MASS

For US imagers as in all of medicine, clinical history is of utmost importance. Before the transducer is placed on the patient, the first step is to take a thorough history about the mass. If the mass is palpable, have the patient point to the area of interest. Examine the area of the mass for skin color changes, dilated vessels, or other findings in a well-illuminated environment. If the mass is not palpable, consult the correlative imaging that triggered the US such as computed tomography, MRI, or PET. It is important to know whether the mass is painful and whether it is growing or stable in size. Gather potentially relevant medical history, including prior malignancy, trauma, surgery, anticoagulation, or systemic diseases.

IMAGING TECHNIQUE

US scanning should utilize a high-frequency linear-array transducer, typically operating within a

---

[a] Department of Radiology, Hospital of the University of Pennsylvania, Philadelphia, PA, USA; [b] Georgetown University School of Medicine, Washington, DC, USA; [c] Washington Radiology, Washington, DC, USA
* Corresponding author. Department of Radiology, Hospital of the University of Pennsylvania, 3737 Market Street, Mailbox #4, Philadelphia, PA 19104.
E-mail address: levon.nazarian@pennmedicine.upenn.edu

frequency range of 12 to 24 MHz. Deeper masses may require a curved linear transducer in the 5 to 9 MHz range to enable better penetration. Generally, the transmit frequency should be set to the highest level which ensures clear visualization of the complete lesion and its surrounding tissues. For larger masses, extended field-of-view technology may be helpful to include the entire mass on a single image to show the relationship of the mass to adjacent structures and enable more precise measurements (**Fig. 1**). Most imaging can be performed with a standard acoustic coupling gel. For very superficial masses a gel stand-off pad can be used, but it is the authors' preference to float the transducer on a large dollop of gel.

The depth of the US image should be minimized while still including the mass and surrounding tissues. If applicable, focal zone(s) should be set at the level of the mass. The gain and time gain compensation curve should be set appropriately—the gain should be low enough to minimize artifacts but high enough so that low-level echoes in the mass are not missed. Once the grayscale characteristics of the mass have been evaluated, the next step is to assess the vascularity in and around the lesion by Doppler. Number and pattern of blood vessels should be assessed by color and/or power Doppler, which should be optimized as follows: depth should be minimized as for grayscale imaging; the color box should be the smallest that still includes the mass; color gain should be set by increasing the gain until there is color noise, then dialing it down slowly until noise first appears; and if applicable, focal zone(s) should be placed at the level of the mass. To optimize detection of slow flow, the scale and wall filter should be at the lowest level that does not cause unacceptable color noise. Spectral Doppler is an important adjunct to confirm the presence of flow within the mass and determine whether it is arterial and/or venous.

Once the mass is identified, it should be measured in 3 dimensions. The longest axis of the mass—which may not necessarily correspond to the long axis of the body—should be measured first followed by the orthogonal dimension on the same image. The transducer should then be rotated 90° and the width measured. Using the same measurement technique each time will facilitate a comparison of the mass size on any subsequent studies. If the mass is not measured the same way each time, the examiner may receive a false impression of either stability or growth.

DIAGNOSTIC PATHWAY

The first step in determining the etiology of the mass is localizing it to its compartment(s) of origin—skin, subcutaneous tissues, muscle, bone—as well as determining whether the mass arises from a specific musculoskeletal structure such as joint, bursa, nerve, tendon, ligament, or fibrocartilage such as labrum or meniscus. Placing the mass in a compartment requires paying attention to the anatomic layers visible on a US image (**Fig. 2**). The beam first encounters the epidermis which creates a specular reflection but is difficult to resolve with routine scanning frequencies. The first discernible layer is generally the dermis which is hyperechoic to subcutaneous fat, which is the next layer. The subcutaneous fat layer is of varying thickness, is normally hypoechoic relative to the dermis and muscle, and often has hyperechoic septations.[1] It is a common misconception that fat is hyperechoic on US, but there is nothing intrinsically echogenic about fat. Echoes are created by interfaces between tissues of differing acoustic impedances. Since subcutaneous fat is relatively homogenous, normal fat contains few echoes. Separating the fat from the muscle is hyperechoic fascia of varying thickness. Deep to

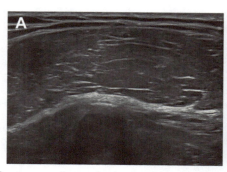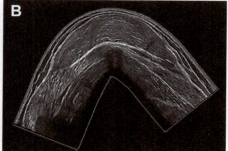

Fig. 1. Subcutaneous lipoma in the shoulder on standard (*A*) and (*B*) extended field of view (EFOV) sonography. The EFOV image allows the entire mass to be depicted, so that it can be more accurately measured and its relationship to the regional anatomy better defined.

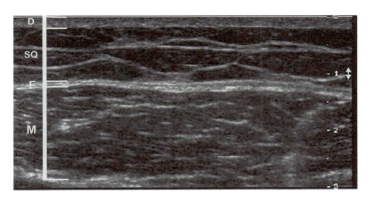

Fig. 2. Normal soft tissues on sonography of the back. D, Dermis; F, Fascia; M, Muscle; SQ, Subcutaneous tissue.

this fascia is muscle which has a typical pattern of hypoechoic muscle bundles separated by hyperechoic fibroadipose septa in a pennate pattern.[2]

The echogenicity of the mass should then be characterized as hypoechoic, isoechoic, hyperechoic, or mixed. Because these terms are relative, there needs to be a standard of reference. The authors recommend comparing the echogenicity to muscle since a regional muscle can almost always be imaged in the same field of view. Next, the borders should be assessed: are the borders well-defined or do they blend in almost imperceptibly with surrounding tissues? It should also be noted whether the mass attenuates the US beam, has no perceptible effect on the beam, or causes acoustic enhancement.

IS THE MASS CYSTIC OR SOLID?

One of the most important functions of US is to determine whether a mass is cystic or solid. Although this task sounds straightforward, it can be tricky. The first thing to do is to evaluate the grayscale appearance. On average, cystic lesions tend to be relatively less echogenic than solid masses, but there are many important exceptions. Cystic masses can have echoes within them because of contents such as hemorrhage, pus, or keratin (Fig. 3). Conversely, solid masses can be relatively hypoechoic or even anechoic if their cellular content is homogeneous with few acoustic interfaces (Fig. 4A).[3] Because the grayscale appearance alone is unreliable, we may need to rely on other clues. Compression should be applied by the transducer in real time. A mass that changes its morphology with compression may be fluid-containing, especially if the internal echoes swirl in real time (Fig. 5, Video 1). The next piece of data is the Doppler evaluation. Doppler flow is more helpful if it is present than if it is absent: internal flow confirms that the mass is at least partially solid (Fig. 4B), whereas flow may not be detectable within a solid mass if the flow is too slow, the internal vessels are too small, and/or the Doppler technique is suboptimal.[4] Spectral Doppler will confirm the types of flow within the mass, arterial and/or venous. However, the shape of the arterial waveform has no predictive value regarding whether the mass is benign or malignant (Fig. 4C; Fig. 8B).[5]

A crucial fact to understand about soft tissue masses is that acoustic enhancement does not mean the mass is cystic. Because acoustic enhancement is commonly used to differentiate cystic from solid masses in organs such as the kidneys, liver, and ovaries, many radiologists incorrectly assume that this finding is also applicable to superficial masses. Unfortunately, that is not the case. In fact, in one series of superficial metastases from melanoma, 71% of the lesions had acoustic enhancement.[3] Homogenous solid masses often attenuate the US beam less than the more heterogeneous adjacent soft tissues. Thus, acoustic enhancement must never be used to differentiate cystic from solid masses (Fig. 6).[3]

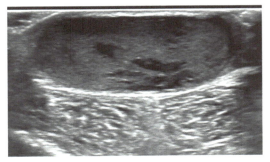

Fig. 3. Epidermoid cyst in the calf. Sonography demonstrates diffuse internal echoes due to keratin accumulation, the so-called "pseudotestis" appearance. There was no internal flow on color Doppler.

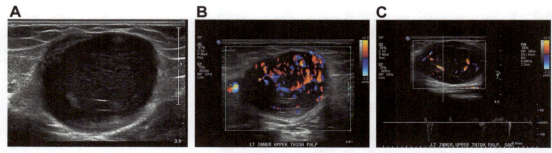

Fig. 4. Soft tissue lymphoma presenting as a subcutaneous thigh mass. Grayscale appearance (*A*) is hypoechoic with low level internal echoes. (*B*) Extensive flow on color Doppler confirms solid nature of the mass. (*C*) Arterial waveform obtained on spectral Doppler. Note the high resistance flow despite the malignant nature of the mass.

DOES THE MASS CONTAIN FAT?

For solid masses the next step is to decide whether the mass is fatty because lipomas are so common, especially in the subcutaneous tissues. The echogenicity of lipomas ranges from hyperechoic to isoechoic to hypoechoic with respect to muscle depending on how many interfaces are created by other components such as fibrous tissue.[6] Lipomas characteristically contain linear echogenic septations that are oriented along the long axis of the lipoma, usually parallel to the skin (**Fig. 7**). There may be a defined capsule around the lipoma, or the borders may blend in with the adjacent soft tissues and be difficult to delineate. When applicable, bilateral comparison can be helpful to differentiate a normal lobulation of fat from a lipoma. Note that on color Doppler lipomas tend to have little or no flow.[6,7] However, there may be exceptions in which a lipoma demonstrates an atypical amount of increased flow (**Fig. 8**). Although the vast majority of fatty masses are lipomas, well-differentiated liposarcomas may look similar to lipomas. Features raising suspicion of liposarcoma include recent rapid growth, deep location (ie, not subcutaneous), and prominent, irregularly branching vessels on color Doppler.[8]

Fat necrosis can present as a palpable subcutaneous nodule virtually anywhere in the body. The nodule may or may not be painful. There is often a history of blunt trauma, surgery, or local injections.[9] On US, subcutaneous fat necrosis has a variable appearance—it can appear uniformly hyperechoic or have a hypoechoic center with peripheral hyperechogenicity (**Fig. 9**). The borders are ill-defined and blend in with the adjacent subcutaneous fat. There is typically no significant vascularity on color Doppler. Compared to lipomas, there tends to be less mass effect on the adjacent soft tissues.

DOES THE MASS ARISE FROM A MUSCULOSKELETAL STRUCTURE?

The examiner should scrutinize the mass for any connection to a musculoskeletal structure since that connection may be the key to the diagnosis. Common examples include the following.

Joints/Bursae

Popliteal (Baker's) cyst

Baker's cyst is a distended bursa that occurs at the medial posterior aspect of the popliteal fossa. To avoid diagnostic errors, it is important to call a

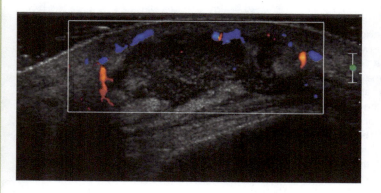

Fig. 5. Infected subcutaneous hematoma in a hockey player who was hit by a puck in the leg. Hypoechoic collection with peripheral color Doppler flow and increased echogenicity of the subcutaneous fat likely reflecting edema.

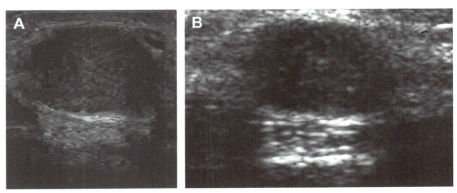

Fig. 6. 2 solid masses that exhibit increased acoustic through transmission. (A) Schwannoma in the hand and (B) Subcutaneous melanoma metastasis in the thigh.

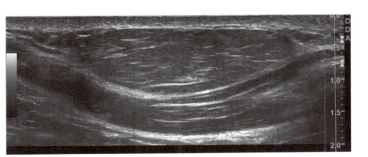

Fig. 7. Subcutaneous lipoma in the supraclavicular space. There was no internal flow on color Doppler.

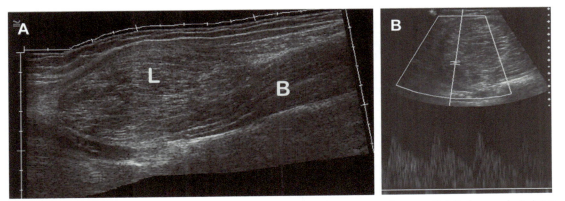

Fig. 8. Lipoma within the biceps brachii muscle. (A) Longitudinal sonogram shows a slightly hyperechoic intramuscular mass with the parallel echogenic lines typical of lipoma. (B) Low resistance arterial flow within the mass on Doppler. Because of the intramuscular location and internal flow, the mass was removed and was benign. L, Lipoma, B, Biceps brachii.

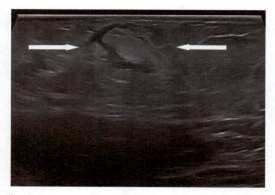

Fig. 9. Fat necrosis presenting as a painless nodule in the arm of a patient with acute myelogenous leukemia. Note that the area is mainly hyperechoic with a hypoechoic component (arrows), and the margins blend seamlessly in with the adjacent subcutaneous fat. Because of the history, the nodule was removed, and fat necrosis confirmed histologically.

Baker's cyst only if it arises between the medial head of the gastrocnemius and the semimembranosus tendon[10] (Fig. 10). Baker's cysts communicate with the knee joint over 50% of the time, so any process that occurs in the knee joint can extend into the Baker's cyst including joint effusions, synovitis, intraarticular bodies, or, rarely, infection.[11,12] A palpable mass in the medial popliteal fossa with typical morphology has no differential diagnosis. However, a popliteal fossa mass without the typical morphology needs to be regarded with suspicion (Fig. 11).

Distended iliopsoas bursa
Analogous to the Baker's cyst in the knee, the iliopsoas bursa commonly communicates with the hip joint and can present as a palpable mass.[13] This bursa also has a typical location: when distended the bursa extends posterior to the common femoral artery and vein at the level of the acetabulum (Fig. 12).[14] More inferiorly the bursa can track along the iliopsoas tendon down to its insertion on the lesser trochanter, where the bursa abruptly ends. Similar to the Baker's cyst the distended iliopsoas bursa is typically anechoic, but can also be filled with thick, echogenic material (see Fig. 12). It can even become so large that it presents as a palpable mass. A distended iliopsoas bursa is generally associated with hip arthritis or iliopsoas tendon pathology, especially in patients who have had a hip replacement.[13,15]

Ganglion cysts or synovial cysts
Ganglion cysts are common in the wrist/hand and ankle/foot but can occur anywhere in the body. Ganglion cysts present as firm nodules that can wax and wane in size and may or may not be painful. When they arise from the volar wrist they can even present as a pulsatile mass if they are deep to the radial artery. Ganglion cysts are most commonly anechoic, either unilocular or multilocular. When a ganglion cyst contains internal echoes, it may be difficult to distinguish from a hypoechoic solid nodule. In such cases, establishing communication to an adjacent joint space or tendon sheath can confirm the diagnosis and help guide surgical resection (Figs. 13 and 14). Synovial cysts are similar in appearance to ganglion cysts but differ in their wall composition and in their contents.[16] Ganglion cysts are filled with a thick, gelatinous material and are relatively non-compressible, while synovial cysts are filled with less viscous fluid extending from the nearby joint and tend to be more compressible.[16] Because they can look identical, whether a cyst is a synovial cyst or ganglion cyst can sometimes be determined by ease of aspiration. There are also characteristic locations where synovial cysts occur, for example, superficial to the acromioclavicular joint (Fig. 15). Cysts can also arise in relation to tears of fibrocartilaginous structures, most common being labral tears in the hip or shoulder or meniscal tears in the knee and are referred to as paralabral or parameniscal cysts, respectively (Fig. 16A, B).

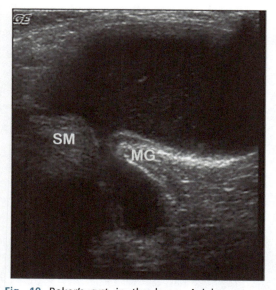

Fig. 10. Baker's cyst in the knee. Axial sonogram shows the origin between the medial head of the gastrocnemius and the semimembranosus tendon. MG, Medial gastrocnemius; SM, Semimembranosus tendon.

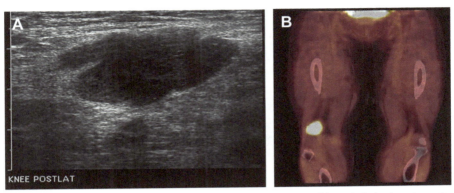

Fig. 11. Recurrent lymphoma in the popliteal space. (A) Axial sonogram. Although Baker's cyst can have internal echoes, this mass is in the wrong location. It is lateral in the popliteal fossa instead of medial, and it does not have the typical anatomy shown in Fig. 10. (B) Coronal PET/CT confirms the hypermetabolic nature.

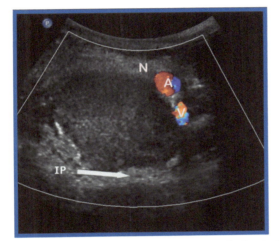

Fig. 12. Distended iliopsoas bursa. Axial sonogram with color Doppler at the level of the right acetabulum shows the distended bursa with diffuse internal echoes. The bursa is in its typical location posterior to the neurovascular bundle. A, Common femoral artery; IP, Iliopsoas tendon; N, Common femoral nerve; V, Common femoral vein.

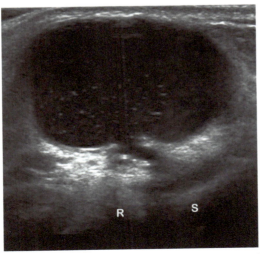

Fig. 13. Volar wrist ganglion with communication to the underlying radioscaphoid joint. R, Radial head; S, Scaphoid.

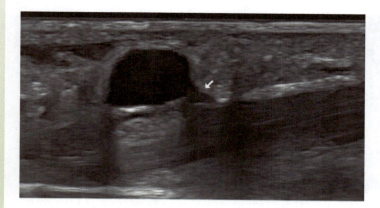

Fig. 14. Ganglion at the volar aspect of the fourth finger arising from the flexor tendon sheath (arrow).

Nerves

Nerve sheath tumors such as neurofibromas or schwannomas characteristically appear as hypoechoic, relatively homogeneous solid masses of varying vascularity. The key to the diagnosis is observing nerve fibers entering and exiting the long axis of the mass, either centrally or eccentrically (Fig. 17). The nerve fibers should be traced to determine which nerve the mass is arising from, understanding that tiny cutaneous nerves may be difficult to trace.[17]

Muscles

Muscle injuries can present as palpable masses either acutely or chronically. Palpable masses at the time of the injury usually represent intra- and/or intermuscular hematomas. Acute hematomas tend to be isoechoic to muscle, but as the hematoma liquefies it becomes more hypoechoic (Figs. 18 and 19). With time, a hematoma can reabsorb, evolve into a seroma, organize and become fibrotic or less commonly ossify, known as myositis ossificans[18] (Fig. 20). Chronic high-grade muscle tears can also present as a palpable mass. The patient may or may not recall the injury. In our experience, the mass is usually due to the patient or physician palpating the healthy, normally contractile muscle that forms a "hill" next to the "valley" which is composed of scarred, atrophic muscle representing the chronic injury (Fig. 21).

The major differential diagnosis for muscle hematoma is a muscle neoplasm. A history of recent trauma suggests hematoma, but occasionally the trauma history is incidental, that is, the trauma draws attention to a pre-existing mass. Neoplasms tend to be better defined than acute muscle hematomas on grayscale and can contain increased vascularity on color Doppler (Fig. 22). In contrast, acute muscle hematomas are more likely to blend in with the adjacent edematous muscle fibers, and if increased Doppler flow is present it tends to be in the adjacent soft tissues, not centrally within the hematoma itself. When differentiation between hematoma and muscle neoplasm is difficult, follow-up US imaging should be performed since hematomas decrease in size and evolve in appearance over time. Correlation

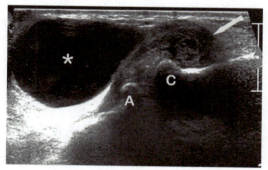

Fig. 15. Synovial cyst (asterisk) arising from the right acromioclavicular joint. The cyst presented as a painless palpable mass. C, Clavicle; A, Acromion; Arrow, Synovial thickening in AC joint.

Approach to Evaluating Soft Tissue Masses

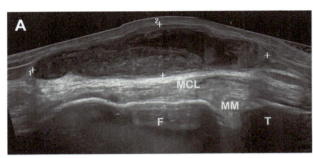
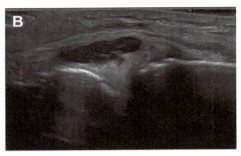

Fig. 16. Parameniscal cyst (A) presenting as a large mass in at the medial knee (between cursors). In (B) the connection to the medial meniscus is demonstrated. T, tibia, F, Femur, MM, Medial meniscus, MCL, Medial collateral ligament.

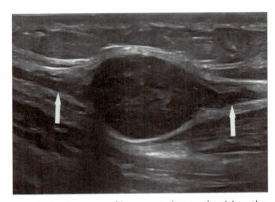

Fig. 17. Sural nerve schwannoma. Note the nerve fibers entering and exiting the nerve (arrows).

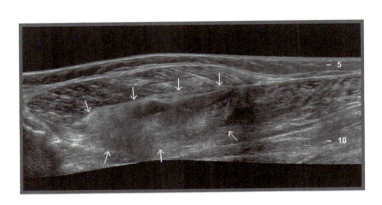

Fig. 18. Acute traumatic hematoma in the soleus muscle (arrows). Note that the hematoma is mainly hyperechoic to the normal muscle fibers, with small isoechoic and hypoechoic components.

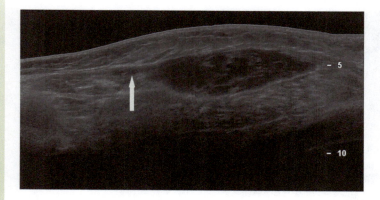

Fig. 19. Subacute hematoma in the gastrocnemius muscle secondary to a muscle tear. The sonogram was performed approximately 2 weeks after the injury. The hematoma is more hypoechoic and well defined than in Fig. 18, and the associated muscle tear is evident (*arrow*).

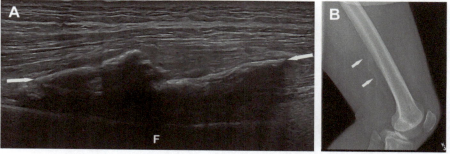

Fig. 20. Myositis ossificans presenting as a biceps femoris mass in this 73-year-old man. (*A*) Longitudinal sonogram shows the echogenic ossification (between *arrows*) with acoustic shadowing. (*B*) Radiograph confirms the diagnosis (*arrows*). F, Femur.

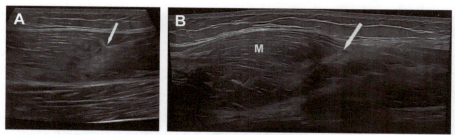

Fig. 21. Chronic rectus femoris tear in this 22-year-old female soccer player with a history of pulled muscle in the thigh. The patient presented for evaluation of a painless mass. (*A*) Longitudinal sonogram shows a contracted hyperechoic scar tissue from prior injury (*arrow*). The palpable "mass" (M) represents the normally contractile muscle fibers at the cephalad edge of the tear (*arrow*) accentuated by muscle contraction against resistance (*B*).

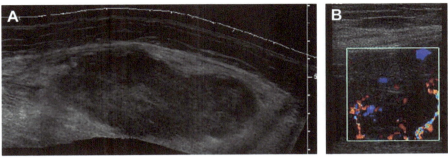

Fig. 22. Biceps sarcoma mistaken clinically for a biceps muscle tear because of arm swelling (A) Longitudinal extended field of view sonogram demonstrates a well-defined hypoechoic intramuscular mass. The mass was nontender. (B) Color Doppler shows irregular internal vascularity.

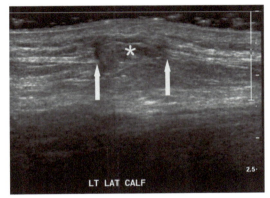

Fig. 23. Muscle hernia (*asterisk*) presenting as a painless calf mass. Longitudinal sonogram shows muscle fibers protruding through a fascial defect (between *arrows*).

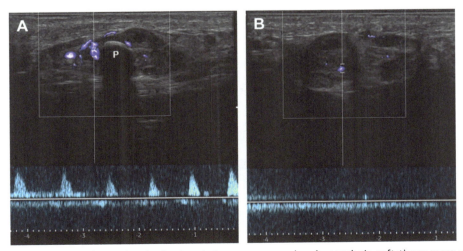

Fig. 24. Arteriovenous malformation in the hand. Sonogram reveals a hypoechoic soft tissue mass with cystic spaces, a phlebolith, and both arterial (A) and venous (B) flow. P, Phlebolith.

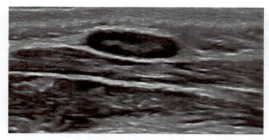

Fig. 25. Normal cervical lymph node.

with MRI can also be helpful in making this distinction.[12]

Injuries to the fascial envelope over the muscle can lead to muscle hernias, which can present as masses that may or may not be painful. The key to the diagnosis is identifying the discontinuity of the fascial layer and showing the muscle tissue that protrudes through the defect. Muscle hernias in the lower extremity may only be evident if the patient stands or contracts their leg muscles. As in hernias elsewhere in the body, the examiner should try to reduce the muscle hernia with probe pressure (Fig. 23, Video 2).[19]

Skin

A wide array of skin lesions can be encountered on US, but a full description is beyond the scope of this article. Because the epidermoid cyst is so common, it should always be considered when there is a well-defined mass located in the dermis and subcutaneous tissues. These cysts are typically hypoechoic but can be more echogenic and heterogeneous if they contain a large amount of keratin, even displaying a "pseudotestis" pattern (see Fig. 3). There is typically no internal flow on Doppler US images.[20,21]

IS THE MASS VASCULAR IN ORIGIN?

Vascular malformations can look nondescript on grayscale but should always be considered when there are prominent vascular spaces and/or phleboliths. On physical examination, there may be bluish or reddish discoloration of the overlying skin. To guide management, it is important to evaluate the amount of flow on color Doppler and to use spectral Doppler to determine whether the flow is arterial and/or venous (Fig. 24). Low-flow vascular malformations include mainly venous, lymphatic, and mixed malformations, whereas lesions that have arterial waveforms are considered high-flow malformations. These include arteriovenous malformations and arteriovenous fistulas. MRI correlation can be done for a broad overview of the vascular extent, the anatomic relationship with adjacent structures, and confirmation of sonographic findings.[22]

IS THE MASS A LYMPH NODE?

Both normal and abnormal lymph nodes can present as palpable masses, so it is important to have a strategy to differentiate benign from malignant lymph nodes. Benign lymph nodes tend to have an oval shape, defined by Solbiati as a length-to-anteroposterior ratio greater than 2.0[23] (Fig. 25. The node should have a homogenous echotexture, uniform thickness, and preserved echogenic hilum noting that certain lymph nodes, particularly in the cervical chain, have a small hilum. Color Doppler flow in benign lymph nodes, if present, enters at the hilum and has a regular branching pattern within the node parenchyma Conversely, malignant lymph nodes often exhibit a rounder appearance, more heterogeneity of the node parenchyma, and/or uneven

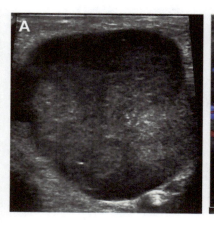
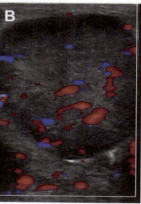

Fig. 26. Malignant inguinal lymph node on (A) grayscale and (B) color Doppler.

thickening. The echogenic hilum is frequently narrowed or obliterated (**Fig. 26**A). On color Doppler, the vessels in malignant nodes often have irregular branching patterns and uneven distribution within the node (**Fig. 26**B). These vessels also tend to enter the node through its periphery rather than through the hilum.[24]

SHOULD THE MASS BE BIOPSIED?

US-guided biopsy is a very important tool because the grayscale and color Doppler characteristics of masses are often nonspecific. When in doubt, percutaneous biopsy is a very safe and effective method for diagnosis.[25]

Figure: Flow chart of ultrasound evaluation of soft tissue masses.

CLINICS CARE POINTS

- Key to differential diagnosis: specific anatomic location.
- Joint and tendon: benign lesion.
- Bursa: unilocular and compressible.
- Ganglion: unilocular or multilocular and not compressible.
- Malignancy: hypoechoic, heterogeneous with blood flow.

DISCLOSURE

The authors have nothing to disclose.

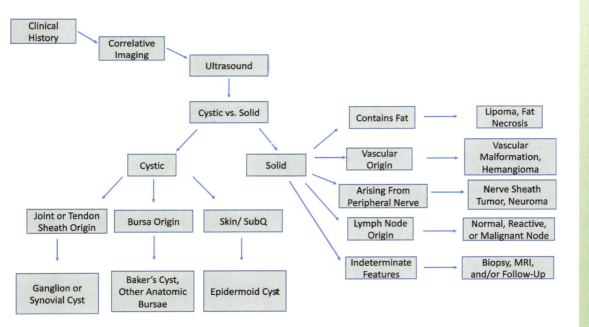

SUMMARY

US is useful in the differential diagnosis of a wide array of superficial soft tissue masses. Applying the systematic approach outlined in this paper can lead to a confident diagnosis in many cases. When US results are inconclusive, and the mass is potentially neoplastic, US-guided biopsy can be an important next step in obtaining a definitive diagnosis. US should have a central role in evaluating superficial masses, leading to effective treatment strategies and improved patient outcomes.

SUPPLEMENTARY DATA

Supplementary data to this article can be found online at https://doi.org/10.1016/j.rcl.2024.08.004.

REFERENCES

1. Mlosek RK, Malinowska S. Ultrasound image of the skin, apparatus and imaging basics. J Ultrason 2013;13(53):212–21.
2. Peetrons P. Ultrasound of muscles. Eur Radiol 2002; 12(1):35–43.

3. Nazarian LN, Alexander AA, Kurtz AB, et al. Superficial melanoma metastases: appearances on gray-scale and color Doppler sonography. AJR Am J Roentgenol 1998;170(2):459–63.
4. Alexander AA, Nazarian LN, Capuzzi DM Jr, et al. Color Doppler sonographic detection of tumor flow in superficial melanoma metastases: histologic correlation. J Ultrasound Med 1998;17(2):123–6.
5. Kaushik S, Miller TT, Nazarian LN, et al. Spectral Doppler sonography of musculoskeletal soft tissue masses. J Ultrasound Med 2003;22(12):1333–6.
6. Wagner JM, Lee KS, Rosas H, et al. Accuracy of sonographic diagnosis of superficial masses. J Ultrasound Med 2013;32(8):1443–50.
7. Jacobson JA, Middleton WD, Allison SJ, et al. Ultrasonography of superficial soft-tissue masses: society of radiologists in ultrasound consensus conference statement. Radiology 2022;304(1):18–30.
8. Shimamori N, Kishino T, Okabe N, et al. Discrimination of well-differentiated liposarcoma from benign lipoma on sonography: an uncontrolled retrospective study. J Med Ultrason 2020;47(4):617–23.
9. Walsh M, Jacobson JA, Kim SM, et al. Sonography of fat necrosis involving the extremity and torso with magnetic resonance imaging and histologic correlation. J Ultrasound Med 2008;27(12):1751–7.
10. Ward EE, Jacobson JA, Fessell DP, et al. Sonographic detection of Baker's cysts: comparison with MR imaging. AJR Am J Roentgenol 2001;176(2):373–80.
11. Handy JR. Popliteal cysts in adults: a review. Semin Arthritis Rheum 2001;31(2):108–18.
12. Carra BJ, Bui-Mansfield LT, O'Brien SD, et al. Sonography of musculoskeletal soft-tissue masses: techniques, pearls, and pitfalls. AJR Am J Roentgenol 2014;202(6):1281–90.
13. Wunderbaldinger P, Bremer C, Schellenberger E, et al. Imaging features of iliopsoas bursitis. Eur Radiol 2002;12(2):409–15.
14. Johnston CA, Wiley JP, Lindsay DM, et al. Iliopsoas bursitis and tendinitis. A review. Sports Med 1998;25(4):271–83.
15. Meaney JF, Cassar-Pullicino VN, Etherington R, et al. Ilio-psoas bursa enlargement. Clin Radiol 1992;45(3):161–8.
16. Giard MC, Pineda C. Ganglion cyst versus synovial cyst? Ultrasound characteristics through a review of the literature. Rheumatol Int 2015;35(4):597–605.
17. Jacobson JA, Wilson TJ, Yang LJ. Sonography of common peripheral nerve disorders with clinical correlation. J Ultrasound Med 2016;35(4):683–93.
18. Paoletta M, Moretti A, Liguori S, et al. Ultrasound imaging in sport-related muscle injuries: pitfalls and opportunities. Medicina (Kaunas) 2021;57(10):1040.
19. Beggs I. Sonography of muscle hernias. AJR Am J Roentgenol 2003;180(2):395–9.
20. Hoang VT, Trinh CT, Nguyen CH, et al. Overview of epidermoid cyst. Eur J Radiol Open 2019;6:291–301.
21. Huang Chung-Cheng, Ko Sheung-Fat, Huang Hsuan-Ying, et al. Epidermal cysts in the superficial soft tissue. J Ultrasound Med 2011;30(1):11–7.
22. Donnelly LF, Adams DM, Bisset GS 3rd. Vascular malformations and hemangiomas: a practical approach in a multidisciplinary clinic. AJR Am J Roentgenol 2000;174(3):597–608.
23. Solbiati L, Cioffi V, Ballarati E. Ultrasonography of the neck. Radiol Clin North Am 1992;30(5):941–54.
24. Ahuja AT. Ultrasound of malignant cervical lymph nodes. Cancer Imag 2008;8(1):48–56.
25. Vasilevska Nikodinovska V, Ivanoski S, Kostadinova-Kunovska S, et al. Ultrasound-guided biopsy of musculoskeletal soft-tissue tumors: basic principles, usefulness and limitations. J Ultrason 2022;22(89):109–16.

Ultrasound Evaluation of the Abdominal Aorta and Mesenteric Arteries

Gowthaman Gunabushanam, MD[a,*], Michelle LaVonne Robbin, MD[b], Leslie Millar Scoutt, MD[a]

KEYWORDS

- Aorta • Abdominal aortic aneurysm • Endoleak • Chronic mesenteric ischemia
- Median arcuate ligament syndrome • Ultrasound

KEY POINTS

- Diameter threshold of 3 cm, or 1.5 times the diameter of the more proximal abdominal aorta, is used to diagnose abdominal aortic aneurysm.
- Treatment using endovascular aneurysm repair or open surgical repair is indicated for abdominal aortic aneurysms 5.5 cm or greater in men, 5.0 cm or greater in women, and/or larger than 4.0 cm with a rapid increase in aneurysm size (1 cm over a 1 year period or 0.5 cm over a 6 month period).
- Endovascular aneurysm repair is often associated with endoleaks, with type II endoleaks being the most common.
- There are no widely accepted peak systolic velocity thresholds to diagnose celiac and mesenteric artery stenosis; however, a peak systolic velocity greater than 200 to 320 cm/s for the celiac artery, greater than 275 to 400 cm/s for the superior mesenteric artery, and greater than 200 cm/s for the inferior mesenteric artery are suggestive.
- Expiratory peak systolic velocity greater than 350 cm/s and deflection angle of greater than 50° are suggestive of median arcuate ligament syndrome.

Abdominal aortic aneurysms (AAAs) are common in the United States with significant morbidity and mortality. It is estimated that close to 200,000 cases are diagnosed per year, and rupture of an AAA is the tenth leading cause of death in men over the age of 55 years. While mesenteric arterial pathology is less common, it also is associated with significant patient morbidity. There is an increased trend toward treatment of AAA and mesenteric arterial stenoses using minimally invasive techniques, and Doppler ultrasound (US) remains the primary screening modality for aortic and mesenteric pathology as well as the initial imaging modality of choice in following patient status post-intervention. This article reviews the US imaging protocol for evaluation of the abdominal aorta and mesenteric arteries, the normal sonographic appearance of these vessels, the US imaging features of the most common pathologies affecting the abdominal aorta and mesenteric arteries, as well as the role of US in follow-up of patients who have undergone therapeutic intervention for AAA or mesenteric arterial stenosis.

AORTA

Scan Protocol

Patients are instructed to fast for 6 hours prior to imaging, as the presence of bowel gas limits evaluation of the abdominal aorta. The aorta is

[a] Department of Radiology and Biomedical Imaging, Yale University School of Medicine, 333 Cedar Street, PO Box 208042, New Haven, CT 06520, USA; [b] Department of Radiology, University of Alabama at Birmingham, JTN 358, 619 S 19th Street South, Birmingham, AL 35294, USA
* Corresponding author.
E-mail address: gowthaman.gunabushanam@yale.edu

scanned throughout its length within the abdomen in both the longitudinal and transverse imaging planes using grayscale and color Doppler. Representative images are saved at the level of the proximal, mid (near the level of renal arteries), distal abdominal aorta, bifurcation, and the bilateral proximal common iliac arteries.[1] The maximal diameter of the proximal, mid, and distal abdominal aorta is measured from the outer-to-outer wall in 2 orthogonal planes (Fig. 1). The anteroposterior outer diameter is preferentially measured on a sagittal image with the plane of measurement-oriented perpendicular to the long axis of the lumen. The transverse outer diameter is measured on a transverse image obtained perpendicular to the long axis of the lumen. If a short-axis transverse plane cannot be obtained, the transverse diameter may be measured from a coronal image. Measurements of the bilateral common iliac arteries should be obtained in a similar fashion, as aneurysms of the iliac arteries are common in patients with AAAs. Note should be made of thrombus/plaque within the lumen of the aorta, if present. If an AAA is noted, the location relative to the renal arteries (suprarenal, juxtarenal, or infrarenal) and the aneurysm shape (fusiform vs saccular) should be described, as both location and configuration will affect patient management. If the origins of the renal arteries cannot be visualized, as a general rule, an AAA that begins more than 2 cm below the origin of the superior mesenteric artery (SMA) is most likely infrarenal.

The normal abdominal aorta is located immediately above or slightly to the left of the spinal column and descends in a straight line parallel to the inferior vena cava from the diaphragm to the pelvis where it bifurcates into the right and left common iliac arteries. The wall of the normal abdominal aorta should be smooth, symmetric, and regular. The diameter should measure less than 3 cm and taper slightly from the diaphragm to the bifurcation. The normal spectral Doppler waveform of the distal abdominal aorta is pulsatile and multiphasic without end-diastolic flow, similar to the waveforms of the common iliac arteries. The normal spectral Doppler waveform of the proximal abdominal aorta at and above the level of the renal arteries typically has a lower resistance pattern with continuous forward diastolic flow.

ABDOMINAL AORTIC ANEURYSM

AAAs are defined as dilatation of the aorta greater than or equal to 3 cm in diameter or 1.5 times the diameter of the more proximal aorta. The incidence of AAA in men older than 60 years is estimated to be 1.7% to 3.4%. Major risk factors for AAAs include older age (>65 years), male gender, smoking, and positive family history (first-degree relative with an AAA). AAAs are 6 times more common in men than in women. Other risk factors include hypertension, atherosclerotic cardiovascular disease, and connective tissue disorders.

Although AAA may rarely present as a pulsatile abdominal mass, AAAs are usually asymptomatic until they rupture, at which time, the risk of death is upward of 80%. Accordingly, the purpose of screening is to diagnose and electively treat AAAs to reduce the incidence of AAA rupture.

SCREENING FOR ABDOMINAL AORTIC ANEURYSM

US screening has a high sensitivity (94%–100%) and specificity (98%–100%) for the detection of AAA. The United States Preventive Services Task

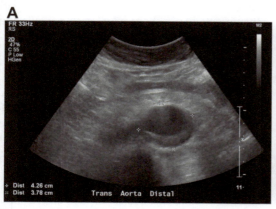
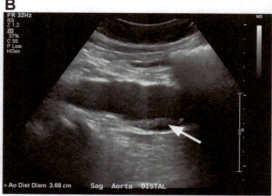

Fig. 1. An 85 year old man with an infrarenal AAA. Transverse (*A*) and sagittal (*B*) grayscale US images show correct placement of calipers from the outer-to-outer wall of the aorta to measure the aneurysm size, which measures 4.3 cm in the transverse dimension and 3.7 cm in the anteroposterior dimension in the sagittal plane. Note the posterior mural thrombus within the aneurysm (*arrow*).

Force (USPSTF) screening recommendations are based on current age, gender at birth, and whether the person has ever been a smoker (defined as ever having smoked 100 or more cigarettes). In 2019, the USPSTF revised its guidelines to recommend one time screening in men aged 65 to 75 years who have ever smoked. Also recommended is selective screening in men aged 65 to 75 years who have never smoked, depending on their family and medical history, other risk factors and personal values. At that time, the USPSTF concluded that the available evidence was insufficient to determine benefit of screening in women aged 65 to 75 years who have ever smoked.[2] However, the Society of Vascular Surgery (SVS) recommends screening aortic US for both men and women aged 65 to 75 years, who have ever smoked or have a first-degree relative with an AAA. Screening is also recommended by the SVS for both men and women aged over 75 years otherwise in good health (ie, potentially interventional candidates) who have previously not been screened.[3]

While patients with AAAs below treatment thresholds (5.0–5.5 cm) traditionally have been followed with yearly US surveillance, the SVS currently recommends follow-up US only every 3 years for AAAs 3.0 to 3.9 cm in diameter with yearly follow-up for AAAs 4.0 to 4.9 cm in size and semiannual follow-up for aneurysms 5.0 to 5.4 cm in size.[3] Additionally, the SVS recommends a follow-up screening US in 10 years when the initial study demonstrates an abdominal aorta 2.5 to 2.9 cm in size.[3] In follow-up studies, an increase in diameter greater than 0.5 cm is usually considered significant. The risk of AAA rupture varies with increasing aneurysm size, growth rate, and gender. Data show that women are at greater risk of rupture at smaller aneurysm size and may have a worse prognosis, even with elective intervention. Endovascular aneurysm repair (EVAR) or open surgical repair is indicated for AAAs 5.5 cm or greater in men, 5.0 cm in women, or larger than 4.0 cm with a rapid increase in aneurysm size (1 cm over a 1 year period or 0.5 cm over a 6 month period). Additionally, treatment is indicated for patients with abdominal or back pain that is attributable to the aneurysm and for all saccular aneurysms. If an AAA extends to the diaphragm, computed tomography (CT) of the chest is indicated to exclude an associated descending thoracic aortic aneurysm.

ENDOVASCULAR ANEURYSM REPAIR VERSUS OPEN REPAIR

Multiple clinical trials have demonstrated similar long-term outcomes for EVAR compared to open repair. However, EVAR has the advantages of being less invasive, with significantly lower short-term morbidity and mortality and shorter recovery times compared to open repair.[4] Therefore, EVAR is preferred wherever the aneurysm anatomy allows for it, which is the case in over 80% of AAAs. However, EVAR does necessitate more frequent follow-up and reintervention, especially in the case of complications, including endoleaks.

POSTTREATMENT ULTRASOUND SURVEILLANCE

Patients with AAAs treated using EVAR need imaging follow-up at regular intervals, usually yearly for life. The most common complication following EVAR is the presence of persistent flow within the excluded aneurysm sac, termed an endoleak. Although surveillance of endografts was initially performed using CT scans, more recently, there has been increasing interest in the use of US for the detection of endoleaks due to the comparatively higher costs associated with CT scans as well as the risks associated with ionizing radiation and iodinated contrast. If the initial CT scan at 1 month following EVAR does not show an endoleak, yearly color Doppler US has been suggested as an alternative to CT scans for imaging surveillance,[5] with subsequent CT or contrast-enhanced US (CEUS) to look for endoleak if aneurysm expansion is detected.[6] Other complications of EVAR include migration of the graft, occlusion of a modular limb (**Fig. 2**), and graft infection.

US surveillance for endoleaks must be performed with meticulous scanning technique, especially if the patient has stacked modules or chimney/snorkel graft extensions with stents placed in the upper aortic branches. Knowledge of the exact details of the endograft repair prior to US evaluation is essential to ensure that all critical components of the endograft are evaluated. The entire abdominal aorta should be evaluated first with grayscale imaging in both sagittal and transverse planes. The location/extension of the endograft should be determined and both the upper and lower landing zones well visualized if possible, assessing for gaps between the endograft and the arterial wall. Careful measurement of the maximal diameter of the aneurysm sac is critical, and the aneurysm sac should be measured at the same location on follow-up examinations. Although not all endoleaks result in continued growth of the aneurysm, increased aneurysm size is one of the most important findings in patients with endoleaks, usually indicating that repair is necessary, no matter the type of endoleak. Anechoic areas within the excluded sac should

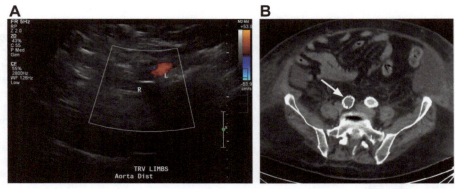

Fig. 2. A 72 year old man who underwent EVAR 8 years prior. (*A*) Transverse ultrasound shows no detectable flow within the right limb of the endograft (R), consistent with occlusion, although color flow clearly fills the lumen of the left outflow limb (L). (*B*) Contrast-enhanced CT scan done for unrelated reasons at a later time redemonstrated thrombosis (no contrast enhancement) of the right limb of endograft (*arrow*). The left outflow limb remains patent.

be assessed with color Doppler and microvascular flow imaging (MVFI), as endoleaks are often anechoic (without thrombus). Subsequently, careful evaluation of the entire aneurysm and endograft in both sagittal and transverse planes should be made with color Doppler and MVFI to document graft and outflow limb patency. Areas of color flow in the excluded aneurysm sac are indicative of endoleak, including at gaps between endograft and aortic/iliac artery wall, retrograde flow in a feeding vessel, or flow extending through the wall of the graft into the aneurysm sac. Color Doppler and MVFI cine clip imaging in both sagittal and transverse planes are very useful.

Types of endoleaks are described in **Table 1**. Type I endoleaks reflect an incomplete seal between the endograft and the vessel wall, most likely due to endograft migration or continued growth or deformation of the aneurysm. A gap between the wall of the aorta or iliac artery and the endograft at the landing zone may be observed on grayscale with flow coursing between the graft and vessel wall on color/power Doppler. A type IA endoleak occurs at the level of the cephalad landing zone and a type IB endoleak occurs at the distal landing zone in the iliac arteries. Type I endoleaks are usually large. Flow may slowly swirl within the endoleak on grayscale and demonstrate a "yin-yang" pattern on color Doppler, similar to flow in a pseudoaneurysm.

Type II endoleaks are the most common type, and these are found in approximately 25% of

Table 1
Types of endoleaks

Type	Cause	Management Considerations
I	Inadequate seal of the endograft to aortic wall	Subtypes IA and IB due to inadequate seal proximally (IA) and distally (IB). Usually treated
II	Retrograde flow in aortic branch arteries, usually inferior mesenteric or lumbar arteries	*Common finding*: Usually treated only if symptomatic, or if the aneurysm increases in size > 5–10 mm
III	Mechanical graft failure with blood flow between graft components, fabric tear, or separation of modular components	Typically require intervention to repair
IV	Graft material porosity	Less commonly seen with current devices. Usually seal spontaneously, and are not treated.
V	Aneurysm enlargement in the absence of an endoleak visible by imaging	Treatment is recommended

patients undergoing EVAR. On grayscale imaging, type II endoleaks often appear as small, round anechoic areas in the excluded aneurysm sac, and will demonstrate flow on color or power Doppler (**Fig. 3**). US can often demonstrate retrograde flow into the endoleak from the patent inferior mesenteric artery (IMA) anteriorly or a lumbar artery posteriorly, confirming a type II endoleak. The spectral Doppler waveform obtained from the feeding branch typically has a "to-and-fro" waveform pattern, similar in appearance to the flow in the neck of a pseudoaneurysm. If persistent forward diastolic flow is observed in the feeding vessel, the possibility of a complex endoleak with either a second feeding vessel or an associated type I or type III endoleak should be considered, and follow-up CT may be helpful.

Type III endoleaks are uncommon and diagnosed when blood is seen flowing directly through a break in the graft structure (**Fig. 4**). Importantly, blood flow seen immediately adjacent to the endograft is not always a type III endoleak but could represent a large type II endoleak. Moreover, type I and III endoleaks may coexist with a type II endoleak, and so need to be excluded in patients with type II endoleaks with increasing aneurysm size.[7]

There is a significant risk of aneurysm rupture with endoleak types I and III, and these require repair. Around 30% to 50% of type II endoleaks resolve spontaneously and can therefore be safely followed if they are asymptomatic, small, and the aneurysm size remains stable or decreases.[8] However, embolization of a type II endoleak is necessary if it is large, symptomatic or if the aneurysm sac increases in diameter by greater than 0.5 to 1 cm.

CONTRAST-ENHANCED ULTRASOUND

There is increasing interest in using CEUS for both on-label and off-label imaging in the abdomen

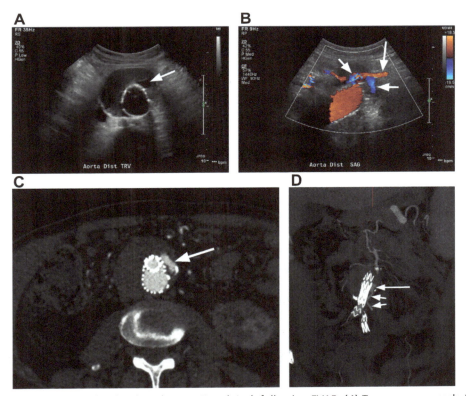

Fig. 3. A 75 year old man who developed a type II endoleak following EVAR. (*A*) Transverse grayscale US image shows a small anechoic region (*arrow*) in the distal aspect of the excluded aneurysm sac that is otherwise filled with low-level echoes, consistent with thrombus. Note that contiguity of the endoleak with the wall of the endograft does not necessarily imply that it is type III endoleak. (*B*) Sagittal color Doppler US image shows the patent origin of the IMA (*long arrow*) supplying the endoleak (*short arrows*) confirming that this is a type II endoleak. (*C*) Axial contrast-enhanced CT scan shows the endoleak (*arrow*). (*D*) Coronal maximum intensity projection reconstructed image from contrast-enhanced CT scan shows the patent IMA (*short arrows*) supplying the type II endoleak (long *arrow*).

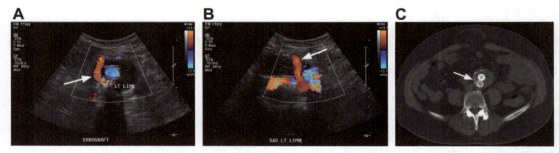

Fig. 4. A 86 year old man who underwent EVAR 6 months prior and developed a type III endoleak. Transverse (A) and sagittal (B) color Doppler US shows a type III endoleak (arrow) with blood flowing directly from the graft lumen through the wall of the left outflow limb of the endograft into the excluded sac of the AAA. (C) Axial contrast-enhanced CT scan shows the endoleak (arrow) as well arising from the left outflow limb situated posterior to the right outflow limb in the infrarenal AAA.

and pelvis, especially when color/power Doppler and MVFI are nondiagnostic, and the AAA has increased in size.[9] Ultrasound contrast agents (UCA) consist of microbubbles of a gas surrounded by an outer shell of lipids, protein, or synthetic biopolymers. Non-linear interactions of US waves with the UCA improve the signal-to-noise of the vessels containing microbubbles as compared to adjacent tissues. CEUS allows continuous monitoring of vascular enhancement of the aorta for up to 5 to 10 minutes after UCA administration.

The timing and location of the appearance of contrast are extremely helpful in endoleak classification. Type I and III endoleaks show immediate contrast enhancement outside of the stent graft within the excluded aneurysm sac, whereas type II endoleaks typically demonstrate delayed contrast enhancement as the UCA needs to exit the aorta and then return to the aorta via retrograde flow through a side branch (Figs. 5 and 6).[9]

CT may be less sensitive than CEUS in cases where flow in the endoleak is delayed and not detected at the preselected CT scan times after contrast administration.[10] A second CEUS injection following the first injection may also be useful to precisely determine the location of the endoleak to facilitate intervention.[9] CEUS can be very useful when a large number of coils in the aorta obscure visualization of the endoleak. Overall, CEUS is considered to be equivalent in diagnostic accuracy to CT angiograms.[11,12] Disadvantages of CEUS include greater operator dependence, limitations secondary to patient factors including bowel gas, large body habitus, and aortic wall calcifications.

ULTRASOUND VERSUS COMPUTED TOMOGRAPHIC SCANS

Both US and CT play complementary roles in the management of patients with AAA. CT scans have the benefit of being less operator dependent, and less susceptible to inadequate imaging due to shadowing from bowel gas, whereas US is less expensive and does not use ionizing radiation or

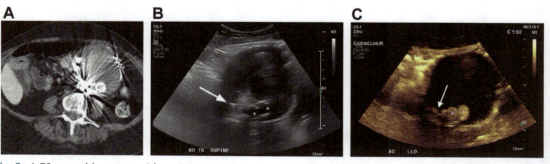

Fig. 5. A 78 year old woman with an 8.1 cm AAA, status post EVAR with type II endoleak. (A) Contrast-enhanced CT is nondiagnostic due to artifact from large number of coils in the aneurysm sac. (B) Transverse grayscale US of the aorta shows the right and left endograft limbs (*) and relatively small amount of artifact from coils (arrow). (C) Although a feeding vessel is not directly visualized, transverse CEUS of the aorta demonstrates a small focal area of delayed contrast enhancement at 1:02 minutes following contrast injection at 7 o'clock position (arrow) within the excluded lumen of the aneurysm sac, consistent with a type II endoleak. Contrast is also noted in both outflow limbs (*) of the endograft.

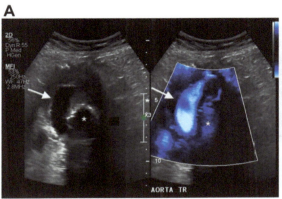
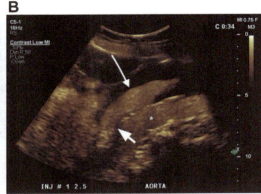

Fig. 6. A 78 year old man with a 5.7 cm AAA, status post-EVAR with type I endoleak. (*A*) Transverse split screen image of the proximal stent graft (*) shows an anechoic region within the aortic lumen on grayscale (*arrow, left*) with blood flow noted on MVFI (*arrow, right*). (*B*) Longitudinal CEUS of the upper edge (landing zone) of the AAA 34 seconds following contrast injection shows contrast within the AAA (*long arrow*) outside the endograft (*) as well as separation of the top edge of the endograft from the wall of the AAA (*short arrow*). Contact with the stent edge and early contrast opacification within an endoleak at the same time as opacification of the endograft lumen is consistent with a type I endoleak.

iodinated contrast. While US is the default modality in the initial diagnosis and surveillance of AAA, CT plays a critical role in treatment planning, especially for determining suitability for EVAR. Both modalities are used in the follow-up of patients following EVAR. Although surveillance protocols vary, most advocate initial follow-up with CT. If on initial and/or 6 month CT scans, no endoleak is seen; there is no increase in the diameter of the AAA; and there are no significant risk factors for endoleak; many believe that further follow-up with color Doppler US alone may be safely performed. While US may have lower sensitivity than CT for the detection of endoleaks, especially when done without US contrast, US is comparable to CT in sensitivity for the detection of endoleaks that are clinically significant and potentially require intervention. Finally, US may not show stent migration and fractures as well as CT scans.

RUPTURED ABDOMINAL AORTIC ANEURYSM

Ruptured AAAs typically present with acute, severe back pain and hypotension. CT angiography is the preferred imaging modality, both to confirm the diagnosis and aid in preoperative planning. In general, US is considered of limited use in the setting of clinical concern for a ruptured AAA due to time constraints. Additionally, hemoperitoneum may cause ileus resulting in significant shadowing from bowel gas, limiting visualization of the aorta and retroperitoneum on US. Abdominal guarding when probe pressure is applied also limits visualization of deep abdominal structures. However, US may be of value in patients with known AAA with clinical suspicion of rupture who are too unstable to undergo CT scan. A focused US scan may demonstrate hemoperitoneum, helping to make a quick diagnosis and expedite emergent EVAR or open surgical repair. Other US findings that have been described in the setting of a ruptured AAA include retroperitoneal hematoma, deformation of the aneurysm, inhomogeneity of the luminal thrombus, and disruption of the aneurysm wall.[13] Rarely, a small focal outpouching of flow into the wall of the aorta on color Doppler may be observed in patients with milder symptoms, indicative of a penetrating ulcer. However, penetrating ulcers are much more frequently visualized on CT scan and may be difficult to differentiate from ulcerated plaque.

CURRENT AND FUTURE DEVELOPMENTS

Three-dimensional US may lead to improved reproducibility of measurement and enables volumetric measurements of aortic aneurysms, both before and after treatment using EVAR.[14] There is ongoing research on applying 4 dimensional US to assess aortic wall strain. This may lead to improved prediction of aneurysm growth rates and potentially assess the risk of aneurysm rupture.[15,16]

DISSECTION

Abdominal aortic dissection may occur secondary to extension of a thoracic aortic dissection, trauma (including iatrogenic causes), and Marfan syndrome (**Fig. 7**). US can demonstrate the echogenic, often mobile, dissection flap, as well as patency of

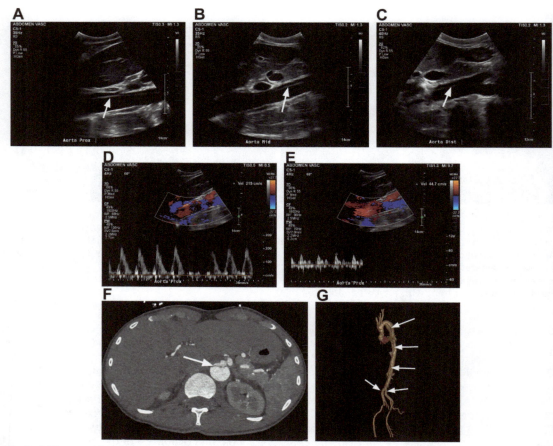

Fig. 7. A 25 year old man with Marfan syndrome and known aortic dissection who previously underwent surgical repair of the ascending aorta. Sagittal grayscale US images of the proximal (*A*), mid (*B*), and distal (*C*) abdominal aorta demonstrate a dissection flap (*arrow*) within the abdominal aorta extending into the common iliac artery. (*D*, *E*) Spectral Doppler images of the proximal abdominal aorta show the true and false lumens. The true lumen is located anteriorly and relatively narrowed with a PSV of 215 cm/s (*D*). The false lumen shows a relatively lower PSV of 45 cm/s with a more abnormal irregular waveform (*E*). (*F*) Axial CECT scan shows the dissection flap (*arrow*). Both the celiac artery and SMA (not shown) arise from the narrowed true lumen. (*G*) Volume-rendered CT image shows the dissection flap (*arrows*) within the descending thoracic aorta, abdominal aorta and bilateral common iliac arteries.

the true and false lumens. Often, the true lumen is compressed anteriorly by the false lumen. The false lumen may be partially or completely thrombosed, in which case it can be difficult to differentiate from an intramural hematoma. Typically thrombus in the false lumen or intramural hematoma is homogeneously hypoechoic, although acute thrombus may be echogenic. The distal extent of the dissection flap should be documented, often extending into one or both common iliac arteries. US can be used to document patency of the major aortic branch arteries and to determine if these vessels arise from the true or false lumen. Depending on patient body habitus, one can determine whether the dissection flap extends into the lumen of the major branches compromising blood flow. CEUS can be useful in assessing patency versus thrombus if CT/MRI is contraindicated.

MESENTERIC ARTERIES
Normal Anatomy

The celiac artery, SMA, and IMA together supply the abdominal viscera, with the exception of the kidneys and adrenal glands. The celiac artery arises anteriorly from the upper abdominal aorta and is readily recognized by its T-shaped bifurcation into the common hepatic artery and splenic artery shortly after its origin. The orientation of the stem of the "T" is quite variable. While it is often directed toward the anterior abdominal wall at a nearly 90° angle from the aorta, it may also curve toward the head or toward the feet, parallel to the SMA. The other branch of the celiac artery, the left gastric artery is less frequently seen in US due to its small size. The SMA also typically originates anteriorly at approximately the 12 o'clock position from the abdominal aorta approximately 1 cm inferior to the celiac artery and gently curves 90° toward the lower abdomen coursing over the mid abdominal aorta for several cm. Occasionally, the celiac artery and SMA will have a common origin. The IMA is smaller in caliber and arises in the distal abdominal aorta anteriorly and slightly to the left of the midline in the 12 to 3 o'clock position, heading almost immediately away from the aorta toward the left lower quadrant. Hence, the IMA is more difficult to visualize. Most stenoses in these arteries occur at the origin and proximal few cm of these arteries and can usually be adequately imaged by US.

Scan Protocol

Images of the origin and proximal segments of the mesenteric arteries should be obtained in the longitudinal plane on both grayscale and color Doppler looking for evidence of atherosclerosis, luminal narrowing, wall thickening, dissections, and aneurysmal dilatation. Gentle graded compression technique is helpful to eliminate shadowing from overlying bowel gas, particularly for visualization of the IMA and distal SMA. Spectral Doppler waveforms should be obtained at a minimum from the origin/proximal, mid, and distal segments. As the trunk of the celiac artery is short, a waveform should be obtained in the common hepatic and splenic arteries, as these vessels are considered the distal outflow of the celiac artery. The celiac artery and SMA have similar, low resistance spectral Doppler waveforms with a sharp systolic upstroke, and continuous forward diastolic flow in the non-fasting state (**Fig. 8**). Peak systolic velocity (PSV) and end-diastolic velocity (EDV) in the celiac artery do not change with food intake. However, PSV and EDV in the SMA are expected to increase postprandial, although the exact degree is unpredictable. Therefore, most protocols no longer advise assessing the SMA following a food challenge. The IMA Doppler waveform typically demonstrates absent or very limited end-diastolic flow.

Chronic Mesenteric Ischemia

Chronic mesenteric ischemia typically requires hemodynamically significant stenosis of at least 2 of the 3 major mesenteric arteries to be symptomatic. Less commonly, however, isolated stenosis of the SMA may lead to symptomatic mesenteric ischemia, especially in patients without well-developed collateral pathways. The most commonly described presenting symptoms are postprandial pain and weight loss. The most common etiology is atherosclerosis, with other etiologies including dissection, fibromuscular dysplasia, and vasculitis. US has a useful role in the diagnosis and management of chronic mesenteric ischemia, unlike cases with suspected acute mesenteric ischemia, which may be a surgical/interventional emergency whereby CT angiogram is the preferred imaging modality due to better assessment of the more distal branches of the SMA and status of the bowel.

There is limited consensus on what PSV thresholds should be used to diagnose hemodynamically significant stenosis of the mesenteric arteries. Factors causing variability in normal PSV include variant anatomy, vessel tortuosity at the arterial origin that makes it difficult to apply appropriate angle correction, and compensatory flow changes due to collaterals. Diagnostic US criteria that have been suggested are quite variable, with PSV thresholds as follows:[17,18]

- *Celiac artery*: PSV greater than 200 to 320 cm/s
- *SMA*: PSV greater than 275 to 400 cm/s
- *IMA*: PSV greater than 200 cm/s

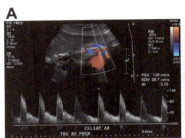 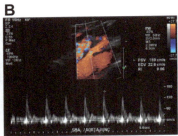 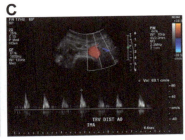

Fig. 8. Spectral Doppler images in two different patients showing the normal appearance of the origin of the celiac artery (*A*), SMA (*B*), and IMA (*C*). Note that the celiac artery (*A*) and the SMA (*B*) have similar spectral Doppler waveforms with sharp systolic upstroke and continuous forward diastolic flow while the IMA (*C*) normally has a high-resistance spectral Doppler waveform pattern with decreased or absent diastolic flow.

A mesenteric-to-aortic PSV ratio greater than 3.5 may also be useful in the diagnosis of stenosis. Given the lack of widely accepted Doppler velocity criteria, the presence of visible narrowing of the lumen on grayscale and color Doppler US, post-stenotic dilatation, and distal tardus parvus waveforms is of particular value in diagnosing significant stenosis and differentiating artifactually elevated PSV from true stenosis. Importantly, the absence of a tardus parvus waveform in the distal mesenteric arteries should not be interpreted as excluding a more proximal stenosis. The decision to treat should be based primarily on clinical assessment of symptoms, not on imaging.

US is particularly helpful in the surveillance of stenosis following endovascular or open surgical intervention. Follow-up is recommended at regular intervals, usually at 1, 6, and 12 months, and annually thereafter. Suggested PSV thresholds that may warrant further workup include a substantial increase in PSV from the baseline post-intervention, or PSV greater than 370 cm/s for the celiac artery and PSV greater than 420 cm/s for the SMA (**Fig. 9**).[5] Stent placement in the mesenteric arteries may result in increased PSV; therefore, narrowing of the residual lumen on grayscale and/or color Doppler, distal tardus parvus waveforms, as well as change over time are extremely helpful in differentiating true in-stent restenosis from elevated PSV secondary to stent placement.

While most cases of mesenteric ischemia are due to atherosclerosis, symptomatic narrowing of the mesenteric arteries may also be caused by arterial dissection or arteritis. Mesenteric dissection may be spontaneous and isolated to the mesenteric arteries or extend from aortic dissections. Risk factors include vasculitis and connective tissue disorders. If a mesenteric dissection is associated with aneurysmal dilatation of the artery, an underlying connective tissue disorder such as Ehler–Danlos or Marfan syndrome should be considered, especially in a young patient. Mesenteric dissection usually results in either an intramural hematoma or thrombosed false lumen. A patent false lumen is rarely seen, although an echogenic dissection flap is usually visualized. While atherosclerosis will cause irregular asymmetric focal narrowing of the residual lumen with heterogenous and/or calcified plaque, a thrombosed false lumen or mural hematoma is typically homogeneously hypoechoic and smooth surfaced. Wall thickening from the

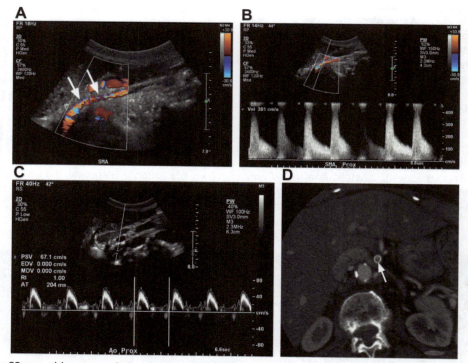

Fig. 9. An 88 year old woman who underwent SMA stent placement 5 years prior. (*A*) Sagittal color Doppler image showing focal aliasing and luminal narrowing in the proximal and mid-SMA (*arrows*). (*B*) PSV is increased in the SMA stent, measuring 391 cm/s. (*C*) PSV in the proximal abdominal aorta measures 67 cm/s, giving a mesenteric-to-aortic PSV ratio of 5.8. (*D*) Contrast-enhanced CT scan shows a crescent-shaped filling defect within the SMA stent (*arrow*), consistent with in-stent restenosis.

thrombosed false lumen or mural hematoma is eccentric rather than circumferential, often spiraling around and compressing the true lumen resulting in increased PSV (**Fig. 10**). The interface between the mural hematoma and true lumen may have either a straight linear or curved crescent configuration on a transverse or short-axis imaging plane, termed the straight line or crescent sign, respectively. In patients with vasculitis, the arterial wall is homogeneously thickened with a smooth surface in a circumferential rather than eccentric, asymmetric configuration.

Median Arcuate Ligament Syndrome

The median arcuate ligament is a fibrous band that connects the right and left crus of the diaphragm along the anterior surface of the aorta at the level of the aortic hiatus. A low insertion of the median arcuate ligament may lead to extrinsic compression of the celiac artery origin, resulting in median arcuate ligament syndrome (MALS). This typically occurs in individuals between the ages of 30 and 50 years and is 4 times more common in female individuals. Common presenting symptoms include epigastric pain, nausea, vomiting, weight loss, and postprandial or exercise-induced abdominal pain.[19] US criteria include[20]

- Increased PSV within the celiac artery greater than 350 cm/s during expiration with relatively normal PSV during inspiration. This helps differentiate elevated PSV due to MALS from elevated PSV due to atherosclerotic stenosis of the celiac artery, which will not vary during the respiratory cycle (**Fig. 11**).
- Deflection angle (celiac artery to aortic angle difference between inspiration and expiration) greater than 50°.
- Hook-like configuration in expiration.

Normalization of velocities with the patient in the standing position has been suggested to improve the specificity of ultrasound.[21] On CT and MRI scans, one would additionally expect to visualize indentation at the superior aspect of the celiac artery, and this can be visible by US. The treatment of MALS is laparoscopic division of the median arcuate ligament without or with celiac ganglionectomy. Persistent stenosis of the celiac artery may require a surgical aortoceliac artery bypass graft, patch or balloon angioplasty, and/or stent placement in the celiac artery.

In summary, US plays an important role in the screening, follow-up, and posttreatment surveillance of AAAs. Although PSV threshold criteria reported in the literature are highly variable, US can

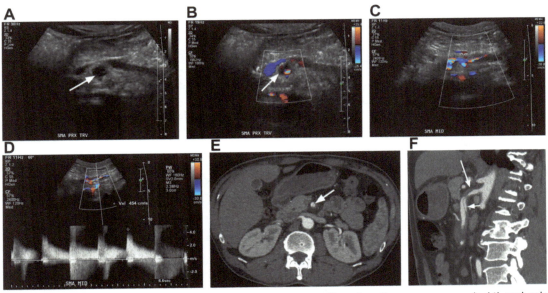

Fig. 10. A 57 year old man who developed a spontaneous SMA dissection. Transverse grayscale (A) and color Doppler (B) images show an echogenic thin linear dissection flap within the SMA (arrow, A), with partial thrombosis of the false lumen (arrow, B) which is homogeneously hypoechoic and with a significantly narrowed true lumen. Note smooth curved interface between the partially thrombosed false lumen and patent true lumen, termed the crescent sign, consistent with dissection. Narrowing of the SMA due to vasculitis or atherosclerosis would result in circumferential wall thickening or irregularly surfaced heterogenous focal plaque, respectively. Sagittal color Doppler image (C) shows narrowing of the SMA with increased PSV of 454 cm/s on spectral Doppler image (D). Axial contrast-enhanced CT scan (E) and sagittal multiplanar reformatted image (F) shows the dissection flap in the SMA (arrow, E and short arrow, F) and partial thrombosis of the false lumen (long arrow, F).

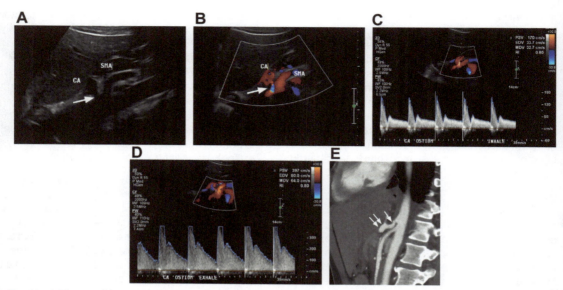

Fig. 11. A 39 year old man with MALS who presented with abdominal pain. (*A*, *B*) Sagittal grayscale (*A*) and color Doppler (*B*) US images show narrowing at the origin of the celiac artery (*arrows*, *A* and *B*), with focal color Doppler aliasing (*arrow*, *B*). CA, celiac artery; SMA, SMA. Sagittal spectral Doppler images of the celiac artery show a PSV of 170 cm/s in inspiration (*C*) and greater than 397 cm/s in expiration (*D*). Note how the celiac artery is angulated inferiorly in inspiration (*C*) and superiorly in expiration (*D*). (*E*) Sagittal reconstructed image of a CT angiogram shows narrowing at the origin of the celiac artery (*arrow*) with a "fish-hook" appearance of the celiac artery and post-stenotic dilatation of the celiac artery (*double arrows*).

also be useful in screening patients with suspected chronic mesenteric ischemia when Doppler velocity criteria are combined with evidence of plaque on grayscale imaging, narrowing, poststenotic dilatation, focal color Doppler aliasing, adjacent soft tissue bruits, and/or the presence of more distal tardus parvus waveforms. Change over time is an additional useful criterion in surveillance of patients following therapeutic intervention. Of note, there are numerous causes of elevated PSV in the mesenteric arteries such as vessel tortuosity, compensatory increased flow, difficulty in obtaining an accurate Doppler angle due to vessel geometry, as well as stent placement. Thus, clinical correlation remains key and should guide recommendations for correlative imaging if US findings are discordant with clinical presentation or pretest probability.

CLINICS CARE POINTS

- Ultrasound is the primary screening modality for aortic and mesenteric pathology as well as the initial imaging modality of choice in following patients post-intervention.
- The Society for Vascular Surgery currently recommends follow-up US only every 3 years for abdominal aortic aneurysms (AAAs) 3.0 to 3.9 cm in diameter, with yearly follow-up for AAAs 4.0 to 4.9 cm in size and semiannual follow-up for aneurysms 5.0 to 5.4 cm in size.
- Ultrasound is comparable to CT in sensitivity for detection of endoleaks that are clinically significant and potentially require intervention.
- Ultrasound numerical criteria for diagnosing mesenteric stenosis are quite variable. Presence of visible narrowing of the artery on grayscale and color Doppler, post-stenotic dilatation and distal tardus parvus waveforms are of particular value in diagnosing hemodynamically significant stenosis.

DISCLOSURE

L.M. Scoutt is an educational consultant for Philips Healthcare (not directly related to this study). M.L. Robbin: Philips Medical, contract, ongoing. Philips Medical Vascular Advisory Board (single session), 2/2023. Jazz Pharmaceuticals, VOD Advisory Board (single session), 6/2023.

REFERENCES

1. AIUM practice parameter for the performance of diagnostic and screening ultrasound examinations

of the abdominal aorta in adults. J Ultrasound Med 2021;40:E34–8.
2. US Preventive Services Task Force, Owens DK, Davidson KW, et al. Screening for abdominal aortic aneurysm: US Preventive Services Task Force recommendation statement. JAMA 2019;322:2211–8.
3. Chaikof EL, Dalman RL, Eskandari MK, et al. The Society for Vascular Surgery practice guidelines on the care of patients with an abdominal aortic aneurysm. J Vasc Surg 2018;67:2–77.e2.
4. Schanzer A, Oderich GS. Management of abdominal aortic aneurysms. N Engl J Med 2021;385:1690–8.
5. Zierler RE, Jordan WD, Lal BK, et al. The Society for Vascular Surgery practice guidelines on follow-up after vascular surgery arterial procedures. J Vasc Surg 2018;68:256–84.
6. Chisci E, Harris L, Guidotti A, et al. Endovascular aortic repair follow up protocol based on contrast enhanced ultrasound is safe and effective. Eur J Vasc Endovasc Surg 2018;56:40–7.
7. D'Oria M, Mastrorilli D, Ziani B. Natural history, diagnosis, and management of type II endoleaks after endovascular aortic repair: Review and update. Ann Vasc Surg 2020;62:420–31.
8. Rokosh RS, Wu WW, Dalman RL, et al. Society for Vascular Surgery implementation of clinical practice guidelines for patients with an abdominal aortic aneurysm: Endoleak management. J Vasc Surg 2021;74:1792–4.
9. Alexander LF, Overfield CJ, Sella DM, et al. Contrast-enhanced US evaluation of endoleaks after endovascular stent repair of abdominal aortic aneurysm. Radiographics 2022;42:1758–75.
10. Karaolanis GI, Antonopoulos CN, Georgakarakos E, et al. Colour Duplex and/or contrast-enhanced ultrasound compared with computed tomography angiography for endoleak detection after endovascular abdominal aortic aneurysm repair: a systematic review and meta-analysis. J Clin Med 2022;11:3628.
11. Harky A, Zywicka E, Santoro G, et al. Is contrast-enhanced ultrasound (CEUS) superior to computed tomography angiography (CTA) in detection of endoleaks in post-EVAR patients? a systematic review and meta-analysis. J Ultrasound 2019;22:65–75.
12. Kapetanios D, Kontopodis N, Mavridis D, et al. Meta-analysis of the accuracy of contrast-enhanced ultrasound for the detection of endoleak after endovascular aneurysm repair. J Vasc Surg 2019;69:280–94.e6.
13. Catalano O, Siani A. Ruptured abdominal aortic aneurysm: categorization of sonographic findings and report of 3 new signs. J Ultrasound Med 2005;24:1077–83.
14. Lowe C, Ghulam Q, Bredahl K, et al. Three-dimensional ultrasound in the management of abdominal aortic aneurysms: A topical review. Eur J Vasc Endovasc Surg 2016;52:466–74.
15. Derwich W, Wittek A, Hegner A, et al. Comparison of abdominal aortic aneurysm sac and neck wall motion with 4D ultrasound imaging. Eur J Vasc Endovasc Surg 2020;60:539–47.
16. Derwich W, Keller T, Filmann N, et al. Changes in aortic diameter and wall strain in progressing abdominal aortic aneurysms. J Ultrasound Med 2023;42:1737–46.
17. Pellerito JS, Revzin MV, Tsang JC, et al. Doppler sonographic criteria for the diagnosis of inferior mesenteric artery stenosis. J Ultrasound Med 2009;28:641–50.
18. AbuRahma AF, Stone PA, Srivastava M, et al. Mesenteric/celiac duplex ultrasound interpretation criteria revisited. J Vasc Surg 2012;55:428–36.
19. Goodall R, Langridge B, Onida S, et al. Median arcuate ligament syndrome. J Vasc Surg 2020;71:2170–6.
20. Gruber H, Loizides A, Peer S, et al. Ultrasound of the median arcuate ligament syndrome: a new approach to diagnosis. Med Ultrason 2012;14:5–9.
21. Wolfman D, Bluth EI, Sossaman J. Median arcuate ligament syndrome. J Ultrasound Med 2003;22:1377–80.

Carotid Ultrasound

Tyler J. Sevco, MD[a,*], Maitraya K. Patel, MD[a], Corinne Deurdulian, MD, FSRU[b,c]

KEYWORDS

- Carotid ultrasound • Internal carotid artery stenosis • Carotid plaque • Spectral Doppler

KEY POINTS

- Most strokes are ischemic, with approximately 15% of embolic strokes originating from vulnerable plaque at the carotid bifurcation.
- Carotid ultrasound (US) is the primary noninvasive method for detecting, grading, and monitoring internal carotid artery (ICA) stenosis.
- The Intersocietal Accreditation Commission Vascular Testing now recommends a modified Society of Radiologists in Ultrasound criteria peak systolic velocity threshold of 180 to 230 cm/s for the diagnosis of 50% to 69% ICA stenosis in the absence of an ICA/CCA ratio greater than 2.0. Peak systolic velocities greater than 230 cm/s remain the primary Doppler US criteria for diagnosing ≥70% stenosis. However, findings should be correlated with grayscale and color Doppler findings as well as secondary parameters, including peak systolic ratio and end-diastolic velocity.
- Carotid spectral waveforms may help diagnose cardiovascular disease as well as nonatherosclerotic pathologic conditions.

INTRODUCTION

In the United States, cerebrovascular disease is a significant cause of morbidity, with stroke being the fifth leading cause of death. In 2020, someone died of stroke every 3.3 minutes on average, and the direct and indirect cost of stroke in the United States was estimated at $56.5 billion.[1] Risk factors for stroke include hypertension, obesity, hyperglycemia, hyperlipidemia, renal dysfunction, and atrial fibrillation, among others.[1]

Approximately 87% of all strokes are ischemic. Significant carotid stenosis is found in 10% to 20% of patients with transient ischemic attack (TIA) or stroke.[2] Most ischemic strokes occur because of atheromatous emboli, with approximately 15% of embolic strokes originating from plaque at the carotid bifurcation. The remaining 13% of all strokes are hemorrhagic, most which are related to hypertension.

In 2002, the Society of Radiologists in Ultrasound (SRU) published specific recommendations on the ultrasound (US) evaluation of carotid artery disease.[3] These criteria were based on a set of Doppler velocity criteria aimed at grading the severity of internal carotid artery (ICA) stenosis according to a method adopted by the North American Symptomatic Carotid Endarterectomy Trial (NASCET).[3,4] As a result, Doppler US has become the primary noninvasive method for detecting, grading, and monitoring ICA stenosis owing to its high sensitivity and specificity, lack of ionizing radiation, widespread availability, and low cost. Carotid Doppler US involves 3 major components: plaque characterization, assessment of ICA stenosis using Doppler velocity criteria, and spectral waveform analysis.

TECHNIQUE

Carotid US is typically performed in the supine position with the patient's neck slightly hyperextended

---

[a] Department of Radiological Sciences, David Geffen School of Medicine at UCLA, UCLA Ronald Reagan Medical Center, 757 Westwood Plaza, Suite 1621, Los Angeles, CA 90095, USA; [b] Department of Radiological Sciences, David Geffen School of Medicine at UCLA, USC Keck School of Medicine, Los Angeles, CA, USA; [c] Department of Radiology, Greater Los Angeles VA Medical Center, 11301 Wilshire Boulevard, Los Angeles, CA 90073, USA
* Corresponding author.
E-mail address: tsevco@mednet.ucla.edu

and turned toward the contralateral side using a high-resolution 5-MHz or greater linear-array transducer.[5] Linear transducers in the 5- to 12-MHz range or 2- to 9-MHz range are often used. The examination should include real-time scanning with grayscale, color Doppler, and spectral Doppler imaging. A 3- to 5-MHz curved array transducer may also be used in patients with a large body habitus or in patients with deep or densely calcified vessels. The vessels can be imaged from an anterior or posterior approach; however, the sternocleidomastoid muscle often provides a good acoustic window. Angulation of the transducer caudally in the supraclavicular area and cephalad at the level of the mandible can also aid visualization.

Carotid US should routinely include assessment of the proximal and distal common carotid arteries (CCAs); the carotid bifurcation; the proximal, mid, and distal internal carotid arteries (ICAs); the proximal external carotid arteries (ECAs); and the mid–vertebral arteries (VAs) in the sagittal and transverse planes using grayscale and color Doppler imaging. In addition, dedicated images of any areas of suspected stenosis or other pathologic condition should also be acquired.

On grayscale imaging, gain is optimized for the assessment of plaque, the vessel wall (such that the normal 3 layers of the CCA wall are clearly depicted), and any other noted abnormalities. When manually placed, the focal zone is placed at the posterior margin of the vessel. Color Doppler is used to identify areas of luminal narrowing or abnormal flow to select regions for spectral analysis. The color gain is adjusted so that color signal remains within the vessel lumen. If no flow is seen, increasing the color gain, decreasing the wall filter, decreasing the color scale, or using power Doppler imaging can improve sensitivity for the detection of flow, particularly in arteries in which near complete occlusion is suspected.

Long-axis spectral Doppler velocity measurements should be obtained at the predetermined sites in all vessels as well as in areas of stenosis or suspected stenosis. If a significant stenosis is found or suspected, images must be recorded at the location of the stenosis with the maximum velocity as well as distal to the site of the maximum velocity to document the presence or absence of poststenotic turbulent flow.[5] The Doppler angle should be between 45° and 60°. The potential velocity error associated with Doppler angle increases with increasing Doppler angle, particularly at a Doppler angle greater than 60°.[5] For this reason, Doppler angles greater than 60° should be avoided whenever possible. The peak systolic velocity ratio (PSVR) is calculated by dividing the peak systolic velocity (PSV) at or just distal to the ICA stenosis by the PSV in the distal CCA. Three measurements of the PSV and end-diastolic velocity (EDV) should be recorded at each vessel. The PSV in the distal CCA should be measured 2 to 3 cm below the carotid bulb where the walls are parallel to one another. For spectral Doppler, the sample gate is placed centrally within the lumen and kept between 1.5 and 2.5 mm in width. The Doppler scale or pulse repetition frequency should be set to maximize the size of the waveforms without aliasing.

NORMAL FINDINGS

Typically, the right CCA arises from the brachiocephalic artery, and the left CCA arises directly off the aorta. Many vascular variants exist, including a common origin of the left brachiocephalic artery and the left CCA (bovine arch), which occurs in approximately 15% of the population. Near the carotid bifurcation, the distal CCA caliber increases slightly to form the carotid bulb. The CCA then bifurcates into its 2 terminal branches, the ICA and ECA. The ICAs supply oxygenated blood to the anterior circulation of the brain, and the ECAs supply the structures of the head, face, and neck. The ECA is most reliably distinguished from the ICA by its branches in the neck (**Fig. 1**) because the ICA does not have extracranial branches. The ICA is also typically larger and located posterolateral relative to the ECA, although these are not reliable distinguishing features because of significant anatomic variation.

The CCA, ICA, and ECA have unique waveform patterns that are related to differences in the tissues they supply. The carotid arteries should demonstrate a sharp systolic upstroke and narrow spectral envelope outlining a spectral window. The ICA typically has a thicker spectral envelope and continuous diastolic flow owing to lower peripheral vascular resistance and higher oxygen consumption of the brain. The ECA waveform typically has a relatively thinner spectral envelope and less diastolic flow owing to higher peripheral vascular resistance and lower oxygen consumption in the head and neck musculature. Because of variable oxygen consumption in the head and neck vasculature, the amount of diastolic flow of the ECA can vary; however, the amount of diastolic flow should be symmetric bilaterally and should be less than the ICA. The CCA has a waveform morphology between that of the ICA and ECA, with PSV ranging from 60 to 100 cm/s and continuous diastolic flow.

PLAQUE CHARACTERIZATION

Plaque characterization is a vital component of the assessment of carotid artery US. The risk of

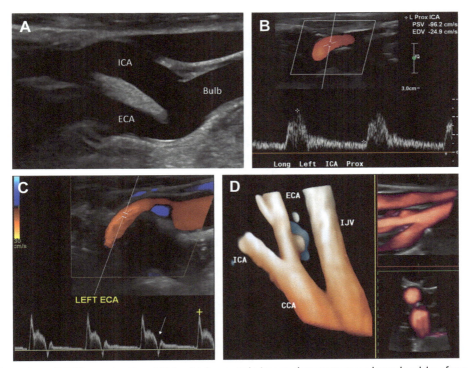

Fig. 1. Normal carotid US examination. (A) Sagittal grayscale image demonstrates a branch arising from the ECA, the ICA, and the carotid bulb. (B) Spectral Doppler of the ICA shows a sharp systolic upstroke, thin spectral envelope, and a larger diastolic flow component than the ECA. (C) Spectral Doppler of the ECA shows a sharp systolic upstroke, thin spectral envelope, an early diastolic notch (*arrow*), and less diastolic flow compared with the ICA. (D) 3D carotid US shows the carotid bifurcation with branches arising from the ECA as well as the adjacent internal jugular vein (IJV).

plaque embolization is directly related to the plaque composition and morphology (Fig. 2). Factors that predispose to plaque rupture include intraplaque hemorrhage, necrosis, inflammation, and thinning of the fibrous cap, which results in the formation of unstable thrombus on the plaque surface. The unstable thrombus may then embolize as it is dislodged by the high-velocity blood coursing through the narrowed lumen. As a result, the degree of stenosis is also indirectly related to the risk of embolization and stroke.[6–8] Ulcerated plaque is also at increased risk of distal embolization owing to exposure of the thrombogenic centrally necrotic core or stagnant flow.[9] Smoothly surfaced

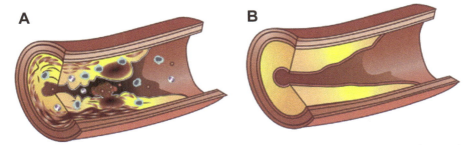

Fig. 2. Plaque. (A) Vulnerable plaque is characterized by neovascularity, inflammation, central necrosis, and thinning of the fibrous cap. Hemorrhage from plaque neovascularity and inflammatory cell death owing to cholesterol and lipid toxicity result in central necrosis, swelling, and ultimately, plaque rupture, exposing the thrombogenic necrotic core to circulating blood. Thrombus forming on the surface of the ruptured plaque or plaque debris is then at risk for distal embolization. (B) Hyalinized, fibrous, or calcified plaque has less inflammation and neovascularity and is less likely to undergo central necrosis and rupture. Thus, unless the surface is irregular, resulting in stagnant flow, thrombus is unlikely to form on the surface of the plaque.

hyalinized, fibrous, or calcified plaque has a lower risk of rupture and distal embolization because of a lack of unstable thrombus on the plaque surface and lack of exposure of the centrally necrotic core.

Plaque burden, echogenicity, and surface characteristics should be assessed using grayscale and color Doppler. Plaque may be described as either hypoechoic or hyperechoic (echogenic), and its composition may be homogeneous, mixed, or heterogeneous. In addition, the plaque surface should be examined and may be either smooth or irregularly surfaced/fissured. Ulcerated plaque is defined as a surface defect greater than 2 mm identified in 2 orthogonal imaging planes and is at increased risk of plaque rupture. Hypoechoic plaque is more likely to be lipid-laden or hemorrhagic and is more likely to rupture.[10–13] As a result, heterogeneous plaque is generally regarded as unstable, as it contains hypoechoic and/or anechoic areas, which indicate intraplaque cholesterol or hemorrhage (Fig. 3). Conversely, echogenic plaque is generally regarded as stable and is unlikely to rupture.

Optimizing carotid US scanning technique is vital in plaque characterization. Plaque may appear falsely hypoechoic or falsely echogenic if the grayscale gain is set incorrectly. Appropriately setting the color gain is also important to avoid obscuring hypoechoic plaque or thrombus, including markedly hypoechoic plaque or thrombus, which may only be seen as a color void on Doppler imaging and not readily detectable on grayscale imaging.

Intima-media thickness (IMT) is an additional parameter that has been proposed as an independent risk factor for cardiovascular disease and a predictor of stroke.[14–17] In 2008, the American Society of Echocardiography issued a consensus statement recommending that the IMT be measured on magnified images along the posterior wall of the distal CCA 1 cm below the bulb using a high-frequency linear-array transducer with the CCA oriented perpendicular to the US beam, avoiding areas of plaque and ensuring not to include the echogenic adventitia in the measurement. An IMT measurement less than 0.7 to 0.8 mm is considered normal, although IMT does vary with age, gender, and ethnicity.[18] Although previous studies have suggested that IMT is an independent risk factor for cardiovascular disease, more recent studies suggest that carotid IMT

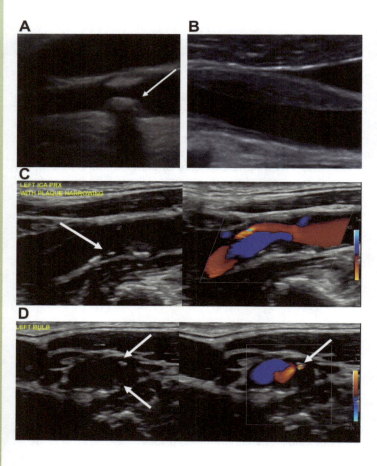

Fig. 3. Plaque characterization. Focal echogenic plaque (A) with posterior shadowing likely representing calcification (arrow), which is unlikely to be vulnerable. Smooth homogeneously hypoechoic plaque with a smooth surface contour (B), also unlikely to be vulnerable. Vulnerable heterogeneously hypoechoic plaque (arrow) with anechoic foci and an irregular surface contour in the proximal left ICA (C). Additional vulnerable heterogeneous plaque (arrows) with anechoic foci and intraplaque neovascularization (D). PRX, proximal.

measurement does not provide meaningful risk stratification for future cardiovascular events.[19,20] A recent international consensus statement defines carotid plaque as diffuse IMT thickening greater than 1.5 mm or any focal protuberant plaque, and repeated follow-up measurements are recommended in these patients even in the absence of symptoms.[21]

Three-dimensional (3D) imaging of atherosclerotic plaque has also been reported to be highly accurate and a predictor of increased risk of cardiovascular events.[22–25] Given that atherosclerotic plaque is a 3D phenomenon, recent studies have suggested that 3D quantification of carotid plaque is more sensitive in the detection of clinically significant stenoses as compared with 2-dimensional imaging.[22] Patients in the top quartile of total plaque area on 3D imaging have also been shown to have a 3 times higher 5-year risk of death, stroke, or myocardial infarction.[23,26] An additional advantage of 3D imaging is an improved ability to evaluate the plaque surface. Patients with a global ulcer volume greater than 5 mm^3 were shown to have a considerably increased risk of stroke, TIA, or death.[27]

Contrast-enhanced ultrasound (CEUS) is an additional technique, which has been shown to be superior to color Doppler imaging in terms of grading stenosis and assessing the plaque surface.[28,29] As US contrast agents are purely intravascular agents, CEUS is also a valuable method for the detection of intraplaque neovascularization, a major feature of plaque vulnerability.[30,31] Delayed phase imaging has also shown increased enhancement of symptomatic plaques relative to asymptomatic plaques, a sign of intraplaque inflammation.[32] However, although CEUS has shown utility in identifying vulnerable plaque and neovascularization, standardized CEUS technique has not yet been established.[33,34] Nevertheless, CEUS could be incorporated into future risk stratification systems for patients with carotid plaques, particularly those with 50% to 69% stenosis.[33,35,36] Superb microvascular imaging (SMI) is an additional novel US technique, which applies an algorithm to differentiate true microvascular flow signals from wall motion artifacts and clutter. Several studies have suggested SMI as a promising noninvasive technique, which can detect neovascularity and assess plaque stability with accuracy comparable to CEUS.[37,38]

INTERNAL CAROTID ARTERY STENOSIS GRADING

In 1991, the NASCET reported that carotid endarterectomy (CEA) was highly beneficial in symptomatic patients with recent hemispheric or retinal TIAs or nondisabling strokes and ipsilateral high-grade ICA stenosis (70%–99%), showing an absolute ipsilateral stroke risk reduction of 17% compared with medical treatment.[4] In the NASCET trial, the percent ICA stenosis was calculated by dividing the narrowest luminal ICA diameter by the luminal diameter of the distal normal ICA (**Fig. 4**). This method has now become widely accepted as the preferred method of grading ICA stenosis, although plaque burden can be significantly underestimated using this method, particularly when there is decreased flow in the poststenotic ICA owing to collateral vessels or tandem lesions.[39] Additional trials also showed a significant but smaller benefit in asymptomatic patients with moderate ICA stenosis (50%–69%).[40,41] Subsequent trials also showed a similar decrease in ipsilateral stroke incidence following carotid artery stent placement.[42,43]

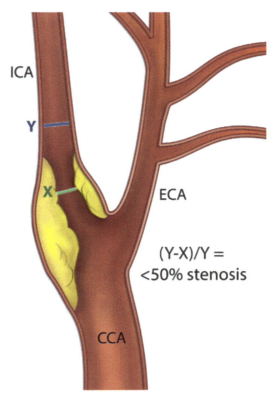

Fig. 4. Calculation of ICA stenosis according to the NASCET method. According to the NASCET study design, percent ICA stenosis is calculated by comparing the diameter of the residual lumen (X) to the diameter of the distal normal ICA (Y). In this schematic image, there is less than 50% ICA stenosis despite the presence of a large amount of plaque. Although the NASCET method reduces interobserver and intraobserver variability, it may significantly underestimate plaque burden.

In 2002, the SRU consensus panel recommended using PSV and the presence of plaque as the primary Doppler criteria for grading ICA stenosis. PSVR and EDV serve as secondary parameters with grayscale and color Doppler correlation.[3,13] Since then, the SRU consensus guidelines have become the most commonly used criteria for assessing ICA stenosis in the United States.

UPDATES

In 2014, the Intersocietal Accreditation Commission (IAC) Vascular Testing issued a White Paper detailing significant variability in the reporting of carotid artery stenosis as well as the potential clinical impact on this variation.[44] The IAC then carried out a research study aimed at assessing validity of the SRU Consensus criteria in an effort to potentially refine the criteria. In this study, the primary parameter for ≥50% ICA stenosis of PSV of ≥125 cm/s did not meet prespecified thresholds for adequate sensitivity, specificity, and accuracy (sensitivity, 97.8%; specificity, 64.2%; accuracy, 74.5%). Test performance was improved by raising the PSV threshold to ≥180 cm/s (sensitivity, 93.3%; specificity, 81.6%; accuracy, 85.2%). These data supported the adoption of a higher PSV threshold of 180 cm/s for 50% ICA stenosis and found the previously used threshold of 125 cm/s to be too sensitive with insufficient specificity and accuracy.[45] As a result, the IAC Vascular Testing now recommends the adoption of modified SRU criteria with a higher PSV threshold value of 180 cm/s for 50% ICA stenosis (Fig. 5, Table 1). However, the IAC continues to recommend correlation with grayscale and color Doppler findings, as there are instances of 50% to 69% ICA stenosis with PSV of ≥125 and less than 180 cm/s. In these cases, the images should demonstrate other sonographic features of stenosis, such as an elevated ICA/CCA PSV ratio greater than 2.0, significant atherosclerotic plaque, and color aliasing at the site of stenosis (Fig. 6). In the event of significant discrepancies between the spectral Doppler and the grayscale and color Doppler findings, an explanation should be sought factoring in individual patient factors, such as the patient's hemodynamics or other factors affecting physiology. If no clinical explanation is evident, additional imaging with computed tomographic (CT) angiography may be of benefit. Although IAC Vascular Testing is now recommending a higher PSV threshold of 180 cm/s for 50% to 69% stenosis, there was insufficient evidence to recommend modification of the SRU Criteria for higher degrees of stenosis (≥70% ICA stenosis) owing to a limited sample size (Fig. 7). However, combinations of PSV ≥230, ≥250, and ≥260 cm/s with ICA/CCA ratio ≥3.3 all met criteria for adequate sensitivity, specificity, and accuracy.[45]

Note that the IAC recommendations have not been uniformly accepted among institutions owing to concerns that have been raised in the published literature. First, the retrospective analysis of the underlying study has been questioned, but it did represent a multicenter trial with catheter angiography as the reference standard. The recommendations underemphasize that the highest accuracy of 87.4% with sensitivity of 94.3% and specificity of 84.3% occurred when both PSV > 125 cm/s AND ICA/CCA ratio >2.0 were required for diagnosis rather than using the isolated

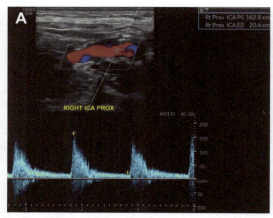 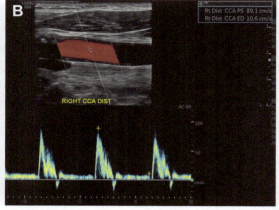

Fig. 5. Less than 50% stenosis of the ICA. (*A*) Small amount of calcified plaque is seen in the proximal right ICA with a PSV of 163 cm/s and a PSV of 89 cm/s in the distal CCA (*B*) for a PSVR of less than 2. By the modified SRU criteria, this would not be characterized as a hemodynamically significant stenosis. ED, end diastolic; DIST, distal; PROX, proximal; PS, peak systolic.

Table 1
Recommended modification of the Society of Radiologists in Ultrasound consensus conference criteria for ICA stenosis

Degree of Stenosis, %	ICA PSV, cm/s	Plaque Estimate, %	ICA/CCA PSV Ratio (Secondary Parameter)	ICA EDA, cm/s (Secondary Parameter)
Normal	<180	None	<2.0	<40
<50	<180	<50	<2.0	<40
50–69	180–230	>50	2.0–4.0	40–100
≥70 but less than near occlusion	>230	>50	>4.0	>100
Near occlusion	High, low, undetectable	Variable	Variable	Variable
Total occlusion	Undetectable	Visible, no detectable lumen	N/A	N/A

threshold PSV > 180 cm/s. The new criteria have also been challenged by the Trial of ORG 10172 in Acute Stroke Treatment, which challenges the assumption that the threshold change has no impact on stroke risk.[46] This is relevant because 50% stenosis is an accepted marker for large-vessel atherosclerosis requiring surveillance.

Using the new criteria, 27.1% of patients would have been removed from surveillance, and these would be lost to follow-up. According to their data, the stroke event rate nearly doubles from the 125 to the 180 cm/s thresholds. The risk of stroke in their study population increased by 89% once the patient has a PSV > 180 cm/s

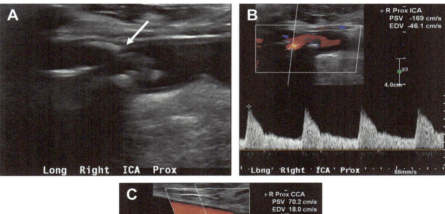
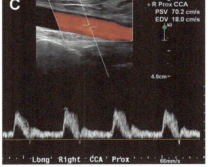

Fig. 6. Stenosis of the right ICA (50%–69%). (A) Sagittal grayscale US of the right proximal ICA shows extensive echogenic plaque (arrow). (B) Spectral Doppler of the right proximal ICA in the region of the plaque shows a PSV of 169 cm/s. (C) Spectral Doppler of the right CCA shows a PSV of 70 cm/s for a PSVR of 2.4. Findings are consistent with a 50% to 69% stenosis of the right ICA when using velocity in conjunction with PSVR and grayscale findings.

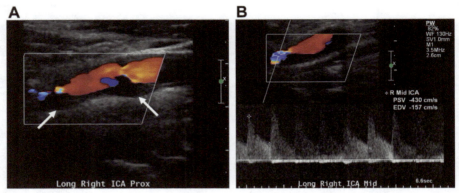

Fig. 7. Greater than 70% stenosis of the ICA. (*A*) Sagittal color Doppler image shows luminal narrowing in the proximal ICA by greater than 70% owing to hypoechoic plaque (*arrows*). (*B*) Spectral Doppler in the right mid-ICA along the distal aspect of the plaque shows an elevated PSV of 430 cm/s, compatible with a greater than 70% right ICA stenosis.

relative to 125 cm/s, and 70% of ischemic strokes thought due to large-vessel atherosclerosis would have been missed by using the new threshold. Future studies will likely be necessary to resolve these concerns.

PITFALLS

Although ICA PSV remains the single most reliable Doppler criterion for grading ICA stenosis, overreliance on this single criterion may overestimate or underestimate stenosis in certain situations. For example, in patients with low-output states, the CCA PSV is often less than 60 cm/s. In these situations, using a threshold of 180 cm/s to diagnose 50% to 69% stenosis may underestimate ICA stenosis if PSV is used as the only criterion to diagnose stenosis. In these situations, correlation with additional grayscale and color Doppler criteria, including plaque burden, PSVR, and EDV, is necessary to accurately quantify stenosis. Conversely, in high-flow states with a CCA velocity greater than 100 cm/s, using a threshold of 230 cm/s to diagnose ≥70% ICA stenosis may be overly sensitive if relying on the PSV alone, potentially leading to a false positive result.

Additional causes of an elevated PSV in the absence of hemodynamically significant stenosis include vessel tortuosity and contralateral ICA/CCA high-grade stenosis/occlusion. Vessel tortuosity may intrinsically increase the PSV and also provides technical challenges to accurate PSV measurement, as it is difficult to orient the Doppler angle correctly in a tortuous vessel. Both of these factors may lead to an overestimation of the PSV. In contralateral high-grade stenosis/occlusion of the ICA/CCA, the ICA and CCA velocities will be increased if these arteries provide collateral flow.[47,48] In either of these instances, correlation with additional spectral Doppler parameters, such as PSVR, as well as grayscale and color Doppler findings is essential to avoid false positive results.

Conversely, hemodynamically significant stenosis can also occur in the absence of an elevated ICA PSV. Long-segment stenosis (>2 cm), tandem lesions, and high-grade nearly occlusive segments may all result in a lower-than-expected PSV, despite the presence of significant stenosis. In these instances, careful assessment of the grayscale and color Doppler findings may assist in the detection of stenosis despite the lack of an elevated ICA PSV.

CAROTID ARTERY WAVEFORM ANALYSIS

Distal to a high-grade stenosis, a tardus-parvus pattern is often observed. The waveform is characterized by a decreased PSV and a slow systolic upstroke with a rounded peak.[49] A widespread tardus parvus throughout the bilateral CCAs, ICAs, and VAs suggests a proximal stenosis, likely at the level of the aortic arch or a moderate to severe aortic valve stenosis[50–52] (**Fig. 8**). Conversely, a unilateral waveform in the distal ICA but with a sharp systolic upstroke in the proximal ICA indicates that the stenosis is in the mid-ICA, which can aid when interrogating this segment. As a result, identifying the distribution and extent of the tardus-parvus waveform or waveforms is crucial in accurately identifying the site of the stenosis.

Proximal to a high-grade stenosis or occlusion, a "knocking" or "staccato" waveform is often observed, which becomes more pronounced closer to an obstructing lesion.[50] The "knocking" or "staccato" waveform is characterized by a sharp systolic upstroke with decreased PSV and decreased, absent, or reversed diastolic flow. For

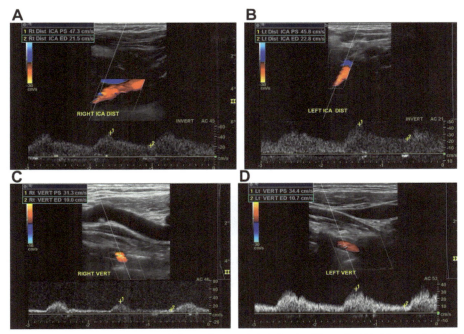

Fig. 8. Aortic stenosis. Spectral Doppler of the right ICA (A), left ICA (B), right VA (C), and left VA (D) shows tardus-parvus waveforms throughout, compatible with aortic stenosis.

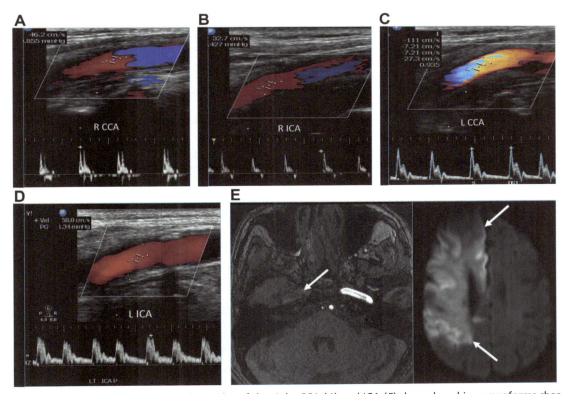

Fig. 9. Knocking waveforms. Spectral Doppler of the right CCA (A) and ICA (B) shows knocking waveforms characterized by high-resistance waveforms, suggestive of a nearby distal complete occlusion on the right. Spectral Doppler of the left CCA (C) and ICA (D) shows compensatory mildly increased velocities with normal antegrade diastolic flow. MR imaging/MR angiography of the brain (E) shows occlusion of the petrous segment of the ICA with a large right MCA territory infarct (arrows). L, left; R, right.

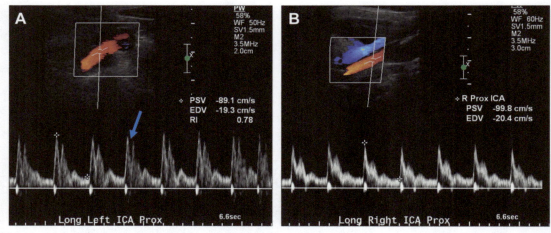

Fig. 10. Severe aortic regurgitation with pulsus bisferiens. (A) Spectral Doppler of the left proximal ICA shows a systolic notch (arrow) or "mid systolic retraction/dip," which is also present but less pronounced in the proximal right ICA (B).

example, a knocking waveform in the proximal ICA suggests a high-grade stenosis/occlusion of the ipsilateral mid/distal ICA. A high-resistance waveform may also be seen in the ipsilateral CCA and ICA in the setting of ipsilateral intracranial ICA or middle cerebral artery high-grade stenosis/occlusion (Fig. 9). Arteritis, vasospasm, or a distal dissection can also rarely cause a unilateral knocking waveform. Increased intracranial pressure can result in bilateral knocking waveforms, often caused by a hematoma, edema, or intracranial mass lesion.[50,53]

Aortic insufficiency can result in a pulsus bisferiens waveform characterized by a systolic notch or "mid systolic retraction" owing to the artery's recoil effect (Fig. 10).[50,53] In patients with a left ventricular assist device (LVAD), a monophasic waveform with a low PSV and marked tardus-parvus morphology is observed (Fig. 11). In patients with an intra-aortic balloon pump (IABP), there will be 2 forward peaks in systole and reversal of flow in diastole. The first forward peak corresponds to systole, and the second peak corresponds to augmented forward flow, which occurs in early diastole when the balloon is inflated (Fig. 12). PSV is variable in the setting of an IABP. As a result, accurate interpretation relies on correlation with grayscale, PSVR, and color Doppler findings in patients with an LVAD or IABP.[53,54]

NONATHEROSCLEROTIC PATHOLOGIC CONDITIONS

The most common cause of carotid artery dissections is trauma, presenting with headache, stroke, or Horner syndrome. Hypertension is the most common predisposing factor for carotid artery dissection. Certain vascular conditions that increase the fragility of the vessel wall, such as Ehlers-Danlos syndrome and Marfan syndrome, also increase the risk for dissection.[55] Dissections most often manifest as an abnormally high-resistance waveform in the proximal ICA because most ICA dissections begin distally at the skull base and extend inferiorly, resulting in stenosis or occlusion of the distal ICA. CCA dissections are characterized by an echogenic intraluminal flap on US (Fig. 13). The true lumen often demonstrates an elevated PSV owing to compression by

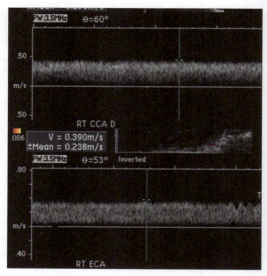

Fig. 11. LVAD. Monophasic blunted waveforms in the right CCA and right ECA with continuous antegrade from an LVAD.

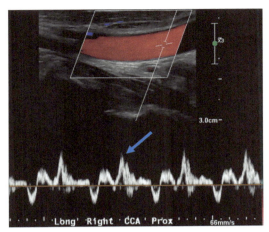

Fig. 12. IABP. Spectral Doppler of the right CCA shows a second antegrade peak (*arrow*) during early diastole owing to inflation of the balloon of the IABP, resulting in augmented flow to the coronary arteries. Transient reversal of flow is noted later in diastole after the balloon is deflated.

the false lumen. The false lumen may demonstrate reversal of flow or could have mural hematoma or thrombosis, characterized by homogeneously hypoechoic thickening of the ICA wall or an eccentric echogenic component.[56] In equivocal cases, MR imaging can also be obtained to readily make the diagnosis.

Fibromuscular dysplasia (FMD) is a nonatherosclerotic angiopathy of small- and medium-sized arteries with the extracranial internal carotid arteries being the second most common arteries affected. On US, FMD is characterized by an irregular beaded appearance of the involved vessels, most commonly affecting the middle to distal ICA. Grading ICA stenosis using the SRU criteria is unreliable in patients with FMD because of the presence of multiple tandem lesions. Takayasu arteritis is a large-vessel vasculitis affecting the aorta and its major branches, which can also extend into the CCA. Associated narrowing of the CCA results in elevated PSV in the CCA; decreased velocities and tardus-parvus waveforms are seen in the ICAs, ECAs, and VAs (**Fig. 14**).[57]

Arteriovenous fistulas can also occur in the carotid arteries, most commonly following trauma or surgical intervention. On US, arteriovenous fistulas are characterized by a direct communication between the artery and vein with markedly elevated PSV and EDV on spectral Doppler. Occasionally, an adjacent soft tissue color bruit is seen due to surrounding tissue vibrations. The draining vein will also show arterialized high-velocity flow.

Pseudoaneurysm (PSA) may also occur following trauma, arterial dissection, or surgical intervention. Vasculitis affecting the carotid vasculature can also rarely cause carotid artery PSA. Like PSAs elsewhere, carotid artery PSAs are characterized by a focal outpouching arising from the impacted vessel on grayscale imaging. On Doppler US, swirling blood flow will be noted in the PSA sac with a "yin-yang" pattern. Echogenic thrombus may also be seen in the PSA sac if it is partially thrombosed.

CAROTID ULTRASOUND AFTER INTERVENTION

Common effective treatments for carotid artery stenosis include CEA and carotid artery stenting (CAS) with similar long-term risk of stroke and restenosis following either procedure. Surveillance US is typically recommended every 6 to 12 months, although the SRU criteria are not applicable due to altered hemodynamics.[58]

During CEA, the vessel compliance and luminal diameter of the carotid bulb both increase, resulting in a decreased PSV. As a result, the PSV indicative of ICA stenosis is likely lower than the native artery; however, there is currently no widely

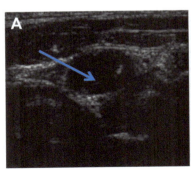
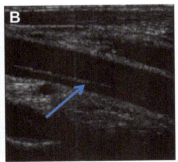
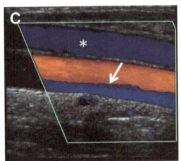

Fig. 13. CCA dissection. Transverse (*A*) and sagittal (*B*) grayscale images of the CCA show an intraluminal flap (*arrow*). (*C*) Normal antegrade flow is seen in the true lumen with reversal of flow in the false lumen. Internal jugular vein (asterisk).

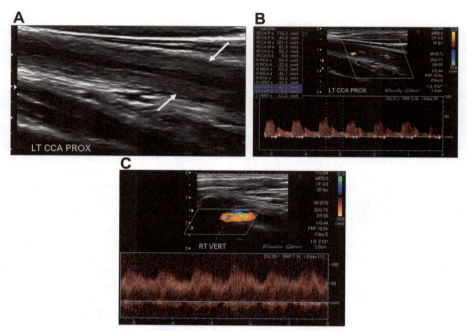

Fig. 14. Takayasu arteritis is in a 21-year-old woman with weak upper-extremity pulses. Sagittal grayscale image shows severe wall thickening (*arrows*) of the proximal left CCA (*A*) with a PSV of 174 cm/s (*B*). Spectral Doppler of the right VA in the same patient (*C*) shows a tardus-parvus waveform. MICA, mid internal carotid artery; PICA, proximal internal carotid artery; VERT, vertebral.

accepted PSV criterion to diagnose stenosis in these patients. Instead, PSVR, grayscale findings, and color Doppler findings in conjunction with PSV changes over time or compared with baseline are used to assess for stenosis following CEA.

CAS placement results in an increased PSV owing to shunting of blood into the ICA from the partially occluded ECA and decreased vessel compliance. External compression from atherosclerotic plaque or incomplete expansion of the stent can also contribute to an elevated PSV (**Fig. 15**). After CAS placement, a PSV greater than 300 to 325 cm/s may represent a ≥70% stenosis, although there is no universally accepted PSV threshold[59,60] (**Fig. 16**). Similar to patients with CEA, correlation with grayscale and color Doppler findings as well as any significant changes in PSV over time or compared with baseline may also aid in the diagnosis of in-stent restenosis. In order to accurately diagnose restenosis, an elevated PSV should typically be accompanied by intraluminal echogenic material representing plaque, thrombus, or neointimal hyperplasia on the grayscale images. These findings can also be

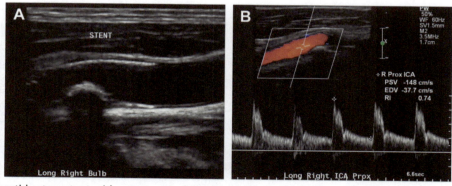

Fig. 15. Carotid artery stent without stenosis. (*A*) Sagittal grayscale image of the right carotid bulb shows less than 50% luminal narrowing related to compression from external calcified atherosclerotic plaque. (*B*) Spectral Doppler of the right ICA within the stent just distal to the area of narrowing shows a PSV of 148 cm/s.

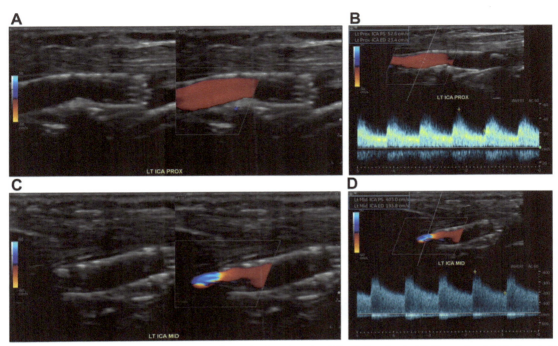

Fig. 16. In-stent restenosis. Sagittal grayscale and color Doppler (*A*) of the stented left proximal ICA shows no luminal narrowing and a PSV of 53 cm/s (*B*). Grayscale and color Doppler (*C*) of the mid-ICA shows greater than 50% luminal narrowing with aliasing and a PSV of 403 cm/s (*D*), compatible with in-stent restenosis. MID, middle.

supplemented by CT angiography findings in select cases.

SUMMARY

Carotid Doppler US is the primary noninvasive imaging method for the detection, grading, and monitoring of ICA stenosis. Recent studies have shown that the previously adopted SRU guidelines for grading ICA stenosis were too sensitive with insufficient specificity and accuracy. As a result, the IAC now recommends a modified SRU criteria with a higher PSV threshold of ≥180 cm/s for 50% to 69% ICA stenosis, or greater than 125 cm/s if there is also an ICA/CCA ratio greater than 2.0. This new threshold should be used in conjunction with grayscale and color Doppler findings, particularly if there are significant discrepancies between the spectral Doppler findings and the grayscale/color Doppler findings. Plaque characterization is also a vital component of the carotid Doppler US assessment, especially in the identification of vulnerable plaque. Techniques including 3D imaging, CEUS, and SMI may help further risk-stratify patients in the future because of their ability to identify vulnerable plaque, particularly in patients with 50% to 69% stenosis.

CLINICS CARE POINTS

- The Intersocietal Accreditation Commission now recommends a modified Society of Radiologists in Ultrasound criteria peak systolic velocity threshold of 180 to 230 cm/s for the diagnosis of 50% to 69% internal carotid artery stenosis.

- Internal carotid artery stenosis of 50% to 69% may still occur with a peak systolic velocity ≥125 and less than 180 cm/s, particularly in cases where other features of stenosis are present, such as an elevated internal carotid artery/common carotid artery peak systolic velocity ratio greater than 2.0, significant atherosclerotic plaque, and/or color aliasing at the site of stenosis.

- Overreliance on the peak systolic velocity as a criterion for grading internal carotid artery stenosis may overestimate or underestimate stenosis in certain situations. For example, a lower-than-expected peak systolic velocity can occur in the setting of hemodynamically significant stenosis in long segment stenosis (>2 cm), tandem lesions, and high-grade nearly occlusive segments.

DISCLOSURE

T.J. Sevco: Nothing to disclose. M.K. Patel: Research grant, Phillips, United States. C. Deurdulian: Book royalties, Elsevier and Jaypee Brothers Medical Publishers.

REFERENCES

1. Tsao CW, Aday AW, Almarzooq ZI, et al. Heart disease and stroke statistics—2023 update: a report from the American Heart Association. Circulation 2023;147(8). https://doi.org/10.1161/cir.0000000000 0001123. Available at: www.ahajournals.org/doi/10.1161/CIR.0000000000001123.
2. Fairhead JF, Rothwell PM. The need for urgency in identification and treatment of symptomatic carotid stenosis is already established. Cerebrovasc Dis 2005;19:355–8.
3. Grant EG, Benson CB, Moneta GL, et al. Carotid artery stenosis: gray-scale and Doppler US diagnosis—Society of radiologists in ultrasound consensus conference. Radiology 2003;229:340–6.
4. North American Symptomatic Carotid Endarterectomy Trial Collaborators, Barnett HJM, Taylor DW, et al. Beneficial effect of carotid endarterectomy in symptomatic patients with high-grade carotid stenosis. N Engl J Med 1991;325(7):445–53.
5. The AIUM practice parameter for the performance of an ultrasound examination of the extracranial cerebrovascular system. J Ultrasound Med 2021;41(4). https://doi.org/10.1002/jum.15877.
6. Hansson GK. Inflammation, atherosclerosis, and coronary artery disease. N Engl J Med 2005;352:1685–95.
7. Ross R. Atherosclerosis-an inflammatory disease. N Engl J Med 1999;340:115–26.
8. Bonati LH, Nederkoorn PJ. Clinical perspective of carotid plaque imaging. Neuroimaging Clin N Am 2016;26:175–82.
9. Fisher M, Paganini-Hill A, Martin A, et al. Carotid plaque pathology: thrombosis, ulceration and stroke pathogenesis. Stroke 2005;6(2):253–7.
10. Bluth EI, Kay D, Merritt CR, et al. Sonographic characterization of carotid plaque: detection of hemorrhage. AJR Am J Roentgenol 1986;146:1061–5.
11. Gerrit L, Sijbrands EJ, Straub D, et al. Noninvasive imaging of the vulnerable atherosclerotic plaque. Curr Probl Cardiol 2010;35:556–91.
12. Polak JF, Shemanski L, O'Leary DH, et al. Hypoechoic plaque at US of the carotid artery: an independent risk factor for incident stroke in adults aged 65 years or older. Cardiovascular Healthy Study. Radiology 1998;208(3):649–54. 14.
13. Gupta A, Kesavabhotla K, Baradaran H, et al. Plaque echolucency and stroke risk in asymptomatic carotid stenosis: a systemic review and meta-analysis. Stroke 2015;46:91–7.
14. Salonen JT, Salonen R. Ultrasonographically assessed carotid morphology and the risk of coronary heart disease. Arterioscler Thromb 1991;11:1245–9. 23.
15. Chambless LE, Heiss G, Folsom AR, et al. Association of coronary heart disease incidence with carotid arterial wall thickness and major risk factors: The Arteriosclerosis Risk in Communities (ARIC) Study 1993-1997. Am J Epidemiol 1997;146:483–94.
16. Bots ML, Hoes AW, Koudstaal PJ, et al. Common carotid artery intima-media thickness as a risk factor for myocardial infarction: The Rotterdam Study. Circulation 1997;96:1432–7.
17. O'Leary DH, Polak JF, Kronmal RA, et al. Carotid-artery intima and media thickness as a risk factor for myocardial infarction and stroke in older adults. Cardiovascular Health Study. N Engl J Med 1999;340:14–22.
18. Coli S, Magnoni M, Sangiorgi G, et al. Contrast-enhanced ultrasound imaging of intraplaque neovascularization in carotid arteries: correlation with histology and plaque echogenicity. J Am Coll Cardiol 2008;52:223–30.
19. Helfand M, Buckley DI, Freeman M, et al. Emerging risk factors for coronary heart disease: a summary of systemic reviews conducted for the U.S. Preventive Services Task Force. Ann Intern Med 2009;151:496–507.
20. Zavodni AEH, Wasserman BA, McClelland RL, et al. Carotid artery plaque morphology and composition in relation to incident cardiovascular events: The Multi-Ethnic Study of Atherosclerosis (MESA). Radiology 2014;271(2):381–9.
21. Johri A, Nambi V, Nappi T, et al. Recommendations for the assessment of carotida arterial plaque by ultrasound for the characterization of atherosclerosis and evaluation of cardiovascular risk: from the American Society of Echocardiography. J Am Soc Echocardiogr 2020;33(8):917–33.
22. Calogero E, Fabiani I, Pugliese NR, et al. Three-dimensional echographic evaluation of carotid artery disease. J Cardiovasc Echogr 2018;28(4):218–27.
23. Johnsen SH, Mathiesen EB, Joakimsen O, et al. Carotid atherosclerosis is a stronger predictor of myocardial infarction in women than in men: A 6-year follow-up study of 6226 persons: The Tromsø study. Stroke 2007;38:2873–80.
24. Schminke U, Motsch L, Griewing B, et al. Three-dimensional power-mode ultrasound for quantification of the progression of carotid artery atherosclerosis. J Neurol 2000;247:106–11.
25. van Engelen A, Wannarong T, Parraga G, et al. Three-dimensional carotid ultrasound plaque texture predicts vascular events. Stroke 2014;45:2695–701.
26. Mathiesen EB, Johnsen SH, Wilsgaard T, et al. Carotid plaque area and intima-media thickness in prediction

26. of first-ever ischemic stroke: A 10-year follow-up of 6584 men and women: The Tromsø study. Stroke 2011;42:972–8.
27. Kuk M, Wannarong T, Beletsky V, et al. Volume of carotid artery ulceration as a predictor of cardiovascular events. Stroke 2014;45:1437–41.
28. Sirlin CB, Lee YZ, Girard MS, et al. Contrast-enhanced B-mode US angiography in the assessment of experimental in vivo and in vitro atherosclerotic disease. Acad Radiol 2001;8:162–72.
29. Kono Y, Pinnell SP, Sirlin CB, et al. Carotid arteries: contrast-enhanced US angiography–preliminary clinical experience. Radiology 2004;230:561–8.
30. Feinstein SB. The powerful microbubble: from bench to bedside, from intravascular indicator to therapeutic delivery system, and beyond. Am J Physiol Heart Circ Physiol 2004;287:H450–7.
31. Xiong L, Deng YB, Zhu Y, et al. Correlation of carotid plaque neovascularization detected by using contrast-enhanced US with clinical symptoms. Radiology 2009;251:583–9.
32. Owen DR, Shalhoub J, Miller S, et al. Inflammation within carotid atherosclerotic plaque: assessment with late-phase contrast-enhanced US. Radiology 2010;255:638–44.
33. Varetto G, Gibello L, Castagno C, et al. Use of contrast-enhanced ultrasound in carotid atherosclerotic disease: limits and perspectives. BioMed Res Int 2015;293163.
34. Saha SA, Gourineni V, Feinstein SB. The use of contrast-enhanced ultrasonography for imaging of carotid atherosclerotic plaques: current evidence, future directions. Neuroimaging Clin N Am. 2016; 26:81–96.
35. Eyding J, Geier B, Staub D. Current strategies and possible perspectives of ultrasonic risk stratification of ischemic stroke in internal carotid artery disease. Ultraschall der Med 2011;32:267–73.
36. Rafailidis V, Charitanti A, Tegos T, et al. Contrast-enhanced ultrasound of the carotid system: a review of the current literature. J Ultrasound 2017;20(2):97–109.
37. Zamani M, Skagen K, Scott H, et al. Advanced ultrasound methods in assessment of carotid plaque instability: a prospective multimodal study. BMC Neurol 2020;20(1):39.
38. Zamani M, Skagen K, Scott H, et al. Carotid plaque neovascularization detected with superb microvascular imaging ultrasound without using contrast media. Stroke 2019;50(11):3121–7.
39. Brott TG, Halperin JL, Abbara S, et al. 2011 ASA/ACCF/AHA/AANN/AANS/ACR/ASNR/CNS/SAIP/SCAI/SIR/SNIS/SVM/SVS guideline on the management of patients with extracranial carotid and vertebral artery disease. J Am Coll Cardiol 2011;57(8):1002–44.
40. Executive Committee for the Asymptomatic Carotid Atherosclerosis Study. Endarterectomy for asymptomatic carotid artery stenosis. JAMA 1995;273:1421–8.
41. Rothwell PM, Eliasziw M, Gutnikov SA, et al. Analysis of pooled data from the randomized controlled trials of endarterectomy for symptomatic carotid stenosis. Lancet 2003;361:107–16.
42. Yadav JS, Wholey MH, Kuntz RE, et al. Protected carotid-artery stenting versus endarterectomy in high-risk patients. N Engl J Med 2004;351:1439–501.
43. Bangalore S, Kumar S, Wettersley J, et al. Carotid artery stenting vs. carotid Endarterectomy: Metaanalysis and diversity-adjusted trial sequential analysis of randomized trials. Arch Neurol 2011;68(2):172–84.
44. Available at: https://www.intersocietal.org/vascular/forms/IACCarotidCriteriaWhitePaper1-2014.pdf.
45. Gornik Heather L, Rundek T, Gardener H, et al. Optimization of duplex velocity criteria for diagnosis of internal carotid artery (ICA) Stenosis: a report of the Intersocietal Accreditation Commission (IAC) Vascular Testing Division Carotid Diagnostic Criteria Committee. Vasc Med 19 2021;26(5):515–25. intersocietal.org/wp-content/uploads/2021/10/IAC-Vascular-Testing-Communication_Updated-Recommendations-for-Carotid-Stenosis-Interpretation-Criteria.pdf.
46. Polak JF. Effect of internal carotid artery doppler peak systolic velocity thresholds for classifying ipsilateral ischemic stroke due to large artery atherosclerosis according to the trial of org 10172 in acute stroke treatment (TOAST) system. J Vasc Ultrasound 2023;47(3):119–24.
47. Grajo JR, Barr RG. Duplex Doppler sonography of the carotid artery. Velocity measurements in an artery with contralateral stenosis. Ultrasound Q 2007;23:199–202.
48. AbuRama AF, Richmond BK, Robinson PA, et al. Effect of contralateral severe stenosis or carotid occlusion on duplex criteria of ipsilateral stenoses. Comparative study of various duplex parameters. J Vasc Surg 1995;22:751–62.
49. Kotval PS. Doppler waveform parvus and tardus. A sign of proximal flow obstruction. J Ultrasound Med 1989;8(8):435–40.
50. Rohren EM, Kliewer MA, Carroll BA, et al. A spectrum of Doppler waveforms in the carotid and vertebral arteries. AJR Am J Roentgenol 2003;181:1695–704.
51. O'Boyle MK, Vibharak N, Chung J, et al. Duplex sonography of the carotid arteries in patients with isolated aortic stenosis: imaging findings and relation to severity of stenosis. AJR Am J Roentgenol 1996;166:197–202.
52. Gunabushanam G, Millet JD, Stilp E, et al. Computer-assisted detection of tardus parvus waveforms on Doppler ultrasound. Ultrasound 2018;26(2):81–92.
53. Scoutt LM, Lin FL, Kliewer M. Waveform analysis of the carotid arteries. Ultrasound Clin 2006;1:133–59.

54. Nuffer Z, Rupasov A, Bhatt S. Doppler ultrasound evaluation of circulatory support devices. Ultrasound Q 2017;33(3):193–200.
55. Flis CM, Jager HR, Sidhu PS. Carotid and vertebral artery dissections: clinical aspects, imaging features and endovascular treatment. Eur Radiol 2007;17:820–34.
56. Sidhu PS. Ultrasound of the carotid and vertebral arteries. Br Med Bull 2000;56:346–436.
57. Deurdulian C, Emmanuel N, Tchelepi H, et al. Beyond the bifurcation: there is more to cerebrovascular ultrasound than internal carotid artery stenosis. Ultrasound Q 2016;32(3):224–40.
58. Scoutt LM, Gunabushanam G. Carotid ultrasound. Radiol Clin North Am 2019;57(3):501–18.
59. Setacci C, Chisci E, Setacci F, et al. Grading carotid intrastent restenosis: a 6-year follow up study. Stroke 2008;39:1189–96.
60. Dai Z, Xu G. Restenosis after carotid artery stenting. Vascular 2017;25(6):576–86.

Peripheral Arterial Ultrasound

Laurence Needleman, MD*, Rick Feld, MD

KEYWORDS

- Duplex Doppler • Ultrasound • Ultrasonography • Peripheral artery • Claudication • Trauma

KEY POINTS

- Peripheral arterial duplex ultrasound with grayscale, color and spectral Doppler can define most extremity stenosis and is helpful for evaluating traumatic lesions.
- Criteria for stenosis differ between native arteries and graft and post intervention examinations.
- Deep arteries, calcified arteries and small calf arteries are more difficult to evaluate with ultrasound.

PERIPHERAL ARTERY

Noninvasive peripheral artery evaluation began as non-imaging physiologic investigations, for example, ankle-brachial index (ABI), to measure disease. Duplex Doppler ultrasound (US) using grayscale, color and spectral Doppler ultrasound directly localizes and measures disease.[1] ABIs are complementary. Spectral Doppler is quantitative while color Doppler localizes the level of disease more efficiently and with confidence.

Most patients evaluated by duplex Doppler have chronic limb ischemia. Acute ischemia is generally evaluated in a more emergent fashion typically by CT or MR angiography rather than US.[2] Arteria duplex has expanded to other processes including traumatic injuries, functional stenotic disease (eg, popliteal entrapment), arteritis, and mappings prior to interventions.[3,4]

Anatomy

The aorta and external iliac arteries are the major inflow arteries.[5] The internal iliac artery is an important collateral pathway from the pelvis to the limb. The common femoral artery originates at the inguinal ligament and after a few centimeters bifurcates into the superficial femoral and the deep femoral artery. The superficial femoral artery travels down the thigh and exits Hunter's canal to become the popliteal artery. The popliteal artery terminates at the junction of the anterior tibial artery and tibioperoneal trunk. The trunk bifurcates into the posterior tibial and peroneal arteries. The posterior tibial artery, located at the ankle behind the medial malleolus and the dorsalis pedis artery (derived from the anterior tibial artery) located on the dorsum of the foot are arteries palpated during physical examination.

The left and right subclavian arteries are usually the first vessels studied during an upper extremity arterial examination. Portions of the arteries are not evaluable due to their relationship to the clavicle. The subclavian artery becomes the axillary artery and then the brachial artery, typically around the antecubital fossa. The bifurcation of the brachial artery forms the ulnar and radial arteries. The arteries at the wrist form several arches before supplying the digital arteries. The radial artery is often chosen for catheterization or even resection (during, for instance, free flap formation), since most patients are not radial artery dependent.

Clinical Overview of Atherosclerosis

Lower extremity atherosclerotic diseases are roughly classified into inflow (aorto-iliac), femoral-popliteal, and/or outflow (calf) disease.

Department of Radiology, Sidney Kimmel Medical College, Thomas Jefferson University Hospital, Thomas Jefferson University, 132 South 10 Street, Suite 763 Main, Philadelphia, PA 19107, USA
* Corresponding author.
E-mail address: laurence.needleman@jefferson.edu

In the earliest stages, atherosclerotic plaques are asymptomatic. As plaque grows, the lumen narrows, which produces stenoses, typically at multiple sites. With progression, symptoms of claudication appear during activity, and eventually progress from mild to disabling pain. In severe cases, resting pain or ischemic changes can result.

Multiple sites of stenosis may be present in a single vessel or at multiple vessels. Progressive stenosis or plaque rupture can lead to complete occlusion. As atherosclerotic disease advances, collateral flow may reconstitute flow, and may mitigate the course of the disease.

Overview of Peripheral Arterial Spectral Waveforms

A recent consensus paper analyzed arterial and venous waveforms.[6] Arterial phases are simplified: If the direction of the outer edge crosses the zero baseline and reverses, it is a *multiphasic* waveform (**Fig. 1**). If it does not cross the baseline the waveform is *monophasic* (**Fig. 2**).

The outline (envelope) of the normal multiphasic peripheral artery spectral waveform is a rapid systolic upstroke (time to peak) and sharp systolic downstroke which crosses the baseline (see **Fig. 1**). The reversal is typically brief followed by a return to baseline. This pattern may be followed by oscillating forward and backward phases. Formerly, describing waveforms as biphasic, triphasic, and so on were used; however, now these waveforms are simply lumped together as multiphasic.

The interior of the waveform (window) under the outside envelope (representing slower velocities) is also evaluated[5,7] (see **Fig. 1**). In a normal straight artery with laminar flow, most of the flow in the center of the artery is traveling near the fastest velocity (see **Fig. 2**). For that reason, the waveform is brightest at the edge, with minimal lower velocities or no flow represented as darker to absent grays. In other arteries with parabolic flow, blood velocity gradually diminishes from the center to the edge and creates a more uniform filling in of the waveform's interior. "Fill in" is termed *spectral broadening*. Spectral broadening also occurs in normal vessels as blood within different regions of the lumen flows at varying velocities, for instance, around a curve or through bifurcations (**Fig. 3**A, B). Technical factors such as an overly large sample volume may also produce broadening. Spectral broadening is an important criterion for abnormal vessels. Irregular flow occurs beyond a stenosis: mild spectral broadening is found with milder stenosis, and turbulent flow appears with more significant stenoses. Irregular currents not aligned with the lumen are seen as multiple velocities and less definition of the edge of the spectrum and simultaneous forward and reversed flow. Vortices with higher velocity spikes may be superimposed on the slower moving blood ("picket fence" appearance).

Spectral Waveforms and Color Doppler Findings in Stenoses

Within a stenosis, narrowing initially produces little change in velocity but as the degree of stenosis increases, the velocity increases related to the drop in pressure through the stenosis.[8] The

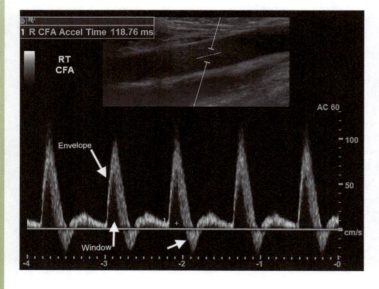

Fig. 1. Normal peripheral artery multiphasic waveform. Spectral Doppler displays the Doppler shift derived velocity versus time. Spectral Doppler waveform of the common femoral artery (CFA) shows antegrade flow in early systole, rapidly decreasing velocity after peak, reversal (*white short arrow*) and return to antegrade flow at the end of the cardiac cycle. The fastest moving blood at the outer edge of the spectrum (envelope) defines peak velocities. The inner aspect of the spectrum (window) shows how the blood velocities are distributed. In this case the absence of signal below the envelope indicating the flood is flowing only at the fastest velocity. During the rest of the cardiac cycle the envelope is thicker (mild spectral broadening) indicating more velocities are present. The time to peak is rapid in normal arteries, (in this case measured 119 ms).

Peripheral Arterial Ultrasound

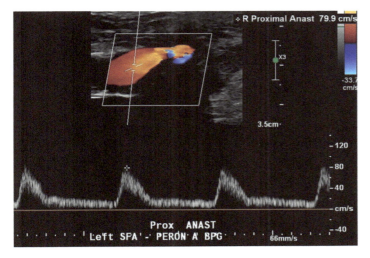

Fig. 2. Monophasic waveform in arterial bypass graft. Spectral Doppler shows antegrade flow throughout the cardiac cycle, a monophasic waveform. There is minimal to no spectral broadening indicating the flow distribution is laminar. Color Doppler shows no narrowing at the site of the spectral Doppler sample volume, although the lumen narrows distal to it, and the color changes (indicating a change in velocity at the narrowing).

increase in velocity is related to the degree of stenosis.

Waveforms within the stenosis are laminar and monophasic with increased systolic and diastolic velocities. In practice, systolic velocity elevation is used as the main criterion for stenosis, although some criteria might also use diastolic velocity or a pulsatility index.

Further downstream from the disturbed flow of stenosis, the flow resumes a laminar profile, but the waveform shape may change to a tardus-parvus (blunted) waveform. The tardus-parvus waveform reflects 2 significant hemodynamic changes created by a significant stenosis. The speed of the systolic upstroke may be diminished ("parvus") and the acceleration is prolonged, taking longer than normal to reach peak ("tardus"). The diminished pressure beyond a significant stenosis reduces the difference between systolic and diastole pressure. The velocity difference in the distal waveform between systole and diastole is likewise reduced creating a less pulsatile waveform.

Arterial stenoses are diagnosed by a profile (**Fig. 4**A–D), with normal or low velocities before the stenosis, elevated velocities within the stenosis, and decreased velocity with post stenotic turbulence beyond the stenosis.[4,7] Relying simply on

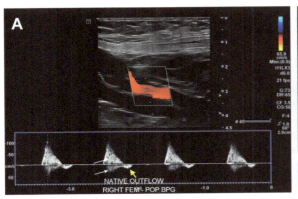
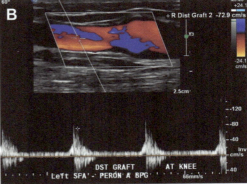

Fig. 3. Spectral broadening. (A) Spectral broadening from normal curvature at bypass graft to native vessel anastomosis. At this anastomosis, a curve creates nonlaminar, spectrally broadened, flow with varying velocities (filling in the window) and directions including toward and away from the transducer (*white arrows*). Later, there is a normal reversed component (*yellow arrow*) in this multiphasic waveform. (B) Spectral broadening from turbulence. In this bypass graft, turbulence downstream from a stenosis creates the typical turbulent spectral waveform of simultaneous forward and reversed flow, shift of velocities to the baseline, and periodic lines in both directions indicating vortices. Bidirectional flow creates deep colors in the forward and reversed direction separated by black lines. There is no aliasing because, though flow is disturbed, the mean velocity (the average of forward and reversed flow) is low.

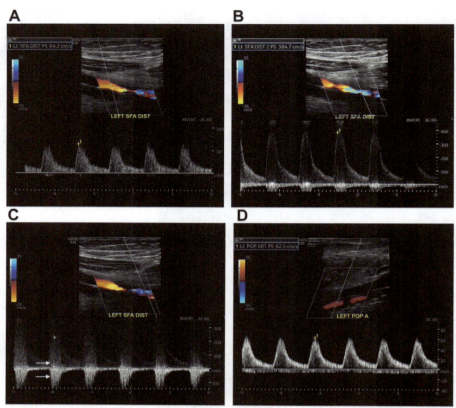

Fig. 4. Profile of a significant native arterial stenosis: The PSV in the stenosis is 384 cm/s, and the PSV ratio is 6. (*A*) Before the stenosis the lumen of the superficial femoral artery (SFA) has normal caliber. The sample is taken from the artery before the stenosis to show its shape (monophasic) and its PSV of 64 cm/s. (*B*) In the stenotic jet, the color lumen is narrowed, and the PS velocity is significantly elevated. The waveform has little fill in of the window because the stenotic jet is laminar. The sample volume size allows some reversed flow to be detected. A bruit (*) created by turbulence creates forward and reversed signals at baseline during systole. (*C*) After the stenosis, flow is grossly turbulent. The flow has different directions and velocities. The waveform shows spectral broadening with poor definition of the spectral envelope, simultaneous forward and reversed flow, and a shift of the average velocity toward the baseline (*arrows*). Superimposed on this is a persistent part of the jet which remains (*). (*D*): Tardus-parvus (dampened) waveform downstream from the stenosis. Distal to the pressure reducing stenosis, the waveform has a slow upstroke with a delayed time to peak and diminished pulsatility (the reversed component is lost; there is too much diastole compared with systole).

the elevated velocity is not as accurate as confirming all 3 waveforms on a duplex examination.

Mild stenoses have no or modest increased velocity with filling in of the spectral envelope or mild bidirectional disturbed flow. Significant stenoses are pressure reducing and flow limiting. These stenoses are associated with significantly elevated (especially systolic) velocities, post-stenotic turbulence beyond the immediate narrowing, and usually tardus-parvus waveforms further distally.

The waveform shape proximal to a stenosis is variable depending on the degree of stenosis, degree of collateral flow, and pressure reduction created by the stenosis.[6] In a normal multiphasic waveform, downstream pressure creates reflected waves from downstream arterioles to produce the reversed phase. A pressure-reducing lesion produces less antegrade pressure and a significantly attenuated reflected wave, thereby reducing or eliminating the reversed components proximal to the stenosis.[9] Vasodilatation distally may also be a factor. Therefore, the waveform before a stenosis may be monophasic with a rapid upstroke unless it has been altered by a proximal obstruction. But, if the degree of stenosis is profound or there is occlusion, the waveform proximally may be excessively pulsatile with only a short forward systolic phase (staccato, water hammer waveform) indicating very high resistance beyond the sample site.

Color Doppler is best considered a pathfinder and shows narrowing at areas of plaque formation (see **Fig. 4**B). The color is not equivalent to an angiogram since the color represents a rough outline of the lumen. Factors such as gain, phase of the cardiac cycle, and low volume may affect the color diameter and intraluminal features. 2 color Doppler criteria are used for stenoses: the size of the color lumen and the change in velocity in areas of narrowing. Elevated velocity in areas of narrowing change the color (appreciated by the color scale next to the image).

Aliasing is an artifact that can help identify high velocity flow. Aliasing occurs when the velocity which is being measured exceeds the sampling rate, so that direction and velocity are misrepresented (**Fig. 5**A, B).[9] Color aliasing has 2 appearances: (1) a series of layers of colors in the proper direction next to color layers encoded in the wrong direction ("onion skin" appearance) or (2) correct and incorrect direction pixels mixed ("mosaic" pattern). Aliasing is also seen in spectral Doppler where the waveform wraps around top of the correct direction and reappears at the bottom in the wrong direction. If the artifact is large enough, the wrap around even returns to the correct direction (albeit with the incorrect velocity). Spectral multiple aliasing is the analog of the mosaic pattern, but aliasing is more common in color Doppler since the sampling rate for color is far slower than spectral Doppler.

Protocols

Lower extremity native arteries

Arteries are scanned with different transducers based on the depth of the artery from the skin.[10,11]

In general, the highest frequency is used, and linear transducers are favored, since this configuration aligns with the vessel wall. Curved array transducers are generally reserved for deep pelvic vessels and where body habitus is adverse. The femoral vessels in the thigh are generally scanned from an anterior position with the leg rotated outward. A posterior approach, sometimes in the decubitus position, is generally needed for popliteal and posterior calf artery evaluation. The anterior tibial artery is small and usually the most difficult calf artery to visualize, optimally imaged from the anterolateral position, although its origin may be seen from a posterior view.

The native arterial duplex mapping protocol[4] consists of mapping from the common femoral to the popliteal arteries (**Table 1**). All accessible portions of the arteries are evaluated since plaque and stenosis, although favoring some locations, may occur anywhere along the artery. In a patient without stenosis, representative segments are documented at selected sites.

If a stenosis is suspected, additional imaging of the area documents the greatest velocity elevation in the stenosis and any post-stenotic changes. If there is an occlusion, an attempt to document the length of the occlusion is made.[4]

Peak systolic velocities (PSV) are sought by interrogating through stenoses.[7] The highest angle-corrected PSV in a stenosis is recorded and compared with an angle corrected PSV taken from a normal vessel 1 to 4 cm before the stenosis. A fixed Doppler angle, such as 60°, is *not* necessary

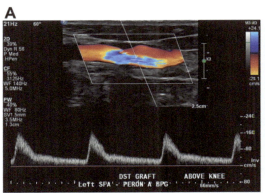
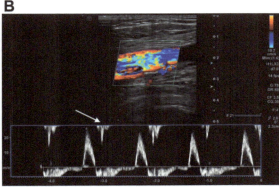

Fig. 5. Aliasing. (*A*) Color aliasing (onion skin appearance) occurs when the speed of blood exceeds the sampling rate and shows the wrong color direction and/or velocity. Aliasing is related to the velocity *not* turbulent flow. Color has a slower sampling rate, so it is aliased while the laminar spectral waveform is not. The aliased color goes from one color to the next and then wraps around to the reversed colors in layers since the color scale of 24 cm/s is too low for the *mean* velocity (approximately 100 cm/s). (*B*) Color aliasing (mosaic appearance) and spectral aliasing are present. When the aliased signal wrap arounds more than once, the color aliasing pattern produced has all available colors mixed together like tiles in a mosaic. There is also some aliasing in diastole in the spectral Doppler waveform. The baseline allows more signal in systole, so it does not alias, but there is less room for retrograde flow and it aliases. The aliased diastolic flow wraps around, appearing falsely antegrade at the top of the spectrum (*arrow*).

Table 1
Native artery protocol sampling sites

- The accessible portion of the entire vessel or the arterial segment of interest is surveyed. This is typically grayscale and/or color.
- Representative areas as noted below are recorded for normal/mild disease.
- Areas of suspected or known stenoses require additional images. Profiles by grayscale, color Doppler, and spectral Doppler before, at and after any area of interest are recorded.

Lower Extremity Arteries	Grayscale ultrasound to document normal or plaque ± calcification, and/or size (if aneurysmal).	Spectral Doppler long axis image. Peak systolic velocity is documented	Color Doppler long axis image
Common femoral	✔	✔	✔
Deep femoral proximal	✔	✔	✔
Proximal superficial femoral	✔	✔	✔
Mid superficial femoral	✔	✔	✔
Distal superficial femoral above knee	✔	✔	✔
Popliteal above knee	✔	✔	✔
Popliteal below knee	✔	✔	✔
If appropriate, external iliac, tibioperoneal trunk, anterior tibial, posterior tibial, peroneal, and/or dorsalis pedis arteries could be perfromed.			
If appropriate, provocative testing, for example, for popliteal entrapment, should be performed.			
Upper Extremity Arteries	Grayscale ultrasound to document normal or plaque ± calcification, and/or size (if aneurysmal)	Spectral Doppler long axis image. Peak systolic velocity is documented	Color Doppler long axis image
Subclavian	✔	✔	✔
Axillary	✔	✔	✔
Brachial	✔	✔	✔
If appropriate, innominate, radial, ulnar arteries, and/or palmar arch could be performed.			
If appropriate, provocative testing, for example, for thoracic outlet syndrome or radial dependence, should be performed.			

Adapted from Ref.[4]

and angles lower than 60 are favored since there is less associated error. Angles above 60° are prone to error and should be interpreted with caution, if at all. Velocities from angles above 70° are not reliable and should not be used. A velocity ratio of the PSV in the stenosis divided by the PSV before the stenosis is calculated. End-diastolic velocity and diastolic ratios are used in some laboratories and are optional. To gain an approximation of inflow disease within the lower extremity, the time to peak of the or so-called acceleration time, may be recorded (normal in the common femoral artery being faster than 144 miliseconds [see **Fig. 1**]).

Longer protocols may be warranted based on the study indication or individual laboratory preferences. A common addition is calf artery evaluation. In some laboratories this may be simply include a grayscale and/or color survey to document stenoses or occlusions. In others, one or more spectral samples from each calf artery may be obtained. A low PSV or a tardus-parvus waveform from a calf artery may be a surrogate for poor flow. Some laboratories, when doing pre-operative calf mapping, scan from distal to proximal until a stenosis or occlusion is found, since bypasses need to be placed beyond the lowest obstructive sites.[12]

In selected patients, such as to evaluate trauma or to resolve an issue from prior imaging, a focused examination may answer specific questions.

Post intervention
Bypass grafts are evaluated along their entire length with grayscale and color Doppler.[4] A series of representative images are recorded with profiling of any suspected or real stenosis. A long axis image of the segment with the highest detected velocity is documented. Additionally, the

proximal and distal native vessels and proximal and distal anastomoses are interrogated, and representative images recorded. Additional imaging of the native circulation can be included per laboratory protocol.

Endovascular intervention sites (eg, angioplasty, stents) are evaluated at the site of the intervention and include evaluation of the native arterial segments proximal and distal to the site to assess stent inflow and outflow. Stents are interrogated as thoroughly as possible. PSVs are recorded: before and distal to the stent and within the proximal, mid and distal stent.

Additional imaging of the native circulation remote from the intervention can be included per laboratory protocol.

Diagnostic Criteria

Arteries have different normal velocities so using a single velocity to determine if a significant stenosis is present is not optimal. Most grading systems use a PSV ratio.[10,13] Grades of native arterial stenosis separate those above and below 50% stenosis since this threshold correlates with a pressure reducing stenosis.

Native arteries

1) Normal vessels: no plaque, no other pathology and no narrowing.
2) Mild stenosis: less than 50% diameter reduction: plaque by grayscale and mild color narrowing, no or modest PSV elevations with PSV ratio of less than 2, mild post-stenotic disturbed flow. Distal waveforms are generally multiphasic.
3) Greater than greater than 50% diameter stenosis: plaque or other process (eg, dissection) producing narrowing, PSV ratio greater than or equal to 2. (Some laboratories lump all significant stenoses together and use ≥ 2 to indicate a 50%–99% stenosis). Distal turbulence is present, and distal waveforms beyond the turbulence are generally monophasic.

Some laboratories also create a grade of greater than 75% when the PSV ratio is greater than 4. In this scheme, a ratio between 2 and 4 is a 50% to 75% stenosis. **Fig. 4** profiles a stenosis with a PSV 385 cm/s and a PSV ratio of 4.8. The degree of stenosis can be reported as "Greater than 75%" or "50% to 99%" diameter reduction.

For iliac arteries, some laboratories use a higher cut-off ratio greater than 2.8 for greater than 50% stenosis.[12]

4) Occlusion: no flow on color Doppler. No flow on spectral Doppler (**Fig. 6**A). Waveforms before a high-grade stenosis or occlusion may show a staccato waveform (**Fig. 6**B).

Post intervention

Failure of endovascular or surgical revascularization can occur at different time points. Early on, typically within the first month, failure is associated with technical factors including residual valves, hypercoagulable states, poor runoff, and dissections. For stents, other factors may include stent recoil or deformity. In the first several years, myointimal hyperplasia is a stenosing process which can cause treatment failure. After that time progression of atherosclerosis around the intervention may lead to recurrent symptoms and/or jeopardize the treatment.

Criteria for stenosis in bypass grafts and endovascular procedures have different cut points (**Fig. 7**A, B).[14] Note elevated velocities may occur across different vessels. In bypass grafts an elevated velocity without stenosis may occur as a larger graft enters a smaller runoff native artery.

1) Normal or mild disease less than 50% diameter reduction.
2) 50% to 70% stenosis (intermediate stenosis): Narrowing with a PSV ratio greater than or equal to 2.
3) Greater than 70% stenosis (severe stenosis): Narrowing with a PSV ratio greater than 3.5.
4) Occlusion: no flow on color Doppler. No flow on spectral Doppler.

These cut points reflect the risk of progression and occlusion and can be used to guide intervention. For bypass grafts, diminishing ABIs along with the elevated ratio, a low average velocity from non-stenotic sites less than 40 cm/s[13] or a staccato waveform suggest a severe stenosis may need even earlier intervention.

Pitfalls

Duplex arteriography has several pitfalls. The most obvious is that a vessel is not entirely evaluable: visualization is worse in the infrapopliteal vessels, followed by the iliac arteries, and sporadically compromised in the femoral and popliteal arteries.[14] Poor runoff has weaker flow which produces diminished Doppler signals and limited imaging. Arterial wall calcifications are another leading reason for compromised studies. Some indirect evidence of the degree of a calcified lesion can be assumed by comparing the waveform and velocities before the calcification to the waveform exiting the calcification. Significant may be suggested by turbulence at the exit point, a change in waveform shape from multiphasic above to monophasic below the calcification, or markedly diminished velocity.[15]

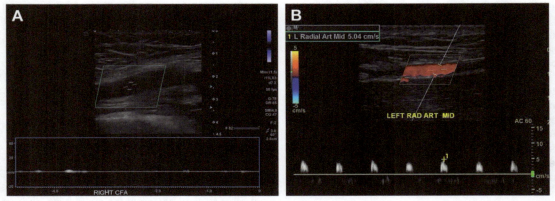

Fig. 6. Occlusion and Staccato Waveform before occlusion. (*A*) There is an occlusion of the common femoral artery (CFA) and no flow by color Doppler or spectral Doppler. A small amount of signal at the spectral baseline is noise. (*B*) Staccato waveform before an occluded distal radial artery (not shown). The mid radial artery waveform is a short forward pulse of blood, generally with low velocity (here, 5 cm/s). The distal occlusion creates high resistance, so flow ceases except at early systole.

Multilevel disease does not appear to affect the accuracy of detecting subsequent stenoses.[16] However, when there are multiple stenoses above 50%, our laboratory practice is to grade them all above 50% and not to determine which of the stenoses is worse than another.

Trauma

Traumatic vascular injury includes blunt and penetrating causes, and iatrogenic complications such as vascular access or angiography.[17] Patients with blunt and penetrating trauma with hard clinical signs after trauma generally need emergent surgical exploration or angiography (eg, CT angiography or intraoperative angiography). Hard signs include pulsatile bleeding, arterial thrill, bruit around the traumatized site, absent distal pulse, or expanding hematoma. An abnormal ABI is helpful to guide management of lower extremity injuries. Those with "soft" findings (significant hemorrhage by history, neurologic abnormality,

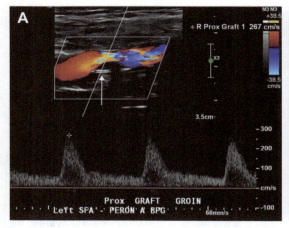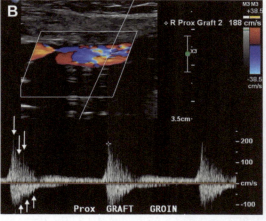

Fig. 7. Bypass graft stenosis. PSV ratio is 3.3 indicating an intermediate stenosis of 50% to 70% (Pre-stenotic segment is **Fig. 2**). (*A*) Stenotic jet. The double wall of the graft material is best seen posteriorly (*arrow*). The stenotic jet is searched for along the narrowed segment of the graft as determined by the narrowing on color and the aliased color. Peak velocity is 267 cm/s. The Doppler angle to determine velocity is set along the walls of the graft or along the color lumen. (*B*) Post stenotic turbulence. The color lumen is normal. The spectral waveform distal to the stenosis has typical features of turbulence: There is simultaneous forward and reverse flow. The envelope is poorly defined, and there are more signals (more brightness) at lower and reversed velocities than along the edge. Periodic lines in the waveform indicate transient vortices (*arrows*). Color aliasing is present related to the high velocity in part of the cardiac cycle.

proximity bony injury, penetrating wound) may be studied by duplex ultrasound if there are available resources. Presence of a normal pedal pulse does not exclude the need for arterial evaluation.

A targeted duplex study is indicated if there are signs of arterial disease after arterial catheter placement and/or catheterization, or IV access. Grayscale ultrasound, and spectral and color Doppler performed above, at, and beyond the site should be performed. While the examination concentrates on arterial trauma, some attention to the veins may uncover venous injuries, such as thromboses or arteriovenous fistulas.

The most common finding in post-traumatic injury is either normal or altered soft tissue echogenicity suggesting ecchymoses of the skin or subcutaneous fat. Abnormal appearance of adjacent muscle may suggest muscle injury.

A hematoma is an avascular fluid collection. The fluid inside has variable echogenicity, but the most frequent appearances are anechoic fluid or fluid with lace-like echoes. Low level echogenicity, a clot ball, or fluid-fluid levels are less common findings. Peripheral color vascularity is not generally present but may develop over time if there is reactive hyperemia around the hematoma or a developing abscess.

A penetrating traumatic injury may cross the walls of an artery and a vein creating an arteriovenous fistula (AVF).[18] This may include an adjacent artery and vein such as the common femoral artery and vein or connect a vein remote from the artery through a via an elongated tract (eg, a femoral artery to saphenous vein branch). Waveform at the fistula has monophasic high velocity secondary to the arterial-venous pressure gradient (**Fig. 8**A). The draining vein may show rapid inflow with each heartbeat or so-called "arterialized" flow (**Fig. 8**B). The feeding artery above it may also be monophasic, but the waveform below the fistula is usually multiphasic. The turbulence through the fistula may cause vibrations in the soft tissue detected as extravascular color in soft tissue ("color bruit" sign). Albeit rare, clinical steal symptoms can occur.

Arterial puncture which creates a walled-off extravascular space with flow is termed a pseudoaneurysm (PsA)[3] (**Fig. 9**A). "Pseudo" applies because unlike a true aneurysm, the blood is not contained by a vessel wall. The connection between the PsA and the native vessel is usually via a thin track of varying length and width (the "neck"). Occasionally a tear in the vessel creates a collection immediately adjacent to the artery without a neck. The color hallmark of a PsA is a collection adjacent to an artery with swirling blood within it that may resemble a yin-yang symbol. The track is seen on color but has a distinctive spectral Doppler appearance: arterial flow during early systole and slow long reversal of flow direction during diastole and part of end-systole ("to-and-fro" flow) (**Fig. 9**B). The waveform reflects the filling of the PsA during systolic pressurization and its emptying when the pressure in the PsA exceeds the artery. A small PsA may occlude on its own, but they are generally treated either by thrombin

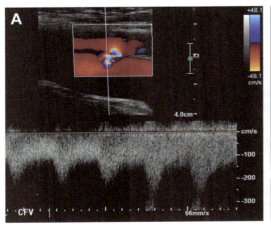 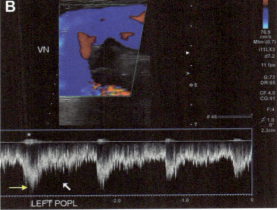

Fig. 8. Arteriovenous Fistula (AVF). (*A*) There is an abnormal connection between the common femoral artery (CFA) and vein (CFV) from prior catheterization. The fistula produces a high-velocity color and spectral jet at the communication. Fistula waveform has monophasic high-velocity flow throughout systole and diastole. Spectral broadening from turbulence is present. (*B*) There is a fistula (not shown) between the popliteal artery and vein from prior trauma. The popliteal vein is dilated. Arterialized flow is high velocity and increases with each beat (*yellow arrow*) and so mirrors the arterial pulse. Turbulence with vortices creates spikes in the waveform (*white arrow*). A bruit with low velocity forward and reversed flow from turbulence is noted during systole (*).

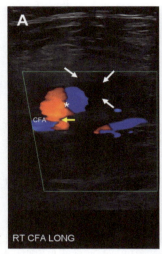
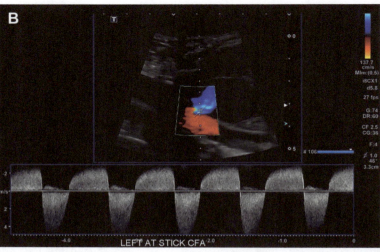

Fig. 9. Pseudoaneurysm (PsA). (*A*) There is flow outside the artery from a contained extra-arterial collection of blood that communicated with the common femoral artery (CFA) through a tract. In this case, the tract is short (*yellow arrow*). The PsA shows twirling forward and reversed color flow around each other resembling a yin-yang symbol (*). There is an anechoic area (*white arrows*) around part of the PsA from partial thrombosis of the PsA. (*B*) In a different patient, the tract (in blue) from the CFA to the PsA shows the typical "to-and-fro" flow, into the PsA during systole, and emptying of the PsA into the artery during diastole.

injection, compression, or surgical or endovascular repair.

Rarely a vessel adjacent to a hematoma or PsA may show a monophasic pattern reflecting reactive hyperemia. This waveform should not be mistaken for a "to-and-fro" waveform or an AVF.

A tear in the vessel wall may create an intraluminal flap known as dissection. A well-defined flap with a true and a false lumen may be present. One lumen may thrombose causing varying degrees of narrowing including occlusion. A well-defined intraluminal thrombosis partially obstructing or occluding the lumen may also form at the site of an injury.

Upper Extremity

Stenoses in upper extremity arteries are evaluated in a similar manner to the lower extremity (see **Table 1**). Some anatomy may be difficult to study due to the overlying chest wall; in those cases, indirect signs of proximal disease may be necessary.

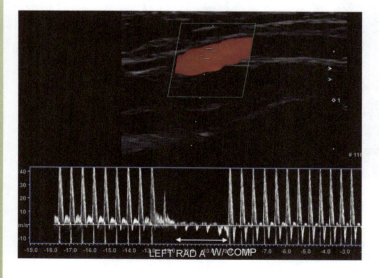

Fig. 10. Duplex test for radial dependence. One of the ways to indirectly evaluate for an intact superficial palmar arch is shown. The proximal radial artery is compressed. While scanning, the distal radial artery flow reverses to create reverse thump (at *double arrow*) that indicates, if the radial artery occluded or resected, the arch could collateralize flow to the radial artery territory.

Thoracic outlet syndrome can be investigated in this manner by evaluating the effect of various maneuvers on the peripheral waveforms. Complications from upper arterial catheterizations are evaluable by duplex as well.[19]

Mapping the radial artery before radial harvest for coronary artery bypass graft and forearm flaps are increasingly used to determine the size of the artery and perhaps to detect if there is radial artery dependence (Duplex Allen test). The deep palmar arch is usually complete, whereas the superficial palmar arch may be incomplete which creates radial dependence in a minority of patients. Radial artery dependence can be determined in a variety of ways including direct evaluation of the palmar arch and indirect evaluation of the radial artery and ulnar artery.[20,21] The radial artery is compressed and flow direction in the arch assessed (**Fig. 10**). After proximal radial compression, a reversal of direction of flow or reversed thump can be found in the normal distal radial artery or arch. The ulnar artery PSV increases, usually above 20%. The test can be complemented with first digit pressures without and with radial compression. Mapping results should report the lumen size in the proximal, mid and distal radial artery segments. The average radial artery lumen measures 2–3 mm. Stenosis and excessive calcifications, if present (medial artery calcinosis) should be reported.

Catheterizations and more frequent deployment of heart failure devices through the upper extremity have also created a need to determine if the arterial size is adequate to accommodate the device. The arteries which need to be measured vary by device. Measurements are taken from short axis images and 2 planes are recorded.

CLINICS CARE POINTS

- Arterial duplex has expanded to other processes including traumatic injuries, functional stenotic disease (eg, popliteal entrapment), arteritis, and mappings prior to interventions.
- Careful attention to technique including profiling stenoses before, at and after the maximal stenosis produces superior results.
- Criteria for stenosis differ between native arteries and graft and post intervention examinations.
- Deep arteries, calcified arteries and small calf arteries are more difficult to evaluate with ultrasound.

REFERENCES

1. Azene EM, Steigner ML, Aghayev A, et al. ACR appropriateness criteria® lower extremity arterial claudication-imaging assessment for revascularization: 2022 update. J Am Coll Radiol 2022;19:S364–73.
2. Gornik HL, Aronow HD, Goodney PP, et al. 2024 ACC/AHA/AACVPR/APMA/ABC/SCAI/SVM/SVN/SVS/SIR/VESS Guideline for the Management of Lower Extremity Peripheral Artery Disease: A Report of the American College of Cardiology/American Heart Association Joint Committee on Clinical Practice Guidelines. Circulation 2024;149(24):e1313–410.
3. Washko PA, Smith SW. Special considerations in evaluating nonatherosclerotic arterial pathology. In: Kupinski AM, editor. The vascular system. Philadelphia: Wolters Kluwer; 2023. p. 251–70.
4. Collaborative Committee AIUM-ACR-SIR-SRU. AIUM practice parameter for the performance of peripheral arterial ultrasound examinations using color and spectral Doppler imaging. J Ultrasound Med 2021;40:E17–24.
5. Fox TB. Ultrasound principles. In: Kupinski AM, editor. The vascular system. Philadelphia: Wolters Kluwer; 2023. p. 11–28.
6. Kim ES, Sharma AM, Scissons R, et al. Interpretation of peripheral arterial and venous Doppler waveforms: a consensus statement from the society for vascular medicine and society for vascular ultrasound. Vasc Med 2020;25(5):484–506.
7. Pellerito JS, Polak JF. Basic concepts of Doppler frequency analysis and ultrasound blood flow imaging. In: Pellerito JS, Polak JF, editors. Introduction to vascular ultrasonography. Philadelphia: Elsevier; 2012. p. 3–19.
8. Kupinski AM. Arterial physiology. In: Kupinski AM, editor. The vascular system. Philadelphia: Wolters Kluwer; 2023. p. 55–62.
9. Zagzebski JA. Physics and instrumentation in Doppler and B-mode ultrasonography. In: Pellerito JS, Polak JF, editors. Introduction to vascular ultrasonography. Philadelphia: Elsevier; 2012. p. 20–51.
10. Armstrong PA, Carroll MI, Bandyk DF. Duplex ultrasound assessment of lower extremity arterial disease. In: AbuRahma AF, editor. Noninvasive vascular diagnosis a practical textbook for clnicians. Cham: Springer; 2017. p. 349–61.
11. Marks N, Hingorani AP, Ascher E. Duplex ultrasound of lower extremity arteries. In: AM K, editor. The vascular system. Philadelphia: Wolters Kluwer; 2023. p. 185–95.
12. Ascher E, Marks N, Hingorani A. Lower extremity arterial mapping: duplex ultrasound as an alternative to arteriography prior to femoral, popliteal, and infrapopliteal reconstructions. In: AbuRahma AF, editor. Noninvasive vascular diagnosis a practical textbook for clnicians. Cham: Springer; 2017. p. 395–408.

13. Hodgkiss-Harlow KD, Bandyk DF. Interpretation of arterial duplex testing of lower-extremity arteries and interventions. Semin Vasc Surg 2013;26:95–104.
14. Sensier Y, Hartshorne T, Thrush A, et al. A prospective comparison of lower limb colour-coded duplex scanning with arteriography. Eur J Vasc Endovasc Surg 1996;11:170–5.
15. Hingorani AP, Ascher E, Marks N, et al. Limitations of and lessons learned from clinical experience of 1,020 duplex arteriography. Vascular 2008;16: 147–53.
16. Sensier Y, Hartshorne T, Thrush A, et al. The effect of adjacent segment disease on the accuracy of colour duplex scanning for the diagnosis of lower limb arterial disease. Eur J Vasc Endovasc Surg 1996;12: 238–42.
17. Dominguez JA, Rowe VL, FA W. Noninvasive vascular testing in the trauma patient. In: AbuRahma AF, editor. Noninvasive vascular diagnosis a practical textbook for clnincians. Cham: Springer; 2017. p. 469–77.
18. Liu JB, Merton DA, Mitchell DG, et al. Color Doppler imaging of the iliofemoral region. Radiographics 1990;10(3):403–12.
19. Steinberg DH. Managing complications of transradial catheterization. Cardiac Interventions Today 2015;58–62.
20. Rodriguez E, Ormont ML, Lambert EH, et al. The role of preoperative radial artery ultrasound and digital plethysmography prior to coronary artery bypass grafting. Eur J Cardio Thorac Surg 2001;19:135–9.
21. Zimmerman P, Chin E, Laifer-Narin S, et al. Radial artery mapping for coronary artery bypass graft placement. Radiology 2001;220:299–302.

Peripheral Venous Ultrasound

Laurence Needleman, MD*, Rick Feld, MD

KEYWORDS

- Duplex Doppler • Ultrasound • Ultrasonography • Peripheral vein • Deep vein thrombosis
- Superficial thrombophlebitis • Chronic venous insufficiency • Venous reflux

KEY POINTS

- Lower-extremity peripheral venous ultrasound when performed as a complete compression ultrasound is an accurate single test to rule in and rule out lower-extremity deep vein thrombosis (DVT).
- Most patients can be assigned normal, acute DVT, or chronic postthrombotic change. A small number of cases will be inadequate, or the findings will be indeterminate.
- Patients with less-comprehensive protocols or technically difficult examinations may require serial or alternative testing.

Compression duplex venous ultrasound (CUS) is the most common test for deep vein thrombosis (DVT). It is sufficiently accurate, superior to venous physiologic tests, better tolerated by the patient, and easier to perform than contrast venography.[1]

CLINICAL OVERVIEW

DVT does have significant morbidity, but its most important complication, pulmonary embolism (PE), means that accurate testing may be lifesaving.[2] The triad of risk factors for DVT has been described by Virchow: stasis, damage to the vein, and a hypercoagulable state. Approximately 69 per 100,000 patients develop DVT or PE, affecting hundreds of thousands of people in the United States each year.[3]

DVT has known signs and symptoms, but these findings are not specific to thrombosis. Therefore, the history and physical examination are not adequate to exclude or diagnose DVT. Hoping to avoid unindicated ultrasound (US) for low-risk patients, many societies have recommended a strategy of clinical evaluation and an assessment of pretest probability before ordering a study.[4] The most common rule set to determine risk is the Wells criteria. This score has 1 point for each major risk factor: active cancer or cancer within 6 months, paralysis, paresis or cast, bedridden for at least 3 days or major surgery within 12 weeks, localized tenderness along the deep venous system, swelling of the entire leg, unilateral calf swelling, unilateral pitting edema, dilation of superficial collateral veins, and prior DVT. Points are subtracted from the score when an alternative diagnosis is at least as likely as DVT. The Wells score is graded as "DVT-likely" or "DVT-unlikely." DVT-likely patients go on to CUS, whereas the DVT-unlikely patients are recommended to get a D-dimer blood test. A negative D-dimer and a DVT-unlikely score effectively excludes acute DVT. Unfortunately, the D-dimer test is sensitive but not specific, and so a positive D-dimer test does not adequately rule in acute DVT. For this reason, patients with positive D-dimer tests go on to CUS. The D-dimer test is frequently falsely positive in inpatients, so the test is only useful for outpatients and emergency room patients.

Department of Radiology, Sidney Kimmel Medical College, Thomas Jefferson University, Thomas Jefferson University Hospital, 132 South 10 Street, Suite 763 Main, Philadelphia, PA 19107, USA
* Corresponding author.
E-mail address: laurence.needleman@jefferson.edu

ANATOMY

The veins of the leg are typically distinguished as deep veins and superficial veins.[5] The deep veins have an accompanying similarly named artery (except for the intramuscular veins of the calf), whereas superficial veins do not have an accompanying artery. Central veins are those located above the knee (popliteal and above), whereas distal veins are in the calf (intermuscular and intramuscular).

The deep veins lie below the muscular fascia and are the major veins draining the lower extremity. The common femoral vein becomes the external iliac vein at the inguinal canal. The common femoral vein is created by the junction of the femoral vein (previously called superficial femoral vein) and the deep femoral vein. The deep femoral vein is usually only evaluated for several centimeters at its termination at the femoral deep femoral confluence. The femoral vein is evaluable throughout its course, although visualization can be challenging at the adductor (Hunter) canal. The femoral vein becomes the popliteal vein as it exits the Hunter canal in the lower thigh. Duplications of the femoral and popliteal veins are not unusual. The popliteal vein is created from the confluence of the intermuscular, typically paired, deep veins in the calf: the anterior tibial, tibioperoneal trunk (formed from the posterior tibial and peroneal veins). There are calf deep veins that lie *within* the muscles of the calf; most importantly, the soleal and gastrocnemius veins. The intramuscular veins are important because they are frequently the earliest site of acute thrombi, and they may be incorrectly considered superficial veins.

US tends to focus on the 2 major superficial veins: the great saphenous and the small saphenous.[6] The saphenous veins lie superficial to the deep muscular fascia but are bounded more superficially by a saphenous fascia. The great saphenous joins the common femoral vein in the thigh. The small saphenous vein runs along the back of the calf with a variable termination either at the saphenopopliteal junction or more superiorly. Perforating veins connect the superficial and deep system.

In the upper extremity, the deep venous system that is evaluable includes the internal jugular, axillary, subclavian, and brachiocephalic veins centrally, and the brachial vein in the upper arm. The upper-extremity examination also includes the superficial cephalic and basilic veins in the upper arm. Extension to the examination to the forearm veins, such as the radial, ulnar, and superficial veins in the forearm, may be performed if there are symptoms.

DEEP VEIN THROMBOSIS PATHOPHYSIOLOGY

The development of DVT depends on baseline susceptibility to thrombosis and the presence of risk factors. Hypercoagulable states may be congenital or acquired.

Lower-extremity DVT frequently begins in the calf, and 50% of these remain isolated. Few, if any, of these small calf clots cause symptomatic PE. Of calf DVT, 10% will propagate more centrally.[7]

Acute DVT in the central veins may be either in isolation or in combination with calf DVT. Central DVT can be in one or more veins. Discontinuous, independent sites of acute DVT are the norm rather than one long thrombus.[8] For this reason, the US examination consists of evaluating all accessible portions of the veins because normal veins may be seen next to affected sites.

Acute thrombus consists of combinations of red blood cells, fibrin, and platelets; it is soft and smooth. DVT typically begins behind vein valves and, as it expands, it enlarges the vein. Complete occlusion by the thrombus is usually short-lived because thrombolysis creates a separation of the clot from the vein wall. This accounts for the outline of DVT around the lumen on color Doppler and venography. Weak attachment to the wall and growth toward the heart may create a "free-floating" appearance.

Embolization occurs in acute DVT and may be clinically symptomatic or silent. Following PE, US demonstrates DVT in approximately 30% to 50%.[9] Contrast venography demonstrates more, in part because of nonvisualized veins on US, such as pelvic and some calf veins.

Even as thrombus is forming, the fibrinolytic system is attempting to remove it. Clot lysis consists of retraction from its edges and recanalization through its substance. Most of the evolution from clot to scar takes days to weeks,[10] with some pathologic changes even noted at months to years.[11] By serial US, half of DVT resolves completely without any evidence by US, and half show chronic changes.

Chronic change is no longer thrombus but rather collagen.[11] Society of Radiologists in Ultrasound guidelines have suggested an alternative name for scarring: chronic postthrombotic change. This nomenclature highlights the mechanism and cause. More importantly, it does not use the word *thrombus*, which can lead to unnecessary anticoagulation if scarring is mistaken for an acute DVT.

LOWER-EXTREMITY VEINS
Protocol

Different specialists evaluate different veins in their protocols, leading to inconsistent care.[1] Historically, US had limited resolution and could only evaluate larger central veins. These limited scans are still practiced in some emergency rooms and medicine practices; they consist of portions of the femoral and popliteal veins at 2 (or 3) areas. Limited scans have a significant limitation: a single negative study is inadequate to exclude some DVT. Therefore, although one test is safe temporarily, an acceptably safe strategy requires 2 negative limited scans 1 week apart to adequately exclude DVT.

Complete compression ultrasound (CCUS) from the inguinal ligament to the ankle is recommended by radiological societies and other organizations.[1,12] CCUS is a safe strategy: one technically adequate normal study rules in most important sites of DVT and effectively rules out DVT. Serial US is unnecessary unless certain conditions are present (**Tables 1** and **2**).

Scanning the groin to ankle overcomes any potential confusion on who needs follow-up after a more limited study. Adding the calf gives more information and detects calf DVT. The treatment of calf DVT is still in evolution.[13] If calf DVT is treated, no short-term follow-up is needed. If not treated, the patient needs a follow-up in 1 week to exclude propagation. If femoropopliteal DVT appears at follow-up, patients are treated. If the calf DVT is gone, no further evaluation is warranted. However, if the 1-week scan continues to show calf DVT, a second follow-up at 2 weeks is needed. If at 2 weeks there is no change, no further imaging is required unless symptoms worsen.

Complete Compression Ultrasound Protocol

Adequately visualized veins are compressed in their short axis at 1- to 2-cm intervals.[12] With modern equipment, calf veins can be seen in most patients, particularly if the calf is well positioned and the veins are distended by elevating the chest and heart above the leg. The anterior tibial vein is not in the standard protocol, as it is rarely isolated. When compressing the intermuscular calf, attention to the adjacent intramuscular veins can frequently identify soleal or gastrocnemius thrombi. Intramuscular veins may be included when symptomatic areas are scanned. If DVT is seen in the common femoral vein, many laboratories extend the examination to the external iliac vein using curved array transducers to determine if proximal thrombus is present.

The protocol also includes Doppler. Color Doppler is used routinely in the common femoral vein and popliteal vein and may be added to evaluate any areas of suspected thrombus or exclude the presence of a filling defect. Spectral Doppler at both common femoral veins and the ipsilateral popliteal vein is used to evaluate for proximal obstruction or excess pulsatility. Both common femoral veins waveforms are used to evaluate symmetry.

Scanning an area of pain may also detect nonvascular causes, particularly musculoskeletal entities that mimic DVT, for example, Baker cysts, muscular or articular abnormalities that may or not warrant additional imaging.

Table 1
Recommended follow-up after initial negative venous ultrasound

Clinical Characteristic	Recommendation
Negative complete duplex ultrasound	
Persistent or worsening symptoms	Repeat scan in 5 d to 1 wk, earlier if concern is high
High risk	Consider repeat scan if cause for symptoms not otherwise elucidated
Technically compromised study	Recommend repeat scan in 5 d to 1 wk if more than minor limitation. D-dimer may be helpful if it is negative
Concern for iliocaval DVT	Pelvic venous imaging, especially CT or MR venography, or iliocaval duplex ultrasound
Negative extended compression or 2-region ultrasound	
Risk of DVT persists or cause of symptoms not elucidated	Repeat scan, preferably complete duplex ultrasound, in 5 d to 1 wk

From: Needleman L, Cronan JJ, Lilly MP, Merli GJ, Adhikari S, Hertzberg BS, DeJong MR, Streiff MB, Meissner MH. Ultrasound for Lower Extremity Deep Venous Thrombosis: Multidisciplinary Recommendations From the Society of Radiologists in Ultrasound Consensus Conference. *Circulation.* 2018;137:1505 to 1515. With permission.

Table 2
Recommended follow-up after initial positive or indeterminate venous ultrasound

Clinical Characteristic	Recommendation
Positive complete duplex ultrasound	
Acute calf DVT, not treated	Repeat scan in 1 wk, earlier if symptoms progress. If progression to femoropopliteal DVT, treat. If normal, stop. If persistent calf thrombus, which is not treated, repeat scan at 2 wk. Scanning after 2 wk is generally not warranted
Acute DVT, on treatment	Repeat not warranted unless a change in the scan will change patient management Follow-up at the end of treatment to establish new baseline
Indeterminate results	D-dimer may be helpful if negative. Recommend repeat scan in 5 d to 1 wk to evaluate for change
Concern for recurrent DVT, equivocal findings for scar vs recurrence at site of scar	D-dimer may be helpful if negative. Recommend repeat scan in 1–3 d and 7–10 d

From: Needleman L, Cronan JJ, Lilly MP, Merli GJ, Adhikari S, Hertzberg BS, DeJong MR, Streiff MB, Meissner MH. Ultrasound for Lower Extremity Deep Venous Thrombosis Multidisciplinary Recommendations From the Society of Radiologists in Ultrasound Consensus Conference. Circulation. 2018;137:1505 to 1515. With permission.

The sensitivity CCUS for acute DVT in the central veins is high, 96.5% (95% CI: 95.1%–97.6%) with high specificity. Calf DVT has lower sensitivity, 63.5% (95% CI: 59.8%–67%) also with high specificity.[14] Calf DVT is more likely to be detected if there are focal calf symptoms.

Normal and Abnormal Ultrasound Findings

DVT US examination determines if the vein is normal, has acute DVT, has chronic postthrombotic change, or is indeterminate (equivocal) (**Table 3**).[1]

Compression Ultrasound

A normal vein will compress completely with apposition of the walls with modest probe pressure. The compression is performed in the short axis so the entire vein can be evaluated during compression. Either paired compression and noncompression views or cine loops may be used as documentation.

The authors' laboratory favors the term normal compression when the lumen is completely obliterated, and the walls of the vein are inapparent or thin (**Fig. 1**A, B). Noncompression is reserved

Table 3
Diagnostic criteria for deep vein thrombosis/chronic postthrombotic change

	Acute Venous Thrombosis	Chronic Postthrombotic Change
Vein size	Enlarged Normal if early, too small to enlarge vein	Small Normal
Vein wall	Thrombus weakly adherent to wall Convex outward	Scar, incorporated into wall Thickening may be focal, broad based, or circumferential Retracted

Intraluminal material with compression the residual lumen will collapse, the intraluminal material will persist	Smooth
	Round
	Soft
	Deformable with compression
	  Oval after compression
	  Narrows anteroposteriorly, bulges laterally
	Free floating
		Irregular
		Flat, rough, or lumpy
		Hard
		Nondeformable with compression
		  Shape does not change
		
		Thin webs (synechiae)
		Flat bands

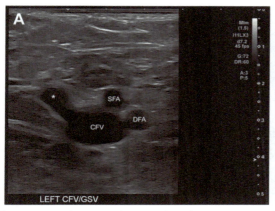 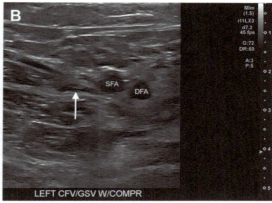

Fig. 1. Normal vein without and with compression. (*A, left*) Transverse view of the common femoral vein (CFV) and the great saphenous vein (GSV) at the sapheno-femoral junction (*asterisk*). The common femoral artery has already bifurcated, and this portion of the CFV is adjacent to the superficial (SFA) and deep (DFA) femoral arteries. (*B, right*) With probe compression (W/COMPR), the vein lumen is completely obliterated and only a thin wall (*arrow*) can be seen.

for any situation where the vein does not compress completely (**Fig. 2**A, B). Noncompressible veins may be due to acute DVT, chronic postthrombotic change, or inadequate compression. "Partial" compressibility is not recommended because it is not descriptive of why the vein does not compress, and this term is not specific enough to describe if there is an acute or chronic process.

Once a vein is noncompressible, further interpretation of the image is required to describe the vein lumen, material inside the vein, and the vein wall to distinguish between acute DVT and chronic postthrombotic change (see **Table 3**).

Acute DVT causes noncompression. Typically, acute DVT dilates the vein. Occasionally small early DVT may not expand the vein. The walls of dilated veins are convex outward, typically smoothly expanding. The material inside the vein is soft and deformable, changing in shape from circular, without compression, to oval, with compression (**Fig. 3**A–D). The material inside the vein is smooth, which is frequently better evaluated in the long axis. Acute DVT is loosely adherent to the wall and extends centrally to appear "free floating" (**Fig. 4**).

Acute DVT is laid down in moving blood, which creates layers of platelets mixed with fibrin and red blood cells. These lines of Zahn have interfaces, and likely, for this reason, the acute DVT is heterogeneous, including anechoic, hypoechoic, and hyperechoic (see **Fig. 4**) on modern US machines. There may be one dominant echogenicity; for instance, some acute DVT is predominantly

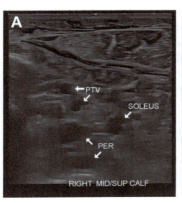 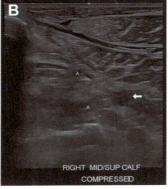

Fig. 2. Calf veins. Acute soleal DVT with normal compression of the paired posterior tibial and peroneal veins. (*A*) Without compression. Calf veins in the mid to superior (MID/SUP) calf show the paired posterior tibial veins (PTV) and the paired peroneal veins (PER). A dilated soleus vein is noted (SOLEUS). The gastrocnemius muscle is under the subcutaneous fat layer and superficial to the soleus at this level. (*B*) With compression. The posterior tibial veins are completely compressible and can no longer be seen. Their adjacent normal arteries are noncompressible (A). The soleal branch remains dilated (*arrow*), indicating it is filled with acute DVT. Reproduced with permission of the American Roentgen Ray Society from Lower Extremity Deep Venous Disease: Current Recommendations, Needleman L, Ultrasound: Core and Emerging Techniques and Concepts, 118-125. Copyright © 2021 American Roentgen Ray Society.

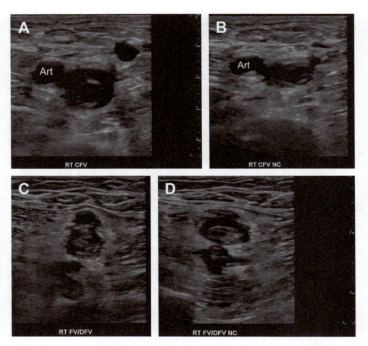

Fig. 3. Acute DVT. (*A, left*) Transverse view of the right (RT) common femoral vein and artery (Art) shows the vein is dilated. The vein is mostly anechoic but contains 2 curvilinear echoes. (*B, right*) After compression, the vein is noncompressible (NC); it does not compress completely. The acute DVT filled vein is soft; it changes shape from circular to oval. The echoes are the edge of some of the acute DVT, but there is also noncompressible anechoic thrombus laterally. Anechoic thrombus is confirmed because there is adequate compression (probe pressure has also deformed the artery). (*C, left*) In the same patient, there is dilatation of the femoral (FV) and deep femoral vein (DFV) compared with their corresponding arteries. The echogenicity of the femoral vein acute DVT is different; it is more echogenic and is heterogeneous. The DVT in the DFV is weakly echogenic. (*D, right*) After compression, both veins are noncompressible but deformable. The acute DVT is deformable and becomes oval shaped. The heterogeneity of the DVT in both veins is more obvious.

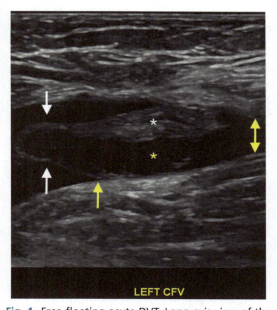

Fig. 4. Free-floating acute DVT. Long-axis view of the common femoral vein shows heterogeneous acute DVT with a free-floating central component (*between white arrows*). The DVT is detached from the vein wall (*yellow arrow*). The DVT dilates the vein; the normal-sized vein is smaller (*yellow double headed arrow*). The acute DVT is heterogeneous; some of the thrombus have a thin echogenic cap (*white arrows*), while the the center of the thrombus has variable echogenicities (*asterisks*).

hypoechoic with an echogenic edge (see **Fig. 3**). Echogenicity and homogeneity are not helpful to distinguish between acute and chronic changes.

Chronic postthrombotic change indicates scarring; the material retracts, and the vein is small or normal size. The collagen is hard and therefore not deformable with probe compression (**Fig. 5**A–C). The wall and/or the material inside generally have irregular margins. Wall thickening is common and may be focal (**Figs. 6** and **7**A, B) or circumferential. In long axis, the material is frequently irregular, flat, or lumpy. With lysis, some clot resorbs along both sides, leading to intraluminal flat bands or fine webs (synechiae) (see **Fig. 7**).

US readers can, in most cases, distinguish acute from chronic in abnormal cases. When there are features of both acute and chronic findings, or the image is inadequate to determine the age, the material is indeterminate (equivocal).

Subacute DVT does not have specific US findings. Rather, the term should only be used at follow-up with differences from a documented recent acute DVT and without completed chronic postthrombotic change. This diagnosis should be rare because most patients do not get short-term follow-up US. Subacute DVT is not a substitute term for indeterminate findings.

Recurrent DVT is a new episode of DVT after a prior episode of DVT. This may be easy to diagnose when the new DVT is in a different leg than a prior

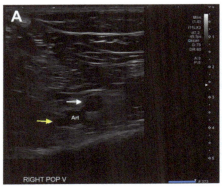 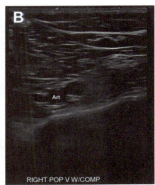 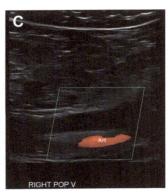

Fig. 5. Chronic postthrombotic change. (*A, left*) Transverse view of the popliteal (POP V) vein (*arrows*) and popliteal artery (Art). The vein is small and has low-level echoes in it (*white arrow*). The popliteal vein is duplicated; a smaller vein is adjacent to the artery (*yellow arrow*). (*B, right*) After compression, the veins are noncompressible and nondeformable. Chronic postthrombotic change is hard, and neither vein changes shape. (*C, right*) Long axis shows occlusion from chronic postthrombotic change. There is no flow by color Doppler. The caliber of the vein narrows compared with the vein inferiorly. The walls are minimally irregular.

case (approximately one-third of patients) or when a baseline study after treatment is available and the vein has undergone changes that are typical of acute DVT. Unequivocal findings of acute DVT, such as a free-floating thrombus or dilated deformable DVT, can be straightforward to diagnose even when scarring is present. Recurrent DVT may be difficult to evaluate because acute DVT may not dilate scarred veins. Swelling also makes evaluation difficult. Some laboratories compare the size of veins with a baseline, but this technique is difficult. If recurrent DVT is equivocal and the patient is a candidate, a negative D-dimer test can exclude recurrent DVT. Alternatively, if not treated, follow-up US can be performed around 3 days, and at 7 to 10 days. No change between examinations argues against recurrent DVT.

Color Doppler

Color Doppler may be used to show or exclude filling defects. By itself, color Doppler is less accurate than CUS to detect DVT, and color Doppler is especially useful when the veins are not well evaluated owing to depth or swelling. If color filling is not apparent at baseline, the flow can be augmented by calf compression to help fill the lumen with color. However, if color is overgained, it can bloom and cover filling defects or overwrite the vein entirely.

Spectral Doppler

The normal lower-extremity vein waveform is respirophasic, phasic variation related to breathing, which makes the velocity increase and decrease (**Fig. 8**A, B).[15] A normal waveform excludes a major obstruction more central to the sample site.

The abnormal Doppler waveform in the lower extremity is continuous without phasic variation (**Fig. 9**A, B) and is due to obstruction, eliminating normal patency from vein to chest. Continuous waveforms have a differential diagnosis: acute DVT, scarring, and extrinsic compression on veins

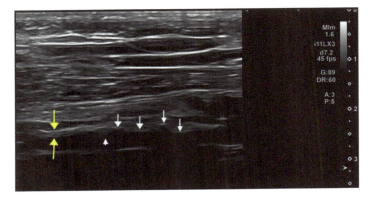

Fig. 6. Chronic postthrombotic change. Long axis of the femoral vein shows a small vein with irregular lumen (*white arrows*) from scarring. The wall is thickened; some are smooth (*between yellow arrows*), and some are more lumpy (*arrowhead*).

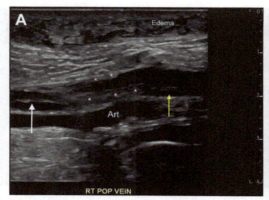
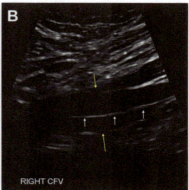

Fig. 7. Chronic postthrombotic change. (A) Long axis of the popliteal shows an irregularly contracted popliteal vein superficial to the popliteal artery (Art). There is extensive mural scarring composed of collagen with long attachments to the wall (*asterisk*). Intraluminal linear fine synechia (*white arrow*) and thicker band (*yellow arrow*) are also present. There is subcutaneous edema from chronic venous obstruction (Edema). (B) Long axis of the common femoral vein (*between yellow arrows*) demonstrates a chronic thin synechia (*white arrows*) composed of collagen within the vein. Although thin, synechia may be extensive and may obstruct the vein.

at or above the sample site.[16] Extrinsic compression may be physiologic, such as from bladder filling or pregnancy, or may be pathologic, such as pelvic masses or adenopathy. A continuous common femoral waveform even with a normal popliteal waveform is abnormal. Continuous waveforms may need further evaluation or follow-up to determine their cause.

Comparison of the right and left can be performed to determine if there is asymmetry. When asymmetry is present, technique is important to exclude false positives; the sonographer should use symmetric leg positions, avoid muscle tensing, and avoid excessive probe pressure.

Continuous waveforms are less sensitive but have high positive-predictive value. Milder loss of phasic variation even with asymmetry has lower specificity and lower-predictive value less than 50%.[17] Nonetheless, it may be helpful to identify mild asymmetry and necessitate further evaluation in selected patients.

Patients with elevated right heart pressure and tricuspid regurgitation may have excessively pulsatile veins. In some patients, the common femoral vein may exhibit pulsatile changes. The authors' laboratory requires seeing abnormal pulsatility in the popliteal vein before cardiac dysfunction is mentioned in the report (**Fig. 10**).

Augmentation of the spectral Doppler by distal compression had been a technique to help the examination. It is rarely useful and is no longer part of the standard duplex protocol.[18]

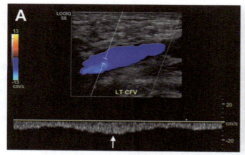
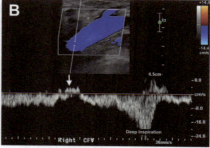

Fig. 8. Normal lower-extremity Doppler. (A) Normal left (LT) common femoral vein (CFV). Spectral waveform shows normal respirophasic variation, which increases mildly during normal inspiration (*arrow*). There is good color filling. (B) Normal common femoral vein waveform. This patient has a short retrograde component during expiration (*arrow*). In the common femoral and iliac veins, this is normal. Later in the waveform, the patient takes a deep inspiration; venous return increases, and the velocity in the waveform increases. Maneuvers to increase venous return, such as deep inspiration or augmentation, are not routine but can be helpful in the rare patient whose waveform is equivocal with normal breathing.

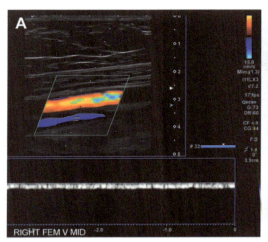
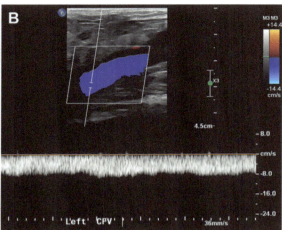

Fig. 9. Continuous Doppler waveforms. (A) Continuous Doppler waveform of right mid femoral vein (FEM V MID). The color lumen is small, and there is circumferential smooth wall thickening from chronic postthrombotic changes. The spectral Doppler waveform is continuous, without respiratory phasic changes. This is abnormal and indicates the scarring has created venous obstruction. (B) Continuous Doppler waveform of left common femoral vein (CFV). The color lumen is normal. The spectral Doppler is continuous. In this case, a pelvic mass has compressed the ipsilateral iliac vein in the pelvis. The continuous waveform indicates obstruction; apart from extrinsic compression from masses, upstream obstructive acute DVT or scarring may cause this finding. In unilateral disease, there will be asymmetry compared with the contralateral leg; in inferior vena cava or bilateral disease, both sides may be abnormal, and asymmetry may not be present.

Pitfalls

Body habitus is the most common reason for an inadequate study. Edema makes compression more difficult and increases the depth to the veins. Switching to a curved array transducer may be helpful. Hunter canal is an area where the muscles at the distal thigh protect the vein and make it difficult to compress. Changing the location of the probe to scan from the posterior thigh while pressing on the anterior thigh may be more effective than anterior scanning. If this is still not adequate, adding color Doppler to document a widely patent vein is reassuring. In difficult cases, if the artery is deformed and the vein does not collapse completely, there is adequate probe pressure (see **Fig. 3**); it is reasonable to determine the vein is abnormal rather than technically inadequate.

A study evaluated equivocal findings.[19] Inability to visualize part of a vein, less than 3 cm, but

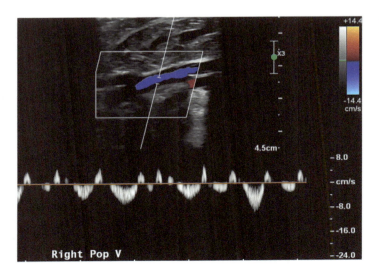

Fig. 10. Pulsatile Doppler waveform. Spectral Doppler of the popliteal vein (Pop V) shows excessive retrograde components. This is produced by elevated right heart pressure, tricuspid regurgitation, and right-sided cardiac dysfunction.

otherwise normal findings was unlikely to be significant (associated with venographically identified DVT). Therefore, sonographers should mention deficiencies and indicate if more than 3 cm of the vein was inadequate. High-probability equivocal studies have a dilated vein with inability to compress and no or reduced color, or inability to completely compress the vein, where it can be difficult. The high-probability finding was usually acute DVT. Based on this study, the patient generally needs something further, either to be treated as positive for acute DVT, followed up with alternative or short-term imaging, or to be evaluated with D-dimer (if applicable). Other intermediate equivocal findings had approximately 10% chance of DVT and may require more evaluation.

Evaluation after an initial positive study is described in **Table 2**. Follow-up several months after treatment is helpful to document scarring, to avoid equivocal results because many patients return for follow-up with DVT symptoms, even after adequate treatment.

Overview of Venous Reflux Evaluation

Chronic venous disease is frequently evaluated with a protocol designed for evaluation of reflux.[6,20,21] The reflux examination has components for the deep system and the superficial system and has specific technical factors that must be met.

The venous reflux examination has 4 components.

1. *A complete compression venous duplex examination:* This is to rule out acute DVT and to determine if venous chronic postthrombotic changes are present. Spectral Doppler can exclude significant obstruction to the deep system. Rarely, the deep system may be congenitally absent. Obstruction in the deep system is critically important because ablation may not be curative.
2. *Superficial venous mapping:* The sizes of superficial veins are used to determine if ablative therapy is indicated. The sizes of the great saphenous and the small saphenous veins are measured along their course from inside the lumen to inside the lumen. Significant accessory veins, like the anterior accessory saphenous veins, are also measured. Areas where the saphenous vein leaves the fascia are noted. Areas of aplasia, thrombosis, and prior treatment are also noted.
3. *Reflux testing:* Reflux is evaluated in selected sites in the deep veins and along the great and small saphenous veins. Reflux is elicited by maneuvers during long-axis spectral Doppler interrogation. The standard maneuver is distal compression, which may be performed manually or by an automated device. Valsalva may be performed at the groin but not more

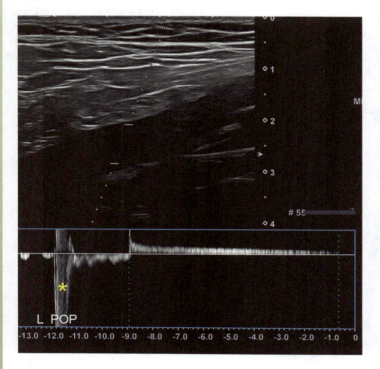

Fig. 11. Reflux in left popliteal (L POP) vein. In long-axis spectral Doppler with a slow sweep speed, augmentation is performed early in the waveform (*asterisk*). After the effect subsides, reflux is elicited (*between dotted lines*). Reflux is toward the foot and toward the transducer, so it is above the baseline. Here, reflux lasts more than 8 seconds. Reflux is diagnosed in deep veins when reflux lasts more than 1 second. Superficial reflux is diagnosed if the reflux is longer than 0.5 seconds.

distally. The patient is preferentially scanned upright but may be at or greater than 45° reverse Trendelenburg if upright is not tolerated. Calf veins can be evaluated while sitting. Abnormal reflux times are reported. Abnormally prolonged reflux times are as follows: greater than 0.5 seconds in the superficial venous system and greater than 1 second in the deep venous system (Fig. 11).

4. *Varicose veins:* Varicose veins are scanned, and the source of the varicosity is sought and recorded. Their entry is usually through saphenous veins or perforating veins.

UPPER-EXTREMITY VEINS

Protocols and evaluation of the upper-extremity veins are significantly influenced by anatomy (Table 4). Some of the veins, particularly the mid-subclavian, central jugular, and brachiocephalic veins, are not well seen because of overlying bone. Grayscale US (with compression, when possible), spectral, and color Doppler are coequals.[22]

Interpretation criteria of upper-extremity grayscale US are identical to lower-extremity criteria (Table 3). Studies with catheters also require evaluation for fibrin sheathing or peri catheter thrombus (Fig. 12). Lines, pacer wires, and prior catheters are often a site for scarring, so identification of obstruction without visible grayscale findings is not unusual.

Spectral Doppler interpretation is somewhat different in the upper extremity (Fig. 13A, B). Veins that are more central, namely the central (medial) subclavian, jugular, and brachiocephalic

Table 4
Vein protocol sampling sites

Lower Extremity	Compression US Short Axis Without and with Compression (Two Images, Dual Image, or Cine Loop)	Spectral Doppler Long-Axis Image	Color Doppler Long-Axis Image
Common femoral	✔	Bilateral At either common femoral or external iliac	Bilateral At either common femoral or external iliac
Saphenofemoral confluence	✔		
Deep femoral proximal	✔		
Femoral vein upper thigh	✔		
Femoral vein midthigh	✔		
Femoral vein distal thigh	✔		
Popliteal	✔	✔	✔
Posterior tibial	✔		
Peroneal	✔		
Symptomatic areas	✔	If appropriate	If appropriate
Upper extremity	**With or without compression, if possible. Otherwise long-axis grayscale**	**Spectral Doppler long-axis image**	**Color Doppler long-axis image**
Internal jugular	✔	✔	✔
Subclavian	✔	Bilateral	✔
Axillary	✔	✔	✔
Brachiocephalic (if seen)	✔	✔	✔
Brachial	✔	Optional	Optional
Cephalic	✔	Optional	Optional
Basilic	✔	Optional	Optional
Symptomatic areas (including forearm veins) when appropriate	✔	If appropriate	If appropriate

NOTE: The fullest visible extent and/or accessible portions of the veins are evaluated by grayscale and compression when possible.

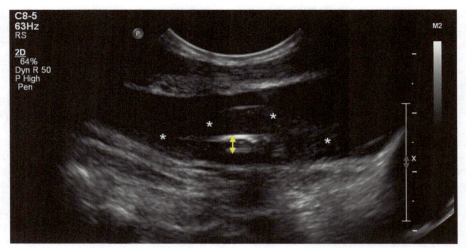

Fig. 12. Pericatheter thrombus. Long-axis view of the internal jugular vein demonstrates mildly echogenic acute thrombus (*asterisk*) attached to the wall surrounding a central line (*double arrow*). The central line extends throughout the vein but is only visible sonographically at the center of the image, where it is perpendicular to the sound beam. Lines are specular reflectors and are only strongly reflective at specific angles. Thrombus is a scatterer and is not angle dependent.

veins, demonstrate pulsatile waveforms (from the cardiac cycle) as well as phasic variation. Veins further distally, such as the mid- and peripheral subclavian and axillary veins, have variable pulsatile changes but do demonstrate phasic variation. For this reason, evaluation of both sides for symmetry at any suspected abnormal site is preferred. Asymmetry and continuous waveforms are abnormal. Mild asymmetry may be significant if technical causes are excluded. Catheters may blunt waveforms and cause obstruction. Bilateral subclavian waveforms at similar spots are standard even if the examination is otherwise normal.

Patient position affects the cardiac and phasic variation. The examination is preferably performed supine, as even modest elevation affects waveform shapes. Relaxation of the arm is also

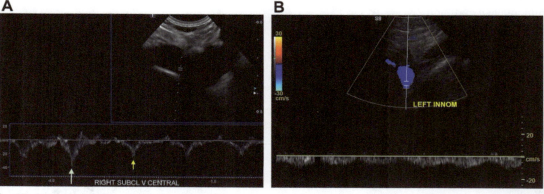

Fig. 13. Normal and abnormal upper-extremity venous waveforms. (*A, left*) The waveform in the central right subclavian vein (SUBCL V) exhibit large variations in velocity, including flow toward and away from the heart. This is termed pulsatile variation and stems from cardiac events. Superimposed on this is respirophasic variation, and the velocities during inspiration (*white arrow*) are greater than at expiration (*yellow arrow*). (*B, right*) The waveform in the left innominate (brachiocephalic) vein (INNOM) shows phasic variation but without pulsatile variation. Without cardiac variations, the waveform is abnormal and indicates obstruction. In this case, the central waveforms on both sides were blunted, which was caused by superior vena caval obstruction from lung carcinoma. Waveforms that would be considered normal in the lower extremity may be abnormal in the central upper-extremity veins. Distal to the thoracic outlet, partial or complete loss of pulsatility can be normal. Asymmetry may be helpful to diagnose subtle alternations in waveform shape after technical causes for asymmetry are excluded.

important, as narrowing of the thoracic inlet may occur in certain positions.

The pulsatile variation may change the direction of flow in the vein over time, which can lead to color Doppler changes in velocity and direction. Good color filling is generally possible with normal veins because the velocities in the vein are greater than in the lower extremity. Careful attention to technique is needed to avoid overwriting small filling defects.

CLINICS CARE POINTS

- Outpatients with low risk for deep vein thrombosis by clinical prediction rules and a negative D-dimer do not generally need venous imaging. Otherwise, venous ultrasound is the imaging test for those with suspected deep vein thrombosis, for those with positive D-dimer test, and for those where the D-dimer is not adequately predictive.
- Lower-extremity peripheral venous ultrasound, when performed as a complete compression ultrasound, is an accurate single test to rule in and rule out lower-extremity deep vein thrombosis.
- Patients with less comprehensive protocols or technically difficult examinations may require serial or alternative testing.
- Most patients can be assigned normal, acute deep vein thrombosis, or chronic postthrombotic change. A small number of cases will be inadequate, or the findings will be indeterminate.
- Color Doppler can distinguish occlusive versus nonocclusive deep vein thrombosis. Spectral Doppler can determine if obstruction is present at or central to the site of an abnormal Doppler signal. This can be especially helpful in the upper extremity because some anatomy is not directly evaluable because of the overlying bony chest.

REFERENCES

1. Needleman L, Cronan JJ, Lilly MP, et al. Ultrasound for lower extremity deep venous thrombosis: multidisciplinary recommendations from the society of radiologists in ultrasound consensus conference. Circulation 2018;137:1505–15.
2. Goldhaber SZ, Bounameaux H. Pulmonary embolism and deep vein thrombosis. Lancet 2012;379: 1835–46.
3. Smith SB, Geske JB, Kathuria P, et al. Analysis of national trends in admissions for pulmonary embolism. Chest 2016;150:35–45.
4. Pyzocha N. Diagnosing DVT in nonpregnant adults in the primary care setting. Am Fam Physician 2019;100:778–80.
5. Kupinski AM. Vascular anatomy. In: AM K, editor. The vascular system. Philadelphia: Wolters Kluwer; 2023. p. 39–54.
6. Min RJ, Khilnani NM, Golia P. Duplex ultrasound evaluation of lower extremity venous insufficiency. J Vasc Intervent Radiol 2003;14:1233–41.
7. Schellong SM. Distal DVT: worth diagnosing? Yes. J Thromb Haemostasis 2007;5(Suppl 1):51–4.
8. Thomas DP. Overview of venous thrombogenesis. Semin Thromb Hemost 1988;14:1–8.
9. Konstantinides SV, Torbicki A, Agnelli G, et al. 2014 ESC guidelines on the diagnosis and management of acute pulmonary embolism. Eur Heart J 2014; 35:3033–69, 3069a.
10. Meissner MH, Caps MT, Bergelin RO, et al. Propagation, rethrombosis and new thrombus formation after acute deep venous thrombosis. J Vasc Surg 1995; 22:558–67.
11. Comerota AJ, Oostra C, Fayad Z, et al. A histological and functional description of the tissue causing chronic postthrombotic venous obstruction. Thromb Res 2015;135:882–7.
12. Collaborative Committee ACR. AIUM practice parameter for the performance of a peripheral venous ultrasound examination. J Ultrasound Med 2020;39:E49–56.
13. Stevens SM, Woller SC, Kreuziger LB, et al. Antithrombotic therapy for VTE disease: second update of the CHEST guideline and expert panel report. Chest 2021;160:e545–608.
14. Goodacre S, Sampson F, Thomas S, et al. Systematic review and meta-analysis of the diagnostic accuracy of ultrasonography for deep vein thrombosis. BMC Med Imag 2005;5:6.
15. Kim ES, Sharma AM, Scissons R, et al. Interpretation of peripheral arterial and venous Doppler waveforms: A Consensus Statement from the Society for Vascular Medicine and Society for Vascular Ultrasound. Vasc Med 2020. 1358863X20937665.
16. Bach AM, Hann LE. When the common femoral vein is revealed as flattened on spectral Doppler sonography: is it a reliable sign for diagnosis of proximal venous obstruction. AJR Am J Roentgenol 1997; 168:733–6.
17. Kayılıoğlu Sl, Köksoy C, Alaçayır İ. Diagnostic value of the femoral vein flow pattern for the detection of an iliocaval venous obstruction. J Vasc Surg Venous Lymphat Disord 2016;4:2–8.
18. Lockhart ME, Sheldon HI, Robbin ML. Augmentation in lower extremity sonography for the detection of deep venous thrombosis. AJR Am J Roentgenol 2005;184:419–22.
19. Norén A, Ottosson E, Sjunnesson M, et al. A detailed analysis of equivocal duplex findings in patients with

suspected deep venous thrombosis. J Ultrasound Med 2002;21:1375–83.
20. Salles-Cunha SX, Neuhardt DL, Houle M. Venous valvular insufficiency testing. In: Kupinski AM, editor. The vascular system. Philadelphia: Wolters Kluwer; 2023. p. 299–316.
21. Zygmunt JA. Duplex ultrasound for chronic venous insufficiency. J Invasive Cardiol 2014;26:E149–55.
22. Talbot SR, Oliver M. Duplex ultrasound imaging of the upper extremity venous system. In: Kupinski AM, editor. The vascular system. Philadelphia: Wolters Kluwer; 2023. p. 271–81.

Moving?

Make sure your subscription moves with you!

To notify us of your new address, find your **Clinics Account Number** (located on your mailing label above your name), and contact customer service at:

Email: **journalscustomerservice-usa@elsevier.com**

800-654-2452 (subscribers in the U.S. & Canada)
314-447-8871 (subscribers outside of the U.S. & Canada)

Fax number: 314-447-8029

**Elsevier Health Sciences Division
Subscription Customer Service
3251 Riverport Lane
Maryland Heights, MO 63043**

*To ensure uninterrupted delivery of your subscription, please notify us at least 4 weeks in advance of move.